Homeland Security
and Emergency Medical Response

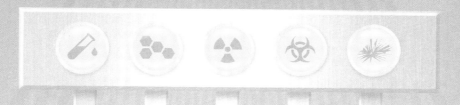

John Campbell, MD, FACEP

Jim Smith, MSS, JD, EdD, NREMT-P

Steve Simpson, BSBA, NREMT-P

Denise Smith, BS, NREMT-P

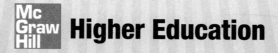
McGraw Hill **Higher Education**

Boston   Burr Ridge, IL   Dubuque, IA   New York   San Francisco   St. Louis
Bangkok   Bogotá   Caracas   Kuala Lumpur   Lisbon   London   Madrid   Mexico City
Milan   Montreal   New Delhi   Santiago   Seoul   Singapore   Sydney   Taipei   Toronto

The McGraw·Hill Companies

Mc Graw Hill Higher Education

HOMELAND SECURITY AND EMERGENCY MEDICAL RESPONSE

ISBN 978–0–07–304437–8
MHID 0-07-304437-7

Publisher: *David T. Culverwell*
Senior Sponsoring Editor: *Claire Merrick*
Editorial Coordinator: *Michelle Zeal*
Senior Marketing Manager: *Lisa Nicks*
Senior Project Manager: *Sheila M. Frank*
Senior Production Supervisor: *Sherry L Kane*
Designer: *John Joran*
Cover Illustration: *©Asylum Studios*
Senior Photo Research Coordinator: *John C. Leland*
Photo Research: *LouAnn K. Wilson*
Compositor: *Techbooks*
Typeface: *10/12 ITC New Baskerville*
Printer: *R. R Donnelley Willard, OH*

The credits section for this book begins on page 256 and is considered an extension of the copyright page.

Library of Congress Cataloging-in-Publication Data

Homeland Security and emergency medical response / John Campbell ... [et al.]. – 1st ed.
  p. cm.
  Includes index.
  ISBN 978–0–07–304437–8 — ISBN 0-07-304437-7 (alk. paper)
  1. Terrorism. 2. Bioterrorism. 3. Emergency medical technicians. 4. Disaster medicine. 5. Civil defense–United States. I. Campbell, John (John E.)

RC88.9.T47H66 2008
363.325'3–dc22

2006052925

John E. Campbell, MD, FACEP

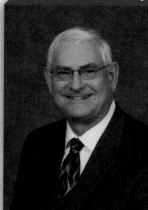

is the EMS Medical Director for the state of Alabama and EMS Program Medical Director at Trenholm State Technical College in Montgomery and Southern Union State Community College in Opelika, Alabama. Dr. Campbell is the President and Editor for International Trauma Life Support, Inc. *Basic Trauma Life Support* published by the Brady Co. is the leading two-day trauma training course for EMT Basics, paramedics and advanced EMS providers and is taught world-wide. His awards include: Ronald D. Stewart Award, National Association of EMS Physicians and EMS Award (first recipient), American College of Emergency Physicians. Dr. Campbell has authored five editions of *Basic Trauma Life Support,* four editions of *BTLS for the EMT-B and First Responder,* and is the editor for *Pediatric Basic Trauma Life Support.*

Jim Smith, BS, MS, EMT-P

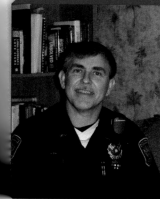

has been employed in public safety for more than thirty years. He currently serves as a certified police chief for a rural southern Alabama town and is a faculty practicioner teaching graduate criminal justice courses for the University of Phoenix. Smith has an Associate in science in emergency medical technology, a Bachelor of Science degree in biology and chemistry along with a Master of Science in safety from the University of Southern California. He also has other advanced degrees. Smith has been a practicing paramedic since 1976 and professional law enforcement officer since 1984. Smith is a graduate of the FBI Post Blast Investigators Course, Level II Certified by the International Society of Explosive Engineers, member of the International Society of Bomb Technicians and Investigators, professional member of the American Society of Safety Engineers, a Certified Emergency Manager, graduate of the U.S. Army Chemical School Domestic Preparedness program and Toxic Agent Training Facility, certified Fire Instructor Level II, and Certified Police Planner. He is a graduate of the FBI Executive Management Program for bomb squads and served as a bomb squad commander for more than ten years along with the supervision a clandestine drug laboratory entry and assessment team. Smith is also a hazardous materials emergency response technician and practiced as a health physics technician at a commercial operating nuclear power facility. He has authored three additional textbooks relating to response to bomb threats, WMD incidents and law enforcement management. Smith has conducted practical research and published data on blast mitigation using specialized equipment, which led to the application for a patent and commercial production of the equipment. He also has published practical research data on pipe bomb fragment propagation and more than fifty other articles in refereed journals.

iv   About the Authors

Steven A. Simpson, BSBA, NREMT-P

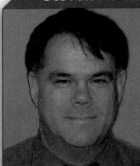

is the EMS & Fire Science Program Director at Southern Union State Community College in Opelika, Alabama. He holds a Business degree with a computer information science major and also holds an Associate of Applied Science degree in EMS. He is the Alabama Chapter Basic Trauma Life Support State Coordinator and is an instructor for BTLS, ACLS, PALS, BCLS, Firefighter I and HazMat Awareness/Operations. He also holds Regional Faculty status with the American Heart Association in ACLS, PALS, and BLS and is currently the AHA BLS National Faculty for the State of Alabama.

Denise C. Smith, BS, NREMTP

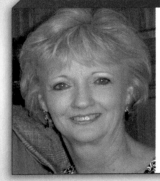

is the Executive Director of the Southeast Alabama EMS Council, Inc in Dothan, Alabama. She is also the Executive Director of the Alabama Chapter of the American College of Emergency Physicians. She received her Bachelor of Science in Health Management from Kennedy–Western University in Agoura Hills, California. She is a nationally registered paramedic, a BTLS instructor, and CPR, ACLS and PALS instructor. She is also on the Board of Directors of the Alabama Poison Control Center.

Dedication

This text is dedicated to all the first responders who daily place themselves in harm's way to serve their fellow man.

Table of Contents

Preface

After the September 11, 2001, attacks, the U.S. government created the Department of Homeland Security. This agency consolidated 22 agencies and 180,000 employees into a single agency whose primary mission is to help prevent, protect against, and respond to acts of terrorism. However, homeland security depends not just on this agency but also on all citizens, especially civilian public safety organizations (law enforcement, fire, and emergency medical services).

This book is part of a 15-hour basic training course. This course consists of a series of lectures about the various terrorist weapons and methods of attack and the proper way to respond to them. Along with the lectures will be demonstrations of various types of equipment needed to identify the weapon being used. The course also consists of four hands-on skill stations to teach how to use personal protective equipment (PPE), how to decontaminate patients, how to use the Nerve Agent Antidote Kit, and scenario exercises in how to respond to the various types of terrorist attacks. These same principles apply to responding to hazardous materials incidents and clandestine drug laboratories.

Though it can be organized in other ways, the 15-hour course is designed to be taught in a weekend. It is admittedly basic and was designed to be that way. There are more advanced courses available, but many emergency responders do not have the time or money to take 5- to 7-day courses. The course goals are to teach you the basic skills needed for your and your patient's survival, and to further stimulate your interest so that you might take more advanced training if you have the opportunity. Although the focus is on emergency medical response, this course is also useful for fire services, and law enforcement. All of these groups have to work together in a terrorist attack or other disaster. Each of these groups also needs to know the basic principles of response, victim rescue, emergency medical treatment, and how to interact with the other groups during a response.

Interested citizens (especially schoolteachers and employees of high-risk organizations—see Chapter 1) will find this book a useful guide to understanding the types of terrorist attacks and the combined emergency response to them. The text manual, while somewhat technical, is basic enough that it can be used for a reference by laypersons.

Acknowledgements

Sincere thanks go to the following McGraw-Hill staff for their considerable efforts, invaluable assistance, and vital guidance during the development of this book: David Culverwell, Publisher, Career Education; Roxan Kinsey, Senior Sponsoring Editor; and Connie Kuhl, Editorial Coordinator. The author would also like to thank Renee Krug at McGraw-Hill for her editorial support, Julie Scardiglia for her assistance in editing the text and CD, and Lisa Whicker, whose contribution made this text a more valuable tool in exam preparation.

Additionally, I would like to exprerss my appreciation to McGraw-Hill for providing the artwork that helped illustrate this book.

REVIEWERS

The author gratefully acknowledges the following advisors and reviewers, whose comments and suggestions helped shape the manuscript into a comprehensive and useful review book.

Dr. Biff Baker
Colorado Technical University
Colorado Springs, CO

E. John Wipfler, III, MD, FACEP
OSF Saint Francis Medical Center
University of Illinois College of Medicine
Peoria, IL

Kristi Koenig, MD, FACEP
Director of Public Health Preparedness
Department of Emergency Medicine
Professor of Clinical Emergency Medicine,
Co-Director, EMS and Disaster Medical Sciences Fellowship,
University of California at Irvine,
School of Medicine
Orange, CA

John Hendrickson, J.D.
Sonoma College
Petaluma, CA

Patrick Cote
Delgado Community College
New Orleans, LA

Robert W. Daly, CPP
Parks College
Denver, CO

C.J. Goldsmith
Kee Business College
Chesapeake, VA

Karla Hirsch Carrigan
Parks College
Thornton, CO

Linda Herrera Mutch
Legal Department Program Director
Blair College
Colorado Springs, CO

Reinaldo Montano
Department Chair, Criminal Justice and Homeland Security
Parks College
Arlington, VA

Bob Jaffin
Department Chair
American Public University System
Charles Town, WV

Dana D. Griffith
Parks College, Corinthian Colleges
Thornton, CO

Mark W. McClintock, M.Ed.
Homeland Security Program Coordinator
Blair College
Colorado Springs, CO

David A. McEntire, PhD
Emergency Administration and Planning
University of North Texas
Denton, TX

Bruce R. Shade, EMT/P, EMS-I, AAS
Cuyahoga Community College
Cleveland, OH

Notes for Students

The Homeland Security and Emergency Medical Response course is a two-day concentrated learning experience. In order to be prepared, you should begin studying the textbook two weeks before the course. During the two days of the course you will review the basic concepts of terrorist attacks and your response to them. This will include demonstrations of use of chemical, biological, and radiological detection equipment. You will have hands-on practice using personal protective equipment (Level C), decontamination of patients, and the nerve agent antidote kit. You will also practice responding to various types of attacks. At the end of the course you should have the basic knowledge needed to properly respond to a terrorist or hazardous materials incident or to a clandestine drug laboratory.

Notes for Teachers

This text is designed to be part of an organized hands-on course. An Instructor's Guide and PowerPoint slides are available to be used in teaching the HSEMR course. If you wish to arrange a course in your area you may write or call:

Tactical Medical Associates and Consultants
C/O Southeast Alabama EMS
2323 West Main Street
Suite 223
Dothan, AL 36301
Phone: 1-334-793-7789
Email: dsmith@seaems.com

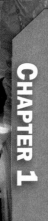

CHAPTER 1

Recognition and Emergency Medical Response

Chapter Objectives

Upon completion of this chapter you should be able to:

1. Discuss the importance of a pre-attack threat assessment and security review.
2. Describe what special protective clothing and equipment may be required for you to perform your duties at the scene of a terrorist attack.
3. Discuss the general emergency response to an emergency call.
4. Discuss how to recognize dangers when surveying the scene.
5. Discuss signs of a possible terrorist attack.
6. Discuss general scene management after a terrorist attack.
7. List and discuss the working zones at the scene of a terrorist attack.
8. Discuss the role of EMS and fire personnel at a crime scene.
9. Be familiar with the National Incident Management System (NIMS) and how it relates to the Incident Command System (ICS).
10. Discuss the role of EMS in a mass casualty situation.

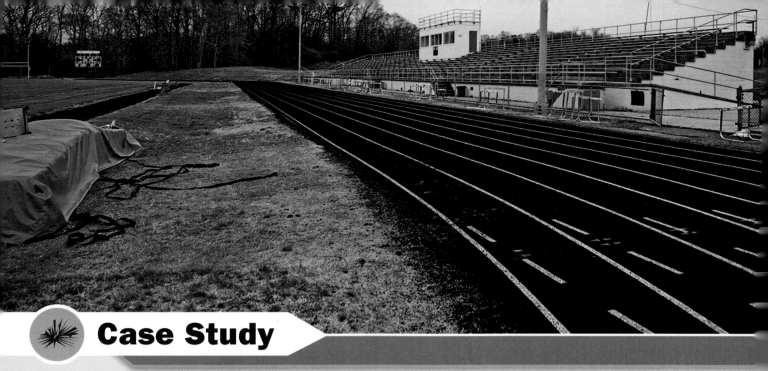

Case Study

You are serving as EMS support during a high school football game with roughly 1,000 people in attendance at a stadium that normally houses up to 5,000. You are somewhat concerned because tensions are high in the community and attendance is off tonight. The two local high schools playing have been experiencing racial unrest, and several fights occurred at the schools prior to the football game. A local white supremist group has recently staged several rallies and a march, further increasing tensions. There have been bomb threats and threats of violence. Because of this, a plan has been made to deal with potential problems and there is a large law enforcement contingent stationed in the stadium and the parking lot. It is a chilly October night and there is a gentle breeze. You suddenly notice many frightened people stampeding down out of the stands on the opposite side of the stadium. Law enforcement officers react. Over the public safety radio channel they tell you to proceed with an evacuation following the bomb threat plan. You follow the plan, quickly exiting the stadium and

going upwind to the prearranged staging area, where you meet incoming fire, law enforcement, and additional EMS units. You hear over the radio that many of the attendees and some officers are experiencing eye pain, tearing, nasal secretions, coughing, and difficulty breathing. You estimate that as many as 100 people are in need of assessment. Some have been injured in the stampede and are unable to leave the stadium.

- What has happened?
- Is a toxic material involved?
- How would you control contamination?
- How would you decontaminate the victims?
- What treatment is indicated?
- Are the EMTs, firefighters, and law enforcement officers on the scene in danger?
- What special protective clothing and equipment is required?

The Case Study will continue at the end of the chapter.

Terrorism is the systematic use of violence against the citizens (or a particular group of citizens) of a country in order to attain some goal. This goal may be granting some demand of the terrorist group, or the attacks may simply be based on hatred.

The term *weapons of mass destruction* (WMD) is used commonly when speaking of terrorist attacks, but such attacks are the exception rather than the rule. The term *WMD* refers to the magnitude of the attack, not the manner of attack. The bombing of the Murrah Federal Building in Oklahoma City in 1995 and the attacks on the World Trade Center and the Pentagon in 2001 are examples of "mass destruction." The damage caused by detonation of a nuclear device would be another example. In actuality most terrorist attacks cause limited damage and death, and the term WMD should not be applied to them.

To achieve their goals, terrorists use a variety of weapons to cause fear. These include:

- CBRNE weapons
  - **C**hemical
  - **B**iological
  - **R**adiological-**N**uclear
  - **E**xplosives
- Incendiary
- Firearms
- Hostage taking
- Computer network intrusion and sabotage (hacking)

Because CBRNE and incendiary are the types of attacks to which you are most likely to respond, they are the focus of this course and text and are discussed in greater detail in Chapters 2 through 6.

Attacks of a larger magnitude (WMD) usually require more money, planning, and organization and thus may run a higher risk of being detected and prevented. It is easier, and usually just as effective in causing terror, to mount an attack that requires a simple weapon that is easy to deploy. For this reason most terrorist attacks (80–85%) are bombings. Most of these bomb attacks, though deadly, affect a limited number of victims. Chemical, biological, and radiological-nuclear weapons can theoretically affect mass numbers of people, but in reality most terrorists do not have the means to disperse these weapons over a large enough area to attain their real potential for causing mass casualties (Table 1.1). However, weapons of less than mass destruction are very successful in causing fear (if not terror) and have certainly had a disruptive effect on our mass transit industry.

Table 1.1	Weapons of Mass Destruction	
Weapon	**Likelihood of Being Used**	**Casualties**
Nuclear weapons	Lowest	Highest
Radiological agents	Low	Low
Biological agents	Low–moderate	Moderate–high
Chemical agents	Low–moderate	Moderate
Conventional explosives	Highest	Low
Incendiaries	Moderate	Lowest

At the present time the threat of more terrorist attacks is very real. Protection from and survival of such attacks depends upon three "P"s and three "R"s: **p**lanning, **p**reparation, **p**revention, **r**ecognition, **r**esponse, and **r**eview.

- *Planning* and *preparation* before an attack happens
- *Prevention* of attacks through the teamwork of alert citizens and law enforcement
- Early *recognition* that an attack is in progress
- Rapid and proper *response* to that attack
- *Review* of the incident and the response in order to improve security measures and response to future attacks

Although increased security measures have almost certainly prevented some attacks, they will not completely deter a patient and determined enemy. Well-planned attacks may occur years apart. Preventing attacks or limiting casualties from such attacks requires *constant vigilance* by private citizens as well as public safety employees (Fire, Emergency Medical Services, Law Enforcement, and Emergency Management).

This chapter briefly covers pre-attack planning, special personal protective equipment that may be needed to enter a terrorist attack scene, response to an emergency event, recognition of a terrorist attack, and management of the terrorist attack scene. The role of EMS and fire personnel at a crime scene and the management of a mass casualty situation, including a review of the incident command system (ICS) and the evolving national incident management system (NIMS), are also included. These principles are integrated into Chapters 2 through 6, which discuss specific responses to different types of attacks.

Pre-Attack Planning: Threat Assessment and Security Review

The assessment of threats is a normal function of emergency planning and should be performed by all organizations and facilities. Threats to assess include not only terrorist threats, but also natural threats, such as the weather, and accidental threats such as fire or a chemical spill. You cannot plan for a situation you have not anticipated, thus it is prudent for each facility and/or organization to review the spectrum of threats they may face. This is called a security review. You can obtain help with this from your local Emergency Management Agency (EMA).

Planning and Preparation

When a security review is performed, the potential for terrorist attack should be evaluated. The review should assess what type of target the facility, institution, or personnel presents. Is the target symbolic, such as a high-value landmark (World Trade Center, White House, Pentagon, etc.)? Is it densely populated, so that an attack could potentially cause numerous casualties (e.g., World Trade Center, Pentagon, soldiers' barracks, shopping mall, school, or office building)? Is it essential to the safety or economic well-being of the community (power plant, water supply, public transportation, public safety personnel, hospital, and so on)? High-value "soft" targets—targets with poor or no security, and a location that is easy to approach and escape from—are more attractive to terrorists than a facility whose construction and security make it a difficult, or "hard," target. The headquarters of the CIA in Langley, Virginia, would be a prime target for terrorists except that its high degree of security makes it extremely difficult to attack. Since 2001 most government and military facilities have been "hardened," thus making soft targets like hospitals, tourist attractions, shopping malls, and schools more attractive.

Each facility should prepare plans that address what to do in the event of either man-made or natural emergencies. These emergencies include such things as fires, power failure, severe weather, earthquakes, medical emergencies, shootings or other acts of violence, abductions, and CBRNE incidents. The plan should clearly define the chain of command and method of notification. Questions to consider include:

- Can the facility's emergency plans operate without power, utilities, communications, or computer systems?
- Who has the authority to activate the facility's emergency operations plan?
- Is there a prompt method for notification of emergencies (and who to notify) as well as a plan for evacuation?
- Does the evacuation plan account for all employees and visitors?
- Does the facility have reasonable levels of internal and external security?
- Does the facility have any special hazards such as hazardous materials (chemical, nuclear, or biological agents)?
- Are realistic emergency drills conducted at least twice a year?

Special Protective Equipment

If you are a public safety responder, you should be familiar with the personal protective equipment (PPE) that you may need to wear to perform your duties in a dangerous environment. Your first line of defense is the protective equipment you wear. Do not enter a hazardous materials scene (which includes many terrorist attack scenes) without appropriate protective clothing and respiratory protection. Not only are you in danger from toxic material at the scene, but you also may be cross-contaminated by patients who have toxic material on their clothes or skin. This is particularly true at a terrorist attack scene if chemical, radiological, or contagious biological agents are involved. Because a bomb may be used to disperse any of the above, all unknown explosion scenes require wearing PPE until contamination is ruled out.

As a general rule, at any terrorist attack scene a hazardous materials (HazMat) team should first evaluate the scene for dangers (CBRNE) and determine the type of protective equipment to wear in order to enter the scene. HazMat teams are usually teams within the fire department. They have had special training in hazardous materials recognition and management and are equipped with special equipment with which to detect chemical, biological, and radiological agents Situations in which HazMat evaluation would be useful include:

- Scenes with multiple people "sick" or "down"
- All explosions of unknown origin
- Bombings
- Suspicious circumstances with an unknown substance, particularly one received by mail or package
- Suspicious scenes in which you encounter mists, smoke, fog, or liquids

In these situations it would be best if you did not enter the scene until the HazMat team evaluates it and determines the correct level of PPE to wear. If you are the first to arrive on the scene and there are obvious living casualties requiring you to enter to *save lives*, you may have to enter before HazMat evaluation. In this situation you should wear at least Level B PPE (Figure 1.1); however, Level C or even firefighter's turnout gear may be all that is available to you.

Normal uniform attire and EMS protective gowns provide essentially no protection against chemical agents and very limited protection against biological or radiological agents. Firefighter turnout gear along with self-contained breathing apparatus (SCBA) will give limited protection against vapor for a short time. Some law enforcement and tactical teams wear charcoal-impregnated outer coverall uniforms that provide chemical protection but are not waterproof or splash-proof. You must be aware of the limitations of your protective equipment. Most chemical and biological agents are dispersed as an aerosol, thus you will need respiratory protection as well as skin protection.

Skin Protection

Most of your skin protection will be from a chemical suit. Most agencies will select a chemical suit resistant to most common chemical hazards (there are multiple choices available). Theoretically, commonly faced chemical hazards should be analyzed (see Chapter 2) and the chemical suit matched to the common threats. Most chemical suits in the medium range (Level B or Level C— made from Tychem, Tyvek, or Tyvek/Saranex) are suitable for law enforcement, medical, and EMS use. These suits provide splash protection and some vapor protection and are commonly used once the chemical threats present have been identified. Fire service personnel who are exposed to a broader range of hazardous materials may elect a higher-grade chemical protective suit (Level A) that is usually made of Tychem. It is important to secure the chemical suit

Figure 1.1
(a) Example of Level B PPE.
(b) Example of Level C PPE.

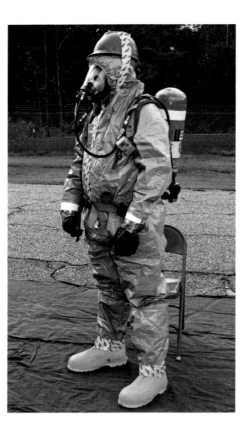 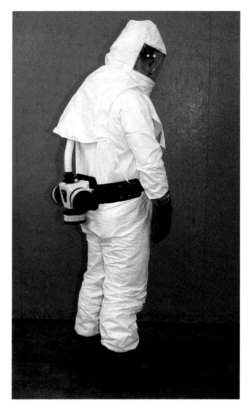

sleeves, cuffs, and face area to vapor. Taping these areas is required. Use chemically rated tape, not duct tape or paper tape. Footwear such as chemical resistant boots (Figure 1.2) is a necessity for law enforcement and fire service personnel, but suits with built-in boots may be adequate for EMS or in a hospital setting (Figure 1.3).

The usual latex gloves provide no chemical protection. Tougher gloves made of vinyl, nitrile, or neoprene provide better protection. Chemical protection may require even thicker nitrile or butyl rubber gloves (Figure 1.4), but these thick gloves limit sensation and fine motor use of the hands. A police officer, for example, could not hold a weapon while wearing these gloves. With an unknown chemical threat you should have the maximum protection, but once the chemical is identified, you *may* be able to change to gloves that allow better use of your hands.

If you find yourself already on a scene (without your PPE) and then find yourself exposed to a chemical agent, you must immediately escape to a safe

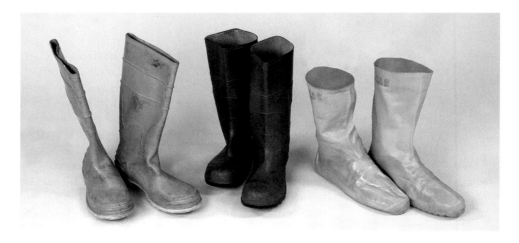

Figure 1.2
Examples of chemical protective boots.

Figure 1.3
Chemical suits with
built-in boots.

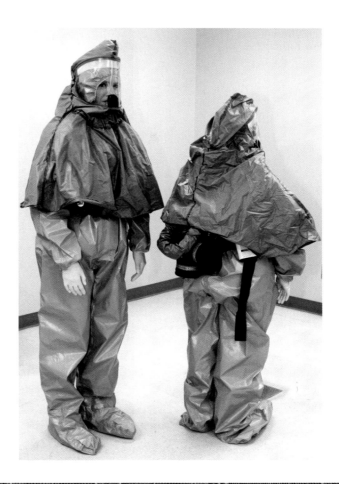

Figure 1.4
Rescuer with butyl rubber
gloves. Notice that he
would be unable to perform
fine motor skills while
wearing these gloves.

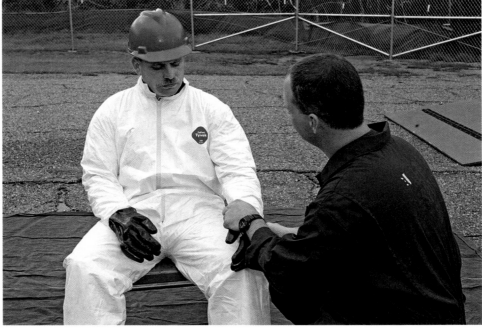

position. Always have an escape route in mind. If you are trapped in such a situation, structural firefighting clothing can afford some protection until you can escape (Figure 1.5). The sleeves, facial area, and legs should be taped if possible. For law enforcement and EMS personnel, rain gear, when taped, will provide some protection against chemical agents. In a situation where you are

Figure 1.5
Example of fire turnout
gear.

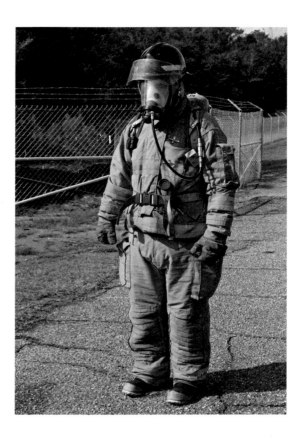

surprised and trapped while under chemical attack, there is little you can do for respiratory protection if you do not have a gas mask or other escape hood close at hand.

Respiratory Protection

Respiratory protection is the most critical aspect of all protective clothing. The most common exposure route is the respiratory system. Most chemical agents are dispersed as an aerosol vapor or, in the case of biological or radiological agents, as small particles suspended in an aerosol. The atmosphere at explosion scenes will be very dusty (fine airborne particles). Working at an explosion scene requires respiratory protection, as this dust may contain asbestos or other toxic materials.

Personal protective gear comes in four levels of protection. Levels A–D are the protection level ratings used by the U.S. Occupational Safety and Health Administration (OSHA), with Level A being most protective and Level D the least. Levels A and B depend on air supplied from a hose or tank, while Levels C and D depend on filtering air through some device.

Level A Protection

Level A OSHA protection is a totally encapsulated chemical suit with a positive-pressure self-contained breathing apparatus (SCBA) worn under the suit (Figure 1.6). This suit is designed to provide the maximum respiratory protection and maximum protection against vapors and liquids. This level of protection is best (though not always available or practical) when dealing with unknown agents. Most Level A suits do not provide thermal protection or protection against direct exposure to flame. Furthermore, this clothing offers no ballistic protection against bullets or fragments from explosions. Because the suit is so bulky, it makes it difficult to move and operate equipment or to maneuver inside buildings. Wearer visibility and manual dexterity are also dramatically reduced. Generally only trained HazMat units operate in Level A PPE. Only the most

Figure 1.6
Example of a Level A suit.

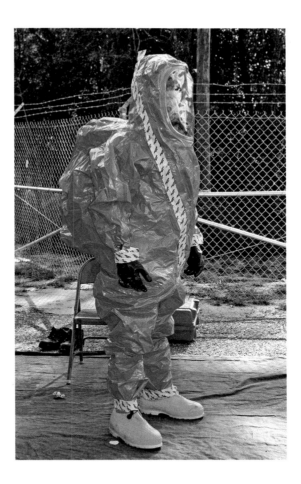

lethal environments require Level A protection, but it is best if the nature of the chemical, radiological, or biological threat is unknown *and a severe risk is anticipated*. Heat stress is tremendous in these suits with the accompanying SCBA. The useful service time is limited to the life of the SCBA air supply and the heat stress on the wearer. Most people cannot tolerate wearing these suits for more than 30 to 45 minutes. This suit is not useful for EMS, hospital, or law enforcement duties, due to these factors, the reduction of dexterity, and the amount of training required to maintain proficiency in their use. People who use these suits must have medical screening and respirator fit testing (see Box 1-1) on an annual basis.

Level B Protection

Level B OSHA protection includes a chemical resistant suit with the SCBA worn externally (Figure 1.7). This provides maximum respiratory protection but less protection against liquids and vapors than the Level A suit. This is adequate protection for most unknown environments when Level A protection is not available or when the situation requires dexterity impossible in a Level A protective suit. Most tasks are performed more easily while wearing Level B protection. Level B is usually adequate for EMS, hospital, and law enforcement settings even when the agent is unknown, as long as there is no strong evidence of a severe risk. However, because of the training, maintenance, and storage requirements of the Level B gear, EMS and Law Enforcement usually choose the simpler Level C PPE. Heat stress is still high in Level B suits. The limited amount of air supplied by the SCBA and the heat load limits this ensemble's usefulness to 45 to 60 minutes. In a facility where air lines are available, only the heat load will be a factor. See "Appendix A" for more detail on donning Level B protection.

Figure 1.7
Example of a Level B suit.

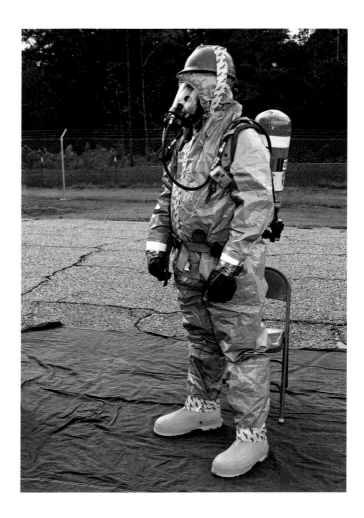

Level C Protection

Level C OSHA protection is a chemical suit worn with an air-purifying respirator (APR) (Figure 1.8). This respirator is commonly known as a *gas mask,* and it uses the negative pressure of breathing to move inhaled air through a filter that can protect against specific hazards (Figure 1.9). The gas mask filter must be matched to the hazard, although standard filters will cover most hazards. These devices are normally limited to use for a known agent with good warning properties such as a characteristic odor. APRs are small and can be easily carried by responders. Responders to any suspicious situation should carry their APRs because they may find themselves in a situation in which an unexpected wind shift places them in a chemical plume (cloud of gas or vapor) requiring immediate respiratory protection to exit the area. APRs do not provide oxygen and are not useful in an area that might be low in oxygen. APRs are not recommended in the presence of gases that have no odor such as phosphine or carbon monoxide, but they are acceptable in the presence of agents with a strong smell such as ammonia (see Chapters 2 and 7). In other words, if the filters fail, the wearer will notice the smell and realize the filters have failed. APRs give good mobility, but they increase the work of respiration and thus cause a significant heat load and workload for the wearer. Though workload and heat load limit the service time for an APR, it is usually longer than that possible in Levels A or B protective suits. Another common version of the APR is a powered air-purifying respirator (PAPR), which uses battery power to drive a fan, which pulls air through filters to provide the wearer with clean air (Figure 1.10). These devices remove the workload of breathing found in a gas mask, but their time of use is limited to the life of the battery. PAPRs are available with either a mask or a hood. A major advantage to the hood-type PAPR is that the hood allows the rescuer to wear glasses (which is not always possible with masks). Hoods are

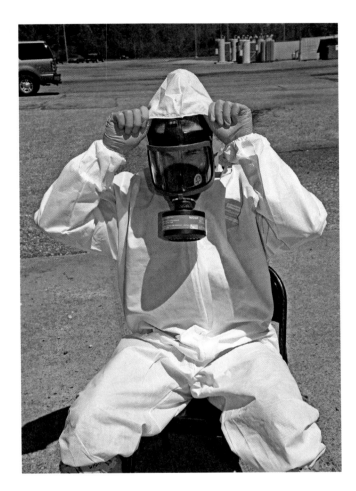

Figure 1.8
Example of Level C PPE
with APR.

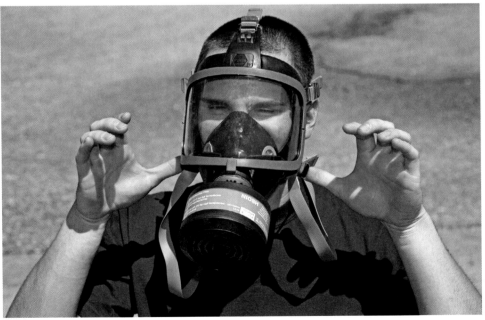

Figure 1.9
Example of a gas mask
(APR). Notice large filter
canister attached to
front of mask.

less claustrophobic, and they are less frightening to victims because the large facial viewing area allows victims to see the rescuer's face. OSHA C-level equipment is commonly used by law enforcement, EMS, and hospitals because it can be worn for a longer period of time and doesn't require as much training to operate and maintain. Another plus is the increased dexterity when compared to Level A or B ensembles. Level C allows users to perform their duties, which they could not do

Figure 1.10
Example of Level C PPE
with PAPR.

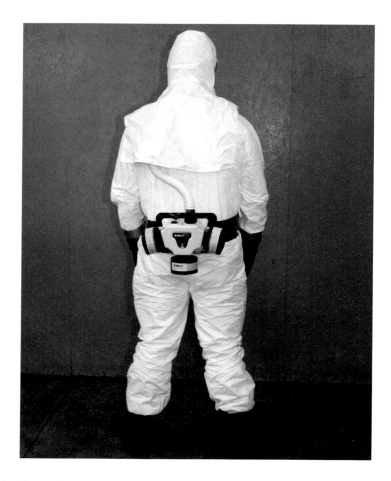

efficiently if wearing Level A or B equipment. The threat hazards to which EMS, hospitals, and law enforcement are usually exposed are less than those faced by the fire service personnel who routinely use Level A or B protection (Box 1-1). See "Practical Skills: 1" for more detail on donning Level C protection.

Box 1-1

All respirators other than some of the hood-type PAPRs require a respirator fit test. All persons wearing a respirator should attend a medical surveillance program to qualify them to wear the device. In some instances, this will necessitate a physical examination and pulmonary function tests. An annual fit test and medical examination is required. Many health care facilities elect to use the hood-type PAPR because it requires no fit test and it allows greater mobility and excellent visibility without a substantial workload (Figure 1.11).

Figure 1.11
Example of medical personnel caring for a patient while wearing Level C PPE with PAPR.

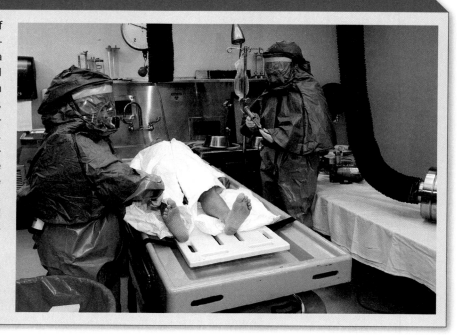

Figure 1.12
Example of Level D PPE.

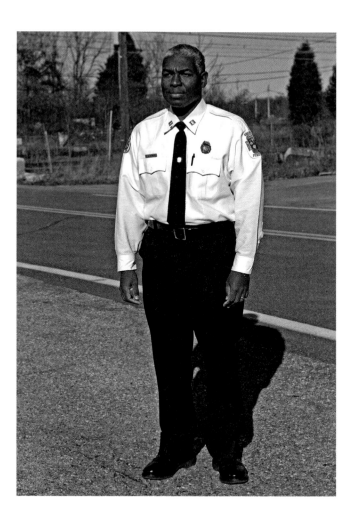

Level D Protection

Level D protection is normal work clothes or the normal uniform or attire worn by the public safety responder (Figure 1.12). This uniform should include an N-95 rated soft mask that covers the nose and mouth (Figure 1.13). This will provide good protection against inhaling biological agents and will also decrease the potential inhalation of radioactive materials. Level D provides excellent maneuverability and dexterity and will provide some protection against skin and

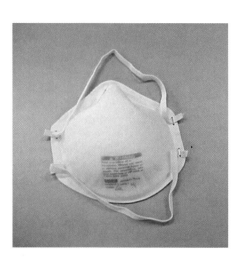

Figure 1.13
Example of an N-95
face mask.

Figure 1.14
Example of a cooling vest that can be worn under PPE.

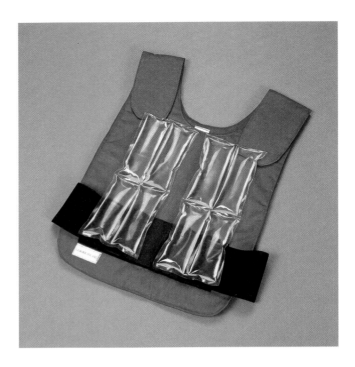

respiratory contamination from biological and radiological agents. Firefighter's turnout gear with an SCBA has been tested against nerve and blister agents and, if taped well, can provide respiratory protection and some vapor protection for up to 30 minutes. Use of this gear in place of higher levels of PPE is not recommended except in immediate lifesaving situations where other PPE is not immediately available.

Heat Stress

Both respiratory protection and chemical protective clothing cause heat stress on the body. The impermeable nature of chemical protective gear makes it retain heat and perspiration, defeating the body's ability to cool itself. The charcoal-impregnated protective suits worn by the military and some law enforcement units allow more vapor and heat loss and may be preferred in some situations. The workload of breathing in an APR or carrying an SCBA plus the heat load of working in the chemical protective gear severely limit the amount of time that providers can perform their duties. Cooling vests are available but add to the weight of the suit (Figure 1.14). Because of the body's inability to cool itself while in chemical protective clothing, heat injuries such as heat exhaustion and heat stroke are common, especially in the summer months. Rescuers working in PPE should be monitored for heat illness.

Body Armor

What about people hazards? In the past, EMS and fire service personnel were rarely attacked. However, assaults on EMS, emergency department staff, and fire service personnel have become more common. When a law enforcement emergency exists, it is now standard procedure for EMS and fire personnel to stage some distance away until the scene is secure. Calls involving assaults, firearms, edged weapons, disorderly persons, or other unusual or suspicious calls, mandate the staging of non-law-enforcement personnel at a distance until the scene is declared safe by law enforcement. Unfortunately, events regularly occur that are not initially considered law enforcement emergencies but evolve into dangerous situations.

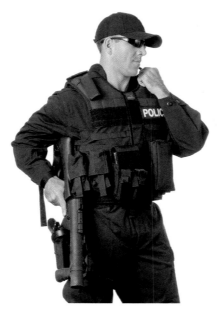

Figure 1.15
Example of vest-type body armor worn by law enforcement personnel. Similar vests are available to EMS personnel.
source: Photo of Cover6 tactical armor courtesy of PROTECH Tactical.

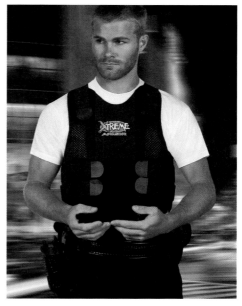

Figure 1.16
Example of concealed body armor. This can be worn under clothing by law enforcement personnel or other emergency responders.
source: Photo of Xtreme body armor courtesy of American Body Armor.

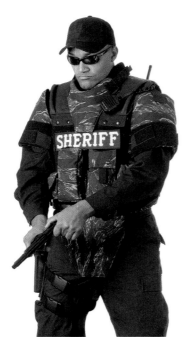

Figure 1.17
Example of Level IV body armor.
source: Photo of TRIMAX tactical armor courtesy of PROTECH Tactical.

In the United States the most common form of lethal assault on law enforcement, EMS, and fire service personnel involves firearms. Knives or other edged weapons are a distant second. Firearm assaults are usually at close range with a handgun. With this in mind, many EMS and fire service personnel are wearing body armor when responding to scenes that involve the potential for assault. Body armor is relatively inexpensive and can be worn externally in an EMS-type vest or concealed under uniform clothing. The most common configuration is the externally worn EMS-type vest that allows the provider to carry equipment in the multiple pockets (Figure 1.15). This form of armor is not easily recognized as a bullet-resistant vest. It is easy to put on and usually does not have to be individually sized for each responder. Concealed body armor must be worn under the uniform shirt and must be custom fitted to each responder (Figure 1.16). It is not easy to put on and is usually worn the entire shift.

Body armor comes in four levels of protection:

- *Threat Level I.* Will stop only low-power handgun rounds, and thus its use cannot be recommended.
- *Threat Level II.* Will protect against most handgun rounds.
- *Threat Level III and IIIA.* Will protect against most carbines and submachine guns that fire pistol-caliber bullets (9 mm is most common).
- *Threat Level IV.* Will protect against most rifle rounds, such as .308 caliber or .223 caliber rounds (Figure 1.17).

Most law enforcement agencies recommended that EMS and fire service personnel have available to them National Institute of Justice certified body armor of at least Threat Level II. The higher Threat Level body armor is available but is more expensive and heavier. Remember that body armor, due to its weight and lack of breathability, results in a substantial heat load to the body. The potential for developing heat exhaustion or heat stroke is increased by the use of body armor.

This is particularly true when body armor is worn under chemical protective clothing and/or used along with an SCBA or APR.

Responding to an Emergency Call

Before getting into the specifics of the various types of terrorist attacks (Chapters 2–6), it is prudent to briefly discuss how to recognize and approach a suspicious event. Such events should be approached and managed in a logical sequence to minimize the number of casualties (especially among responders).

The initial reports of an unusual incident should arouse the suspicion of the Emergency Communication Center (911). If there are any suspicions, the dispatcher should report a possible terrorist attack or at least an unusual event to public safety responders so they can be prepared. When the unit is dispatched, the dispatcher should advise them of any significant call history or advisories attached to the location (prior attacks on responders, known location of dangerous group). Computer Aided Dispatch (CAD) can facilitate this data. Those agencies without CAD will have to rely on dispatcher or responder memory. However, initial reports may not be suspicious and first responders to a terrorist attack may not be aware of the danger.

Situations will vary and are not predictable. Many high-risk calls resolve into a non-event, whereas routine calls can evolve into a life-threatening scenario. *The key is for all responders to practice the same initial approach to calls regardless of the call's apparent nature.* Every call or incident should be assessed in the same manner, with appropriate tactics practiced as needed. Any hazardous materials incident is a possible terrorist attack, especially if multiple casualties are involved. Also, any multicasualty incident that appears unusual, or any report of unusual casualties from an unknown source, should raise a red caution flag and be approached as a possible terrorist attack (Box 1-2).

Box 1-2 Threats and Hoaxes

In most communities the most common call for a possible terrorist incident is not to an actual event but rather to a threat or a hoax. When a threat is called in or a suspicious package is found, the probability of an actual event is low, but you must presume that a device or event is real until proven otherwise. The most common threat is the prank call stating that a bomb is on the premises of a school or other public place. Another common scenario is the discovery of a suspicious device, letter, or package with a threat. In some circumstances the item will contain a powder along with a threat or extortion demand. A similar scenario is the introduction of a hoax substance into a ventilation system of a structure, followed by a threat causing evacuation of the facility. The fact that most of these events are hoaxes must never lull you into dropping your guard and ignoring protocols. If you make a habit of treating every response as a dangerous situation, you will be prepared if the event turns out to be an actual terrorist attack. After the event (hoax or real), take time to evaluate your agency's response and make a concerted effort to correct mistakes and improve your performance.

Approaching the Scene

Scene approach should consist of several stages. On all calls you should turn off emergency lights and sirens as you near the scene. It is not wise to announce your arrival before you have made a careful "through the windshield" scene survey for danger. It is important to practice the same protocol each time so that the practice becomes automatic behavior. *Never assume that the dispatch information regarding the call is accurate and that the scene is safe.*

If the call is high-risk or in a high-crime area, fire service and EMS responders may need to wait for law enforcement to secure the scene. This procedure should be followed only in extreme circumstances and after careful consideration, since the delay could cost the life of a critical patient. If the danger level is so high that you must follow this procedure, then staging some distance away is important. Normally it is advisable to stay out of visual contact with the scene. If persons on the scene can see you, you are within firearms range and potentially at risk. Furthermore, staging in view of the scene can present a public relations disaster.

With every call you should make a cautious approach and not exit your vehicle until you have surveyed the scene through your windshield. If the call is suspicious, it is wise to use binoculars to observe from a distance, especially if there is danger of explosion or hazardous material. Try to make your approach from upwind, uphill, or upstream, avoiding fumes, smoke, mists, and liquids that might be toxic. Do not park directly in front of the scene but rather adjacent to it and a safe distance away. Park with your ambulance facing away from the scene so a rapid retreat can be made if necessary. If there is any danger of CBRNE attack, it is best to stage at a safe distance and then move forward after the HazMat team has deemed the scene safe or determined what level of PPE you should wear to enter. However, if your survey reveals injured patients who may be dying, you will not be able to wait for HazMat but will have to respond and use the highest level of PPE you have available. This is why you should carry your PPE at all times.

If you determine that there is a HazMat emergency or that a terrorist attack has occurred, you should immediately (before leaving the vehicle) notify dispatch and have them contact needed resources. The following may need to be called:

- The nearest HazMat team
- The nearest bomb squad
- The local and state public health departments
- The FBI (the lead federal agency for terrorism)
- Local nuclear regulatory or safety organization
- The local medical facilities that possess the capability to treat patients injured in a WMD incident
- Mutual aid support that is available from local, state, and federal agencies

All of the above should be cataloged and contact numbers recorded (and frequently updated) so they are immediately available. Until federal resources arrive, the coordination point for these events will be the local and state Emergency Management Agencies (EMAs). Expect a delay of several hours for mutual aid resources and up to 24 hours for federal assistance. If there have been multiple coordinated attacks, there may be even further delays of outside assistance.

Remember that terrorists may make an initial attack to draw you to the scene and then have a bomb or ambush set for when you arrive.

Recognition of Danger

Once you leave the vehicle and approach the scene on foot, you should keep an escape route in mind. Constantly look for signs of danger. Try to avoid situations in which there is only one path of escape. Calls involving numerous persons being sick, having difficulty breathing, having seizures, or fleeing the scene should heighten your sense of caution.

Danger can come from a variety of sources. Look for physical hazards and people hazards. Persons hiding, attempting to conceal their presence, or fleeing

It Happens...

The 2002 bombing on the Indonesian island of Bali began as a single suicide bomb (concealed in a backpack) that was detonated in a bar, but when rescue personnel arrived, a second much larger bomb (concealed in a van) exploded. This second explosion killed the majority of the victims, which included many rescue personnel.

Figure 1.18
Always be alert for danger.

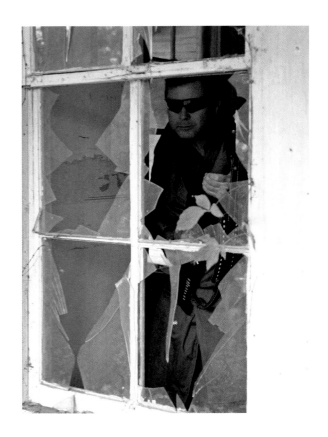

the scene should be considered dangerous. Be alert to vehicles, containers, LPG tanks, or boxes that seem out of place; they may contain a bomb. Carry a flashlight and watch where you step in low-light situations. Many older structures may have poor lighting with dilapidated stairs or steps. Hold the light out to your side. Armed attackers will usually aim at the light. High-intensity tactical lights are best and are small enough to *always* carry in your shirt pocket or on your belt. Listen for sounds of an altercation or persons opening doors or windows. Do not forget to look at windows to see if you are being observed from within the structure (Figure 1.18).

Think about chemical agents if there are complaints about persons down, difficulty breathing, seizures, or other unusual problems. Note any unusual smells. Dead animals or insects or brown vegetation can be an indication of chemical or biological agent exposure. Learn to trust your instincts. If you have a "gut" feeling that something is wrong, most of the time something is wrong. In this situation, withdraw and approach the scene again from a different direction or with additional help (such as HazMat and/or law enforcement).

Basic Scene Management

The initial responders to a contaminated scene should stage at a safe distance and immediately call for the HazMat team to enter the suspicious area to identify the chemical or biological agent(s) present. However, there may be times when you cannot wait for HazMat to arrive. For this reason you should have at least Level C (and preferably Level B) PPE on the response vehicle and available for immediate use.

Once you determine there is a HazMat emergency or a terrorist attack and there are casualties, you should have one member of your team immediately notify your supervisor, dispatch, law enforcement, all other responders, EMA, and medical direction. Your team leader will serve as temporary incident commander until the incident commander arrives on scene. As temporary incident commander, your initial action should be to designate a second member of your team as the triage officer. He or she should don the highest level of protective equipment available and begin triage of ambulatory patients. You should immediately select a safe staging/decontamination area several hundred feet upwind of the scene (see the next section, "Working Zones") and also select a place for the Incident Command Post. Having done this, you should also put on PPE and begin directing the ambulatory patients to the staging/decontamination area. Unless you already know the delivery device for the attack, you should not allow the ambulatory victims to carry anything with them (handbags, briefcases, backpacks, shopping bags, baby carriages, etc.) that could hide a delivery device. Law enforcement help may be needed. Because this may separate victims from their identification, they should be tagged with their personal information as soon as possible. If the HazMat team is not immediately available, you should enter the contaminated area and rapidly rescue the nonambulatory patients.

Backup EMS or HazMat personnel should set up a decontamination tent at the staging area and have the ambulatory patients remove their contaminated clothing and take a shower. These patients should then be given paper coveralls to wear until they can get fresh clothes. Once the patients have been decontaminated (see "Practical Skills: 2"), you should perform a rapid assessment and triage. Most of the ambulatory patients will be triaged priority three ("green tag," or delayed). You may find a few priority two ("yellow tag," or potentially unstable). Your nonambulatory patients will usually make up your priority one ("Red tag," or critical), the majority of your priority two, and all of your priority four ("black tag," or critical but unsalvageable).

As more help arrives, you will be able to use various detecting devices to pinpoint the manner of attack (see "Practical Skills" 3–6) and better plan your further response and treatment.

Working Zones

When responders first arrive at a CBRNE site, they should have the HazMat team evaluate the area for the agent used, and depending on weather conditions and the properties of the agent, they should set up working zones. These working zones are called the hot zone, warm zone, cold zone, and exclusion zone (Figure 1.19).

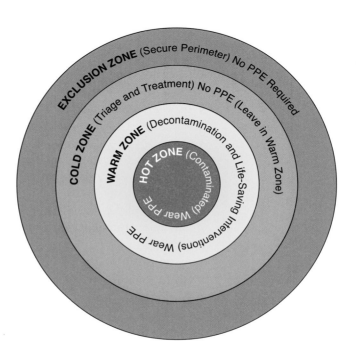

Figure 1.19
Working zones of a contaminated or dangerous site.

Hot Zone

The hot zone is a contaminated area. Everyone who enters this zone must wear the appropriate PPE, and the persons entering must be kept to a minimum. Victims who are still alive must be removed from this area as soon as possible. Bystanders (or anyone else who does not have a specific role) are not allowed into the hot zone.

Warm Zone

The warm zone is the control area immediately outside of the hot zone. Those entering the warm zone must wear the appropriate PPE. Within this zone the decontamination and lifesaving emergency treatment of victims are performed. Bystanders (or anyone else who does not have a specific role) are not allowed into the warm zone.

Cold Zone

The cold zone is the "safe area" where triage, patient evaluation, and treatment are performed. Rescuers coming from the hot or warm zones must themselves be decontaminated and leave their contaminated gear before entering the cold zone. Bystanders (or anyone else who does not have a specific role) are not allowed into the cold zone.

Exclusion Zone

The exclusion zone is a secure perimeter designated for public safety personnel. Law enforcement should secure this area and not allow bystanders (or anyone else who does not have a specific role) into the exclusion zone.

Crime Scene Considerations

All terrorist incidents are crime scenes. Your safety and the safety and care of your patients remain the top priorities, but preservation of evidence is important also. Fire or EMS personnel should not approach any scene suspected of involving violence unless law enforcement officers are on the scene and the scene is reasonably secure. Do not approach any known crime scene in which law enforcement officers are not present, in which the officers are in defensive positions, or when they are holding their weapons. If the scene appears suspicious or dangerous when you perform your windshield survey, call for law enforcement and withdraw until they arrive and secure the scene. On all scenes, use caution when approaching buildings and never stand directly in front of a door when knocking for entrance. If you find your life in danger, you must withdraw immediately even if it means leaving your patient.

To preserve evidence at a crime scene, you should do the following:

- In a terrorist attack, establish and have law enforcement secure scene boundaries (working zones).
- If the delivery device for the attack is unknown, do not allow the ambulatory victims to take anything with them (handbags, briefcases, backpacks, shopping bags, baby carriages, etc.) that could conceal a delivery device.
- When approaching a crime scene, ask law enforcement for the best route to approach (you will leave the same way) so as not to disturb evidence.
- Avoid disturbing possible tire tracks and footprints.
- Avoid touching blood you see on any environmental surface.
- Do not disturb items present on the scene unless absolutely necessary.
- Do not cut or treat through holes in clothing made by projectiles or other objects.

- Remove any medical items brought into the scene.
- When possible, place on a clean sheet any victim to be transported. When the victim is transferred to the hospital bed, retain the sheet for law enforcement investigators to examine for trace evidence.
- Retain, preferably wrapped in a clean sheet or placed in an unused *paper* bag, any clothing or other items removed while in the ambulance.
- Do not place blood-contaminated items in a plastic bag, as this may ruin their value as evidence.
- Do not touch or handle items (particularly weapons) found at a crime scene unless absolutely necessary.
- If expended bullets or casings are found in clothing or on a sheet, do not handle them with metal forceps. Retain them in the sheet or clothing in which they are found and notify law enforcement investigators.
- In a terrorist attack, leave the dead undisturbed on-scene. EMS personnel must enter a crime scene to confirm obvious death. This should be accomplished with minimal scene disturbance. Coordinate with law enforcement personnel.
- Because you may be called upon to testify in court, when any crime scene incident *is completed*, you should write a report that covers all aspects of your involvement at the scene. This report should contain:
  - The name, unit, and phone number of every responder who entered the scene
  - The names of all victims and where they were transported to
  - Your observations and conversations with the family or persons present at the scene
  - Statements made by victims, suspects, or others present at a crime scene
  - How the scene appeared upon your arrival, and also any changes made to the scene during patient assessment and treatment
  - The location of response vehicles and equipment, furniture, weapons, or clothing that was moved
  - The items that you handled
  - Your route to the victim(s)

Medical Management of a Disaster or Mass Casualty Event

In the day-to-day operation of Emergency Medical Services it is not uncommon to have to care for more than one patient at a scene, but in actuality most treatment protocols are designed for single-patient encounters. These protocols will still work if there are few patients or if adequate backup units are available. However, at some point the number of patients will overload the system's ability to provide adequate care. When this happens the situation becomes a "disaster." By definition a *disaster* is an event that overwhelms the ability of the system to respond appropriately. Ability to respond varies from system to system, depending on the availability of resources.

Incident Command System

All EMS activities depend on effective organization, communication, and cooperation. This is even more important when there are multiple patients. In a mass casualty incident, inexperienced rescuers may develop "tunnel vision"

Figure 1.20
Incident Command System.

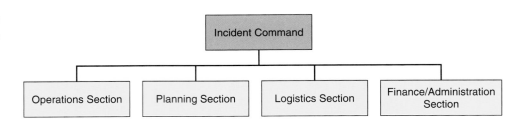

and their actions may hinder patient care. It is easy to forget about triage and concentrate on one critical, but unsalvageable, patient at the expense of multiple others who might be saved. Ambulances may be staged in the wrong area and cause traffic jams, or not be available where needed. Patients may be transported with no record made of who they are and where they were taken. All patients might be taken to one hospital, overwhelming its ability to care for them. Without organization you have chaos, and in a medical situation chaos can cost the lives of your patients. Organization comes from training and experience.

The Incident Command System (ICS) was developed in southern California in the 1970s after a devastating 13-day wildfire that claimed 16 lives and over a half-million acres of land. In the post-incident review it was noted that even though all of the responding agencies cooperated to the best of their abilities, there were numerous problems with communication and coordination. The U.S. Congress mandated that the U.S. Forest Service design a system that would effectively coordinate interagency action and allocation of fire suppression resources in dynamic, multiple-fire situations. From this mandate came a system for coordinating firefighting efforts (FIRESCOPE). This Incident Command System was soon recognized as useful not just for fires but also for management of a wide range of situations, including floods, hazardous materials incidents, earthquakes, and aircraft crashes. By the 1990s the ICS system had continued to evolve and was recognized as being flexible enough to be used by all public safety organizations.

For any system to work in an emergency situation, it must be simple enough for personnel in the field to remember it and flexible enough to adapt to varied and changing situations. The ICS provides a template for organizational control that is simple and flexible enough to adapt to all types of emergencies: fire, rescue, law enforcement, multicasualty, and disaster situations. Under the ICS, most personnel will require little training and will continue doing their jobs much like always. There are key personnel who must be thoroughly trained and must possess a complete understanding of how the system works. Prior planning and on-scene cooperation are the keys.

The components of the ICS are Command, Operations, Planning, Logistics, and Finance/Administration sections (Figure 1.20). One person or a small group (unified command—usually made up of the commanders of the different public safety organizations) assumes overall command and along with the command staff will oversee and coordinate the various sections. This is discussed in the next section, "National Incident Management System." The on-scene components of ICS (under Operations) are Command, Fire Suppression, Rescue/Extrication, Law Enforcement, and Medical branches (Figure 1.21).

National Incident Management System

In response to the terrorist threat, the Department of Homeland Security (DHS) developed the National Incident Management System (NIMS). This system makes use of the ICS but expands it so that federal, state, and local governments can work together, not only to respond to a terrorist attack (or other natural

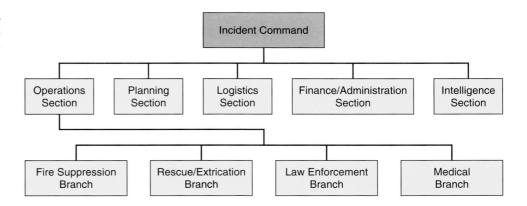

Figure 1.21
National Incident
Command System.

disaster), but also to prepare for and recover from such events. The components of NIMS are:

- Command and Management
- Preparedness
- Resource Management
- Communications and Information Management
- Supporting Technologies
- Ongoing Management and Maintenance

The ICS organization falls under Command and Management. To encourage every agency to learn the NIMS, beginning in 2006 all federal funding for state, local, and tribal preparedness grants will be tied to compliance with the NIMS. Hospitals will not be required to use NIMS but will continue to use HEICS (Hospital Emergency Incident Command System), their version of ICS. Like the ICS, the Incident Command Section of the National Incident Management System will have either a single incident commander or a unified command team. The management sections of the NIMS are the same as for the ICS (Command, Operations, Planning, Logistics, Finance/Administration), but NIMS also includes a potential sixth section (Intelligence/Information) (Figure 1.21). The responsibilities of the various sections are as follows:

- *Command Section.* The Command section is made up of the incident commander (or unified command) and the Command staff. The Command section is responsible for overall management of the incident.

- *Operations Section.* The Operations section is responsible for all activities focused on reduction of the immediate hazard, saving lives and property, establishing situational control, and restoration of normal operations. Local public safety personnel will fall under this section.

- *Planning Section.* The Planning section develops and documents the incident action plan and in most cases is responsible for gathering and disseminating information and intelligence critical to the incident. This includes keeping up with resources assigned to the incident.

- *Logistics Section.* The Logistics section is responsible for all support requirements. This includes facilities, transportation, supplies, equipment maintenance and fuel, food services, and medical supplies.

- *Finance/Administration Section.* The Finance/Administration section, if needed, is responsible for managing the financial and other administrative support services. This section would not be needed in a small incident but would come into play in situations like the bombing of the Alfred P. Murrah Federal Building in Oklahoma City or the collapse of the World Trade Center.

- *Intelligence/Information Section.* The Intelligence/Information section is responsible for gathering intelligence about the incident. This includes not only national security and other classified information, but also other operational information such as risk assessments, medical intelligence (disease surveillance), weather information, toxic chemical or radiation levels, and any other important data. This section can be separate or can be placed within Command, Planning, or Operations.

Other than the medical response, we will not go into further detail on NIMS because the Department of Homeland Security makes such training available through the Federal Emergency Management Agency (FEMA) (see Internet Sources at the end of this chapter).

Medical Incident Command System (MICS)

Medical response falls under the Operations section of NIMS. In general, the first arriving responders to a terrorist or mass casualty event notify dispatch of the situation and the senior person assumes the role of temporary incident scene commander. Another member becomes the initial triage officer. The team dons PPE, if appropriate, and the incident commander quickly surveys the whole scene for dangers to responders, need for special rescue equipment, and possible locations for ambulance staging, command post, and decontamination/treatment areas. At the same time the triage officer does an initial survey for total number of victims and severity of injuries and reports to the scene commander, who then reports to dispatch that ICS is being initiated and what resources are needed. While awaiting help, the team continues triage/treatment of the critical patients.

The Medical branch of the ICS is further divided into Medical Direction, Triage, Treatment, Transport, and Staging groups (Figure 1.22). The number of people needed in each group depends on the scope of the situation. The general rule is to have one person supervise five subordinates. This is

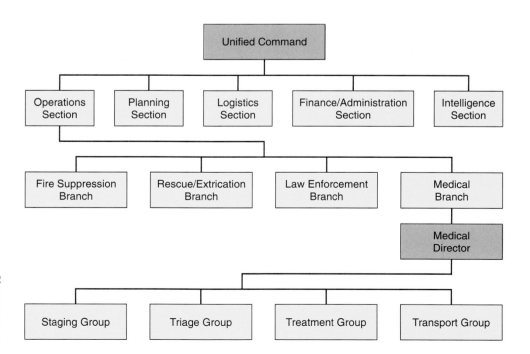

Figure 1.22
National Incident Command System and Medical Incident Command.

Box 1-3 General Responsibilities of Medical Branch Officers

Medical Branch Director

- Establishes liaisons with Incident Commander or Unified Command
- Establishes a working MICS with appropriate sections
- Ensures that proper rescue/extrication services are activated
- Ensures law enforcement involvement as necessary
- Ensures that helicopter landing zone operations are coordinated
- Determines the amount and types of additional medical resources and supplies
- Ensures that area hospitals and prehospital medical direction physicians are aware of the situation so they can prepare for casualties
- Designates assistance officers and their location
- Maintains an appropriate span of control
- Works as a conduit of communications between subordinates and the Incident Commander

EMS Staging Group Supervisor

- Maintains a log of available units and medical supplies
- Coordinates physical location of incoming resources (such as ambulances and helicopters)
- Coordinates incoming personnel who wish to help at the scene
- Provides updates to Medical Director as necessary

Triage Group Supervisor

- Ensures proper utilization of the Initial Assessment triage system or other local protocol
- Ensures that triage tag or other visual identification technique is properly completed and secured to the patient
- Makes requests for additional resources though Medical Director
- Provides updates to Medical Director as necessary

Treatment Group Supervisor

- Establishes suitable treatment areas, including segregation areas for decontamination
- Communicates resource needs to Medical Director
- Assigns, supervises, and coordinates decontamination and treatment of patients
- Provides updates to Medical Director as necessary

Transport Group Supervisor

- Ensures the organized transport of patients off-scene
- Ensures an appropriate distribution of patients to all local hospitals to prevent hospital overloading
- Completes a transportation log of patients and where they were taken
- Contacts receiving hospitals to advise them of the number of patients and their condition (may be delegated to a communications officer)
- Provides updates to Medical Director as necessary

called *span of control*, and it may vary from one person supervising three others in a complex situation to one person supervising seven others in a simple situation. Each person in the MICS will answer to only one supervisor. The general responsibilities of the medical group supervisors of a MICS are listed in Box 1-3.

Triage

Triage is the sorting of patients in order to provide the most care to the most patients. Triage will be different for a small group of patients than for a mass casualty event in which the number of patients exceeds the care available. When there are few patients, the main decision is which patient is to be treated and transported first, whereas in a mass casualty situation the decision must be made as to who will receive care and who will not. The triage officer should spend less than one minute doing an initial assessment to determine the priority of a patient. It cannot be overemphasized that the person doing the triage does *not* render any treatment to a patient other than opening the airway or applying pressure to an obvious external hemorrhage (if the treatment team is not immediately available). Treatment is to be done by the treatment group of the MICS. A triage officer who allows himself to begin treatment of victims is no longer a triage officer, and the function of triage must be reassigned. Once the medical priority of a patient has been determined, using the Triage Decision Tree (Figure 1.23), the

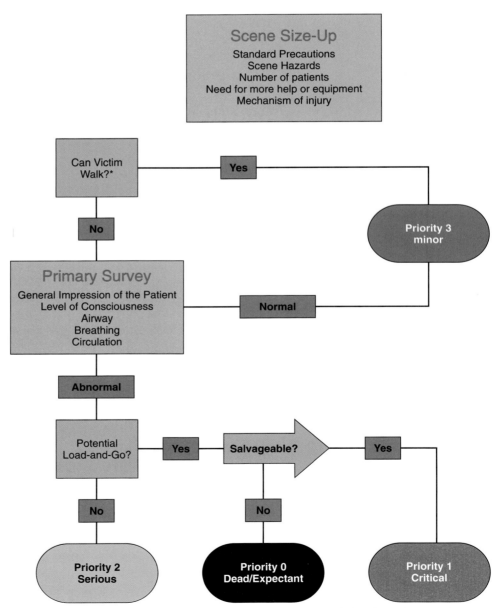

Figure 1.23
Triage decision tree.   *In large-scale incidents with a great number of patients, have those who are able walk to a designated area to be assessed.

Figure 1.24
Example of triage tag with space to record nerve agent antidote injections. Photo: Courtesy of Disaster Management Systems, Inc., www.TriageTags.com.

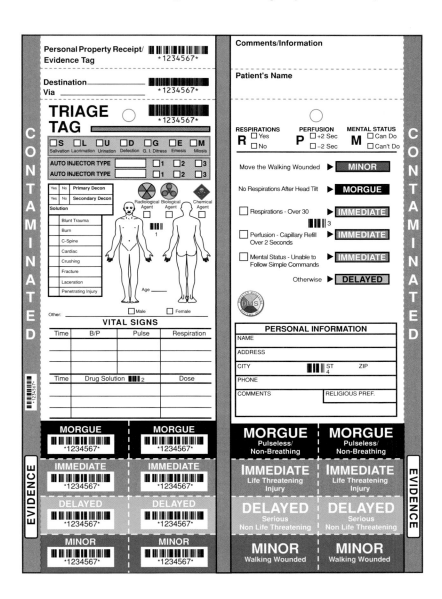

triage officer should affix an appropriately completed triage tag (Figure 1.24) or other visual identification technique to the victim and move on to the next victim to be assessed. Because victims may require wet decontamination, you should use tags that are still functional when wet.

Typically, patients are prioritized into four categories that determine their order of treatment and transport:

- *Priority 1*: Red tagged—critical condition, unstable but salvageable (load-and-go—treat these immediately).

- *Priority 2*: Yellow tagged—serious condition, potentially unstable (treated and transported after Priority 1 patients—treat within 1 hour).

- *Priority 3*: Green tagged—stable condition, minor injuries, "walking wounded" (treated and transported after Priorities 1 and 2—may be transported to the hospital by bus—treat within 3 hours).

- *Priority 4*: Black tagged—dead or alive but with fatal injuries (transported last). If resources are available without taking needed resources away from a salvageable patient, those tagged "alive but unsalvageable" may be grouped with the Priority 1 patients.

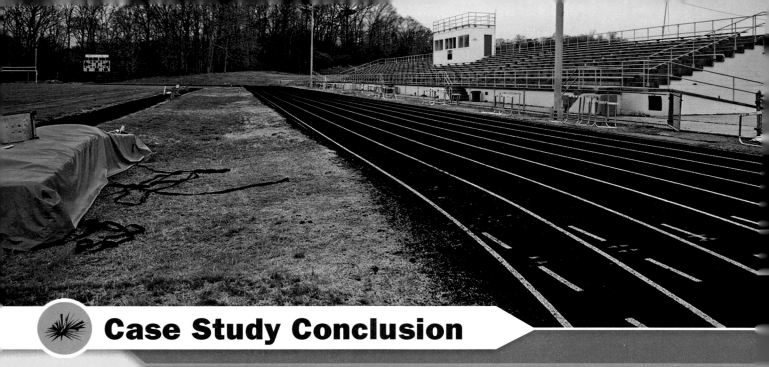

Case Study Conclusion

Many of the injured victims approach the area of the parked public safety vehicles. Police officers, being careful to remain upwind and avoid direct contact with victims, direct the people to segregation areas identified in the stadium disaster preplan. You put on Level C protective clothing and begin to triage the more than 30 ambulatory patients. You note that all of them have tearing and rhinorrhea. The patients also complain of burning of the eyes and difficulty breathing. You note no miosis (pinpoint pupils of the eyes). In the fresh air of the triage area, most of the victims report they are beginning to feel somewhat better but continue to complain about eye pain.

Some of the police officers that were initially in the area where the chemical exposure occurred report that they recognized the odor of ammonia. They are familiar with the effects, smell, and taste of the agent from clandestine drug laboratories. A HazMat team enters the area in Level A protective gear and reports chemical detection of low levels of ammonia with no other agents detected.

Public safety personnel in Level C protective gear enter the stadium to begin treatment of those injured. Patients in segregation/decontamination areas are directed to remove their clothing and receive a fire hose rinse. They are provided paper coveralls. All of the ambulatory patients require transport due to continued shortness of breath and eye pain. Within the stadium those remaining victims who are ambulatory are moved to the decontamination area. Seventy-three patients require stretcher transport for musculoskeletal injuries or severe respiratory difficulty. Two received closed head injuries with skull fractures. Their expedient decontamination is removal of their clothing. Eight patients have severe airway problems, and one has an asthma attack and suffers cardiac arrest. The resuscitation attempt is not successful.

The local hospital emergency department was initially notified early into the incident. They report that more than 100 patients have transported themselves to the emergency department for medical care. The patients are triaged outside the emergency department to avoid cross-contamination. Those in need of immediate treatment (15 patients having asthma attacks or severe respiratory distress) receive expe-

dient decontamination by removal of their clothing followed by medical treatment. Fans are set up in this area to blow contaminated air out of the department. Hospital personnel are in Level C garments using powered air-purifying respirators. Initial treatment consists of high-flow oxygen and flushing of the eyes with water. Anhydrous ammonia has an affinity for moisture and commonly causes eye and respiratory injuries.

The other ambulatory patients are required to remove their clothing and are showered in a decontamination area and then seen by the augmented emergency staff recalled by the implementation of the local disaster plan. The local hospitals dismiss noncritical patients in order to free beds. Local and state Emergency Management Agencies activate the regional medical disaster plan and coordinate the transport of patients to outlying medical facilities and request medical assistance from the state and regional level. Aeromedical support is used to airlift critical airway injuries to a tertiary medical facility. Surrounding hospitals are sent patients who are stable enough for transport. In spite of these measures, local medical and EMS resources are overwhelmed. The governor deploys local National Guard troops, and a regional military facility uses its MAST helicopters (military medical evacuation helicopters that assist in civilian emergencies) to help transport the injured.

Meanwhile, police officers find, on the upwind side of the stadium in the parking lot, three 5-gallon LPG (liquid propane gas) tanks with bluish corrosion on their brass valves. The containers are X-rayed by the bomb squad. It is determined that they are empty and contain no explosives. Tests by hazardous materials technicians note no toxic materials other than low levels of ammonia.

A total of seven persons succumb to respiratory-related injuries, and one of the patients with a closed head injury dies.

A homicide investigation is initiated and local police request FBI assistance. Federal law enforcement personnel begin to arrive within 8 hours. The national media report the story and later that evening begin arriving. A joint operations center is established in the county emergency operations center, and the local town civic center is used as a joint information center. Federal and state EMAs assist with assets to accommodate the media and with victim assistance. More than 100 federal law enforcement agents are involved in the investigation.

The propane gas tanks are recovered and processed for latent fingerprints by the FBI. Several latent prints are recovered and a comparison using the automated fingerprint identification system yields matches to two area residents affiliated with a radical right-wing group. The FBI assumes the lead role in the investigation because this is a terrorist event using WMD. The offenders are arrested without incident and are prosecuted for murder and use of a weapon of mass destruction. They are convicted and sentenced to prison for life without parole.

The direct cost of the incident exceeds $25 million. Some 27 victims have permanent eye injuries and another 8 have serious respiratory injuries that disable them. The final death toll remains at 9. The indirect costs are estimated at more than $250 million.

Case Study Discussion

This is an example of domestic terrorism, and it could happen in almost any community. Anhydrous ammonia is commonly used in agriculture, in the refrigeration industry, and in fertilizer production. It is also used in the manufacture of methamphetamine, so it is commonly in the possession of criminals. Anhydrous ammonia is extremely caustic to the eyes and respiratory system. People with respiratory disease are especially in danger from this chemical.

The scene was managed by a planned response. Patients were directed to a safe area upwind, and EMS personnel in Level C PPE performed initial evaluation and found signs and symptoms of a chemical attack. They initially decontaminated the patients by having them go to a safe area and disrobe. The patients were then wet decontaminated by being sprayed with a fire hose. Public safety personnel who were not attired in protective suits received the same chemical injuries as the football fans. All victims eventually required irrigation of their eyes to remove the caustic anhydrous ammonia. Treatment varied depending on injuries that ran the gamut from chemical exposure to asthma attack to cardiac arrest, as well as head and extremity injuries.

All public safety personnel were exposed to the same chemical attack as the civilians, but most were prepared to rapidly retreat to a planned staging area that was upwind. EMS had Level C PPE available to them so they did not join the ranks of victims but were able to continue performing their duties.

In this particular attack Level C attire was sufficient for protection, but Level A or B would have been better until the agent was identified.

It is always better if you have some warning that an attack might occur so that you can plan how to respond. This is why organizations and facilities should perform a security review. If you identify potential attacks, you can make plans to deal with them. When there is no prior planning or training, the number of dead and injured (especially of public safety and emergency department personnel) tends to be higher.

Pearls

- PPE must be immediately available! Keep your protective equipment in your patrol car, rescue vehicle, or ambulance. If you keep your PPE back at the station, it will be of no use to you when you need it.

- Do not enter a potentially contaminated area without proper protective equipment.

- Better to put on protective equipment and not need it than to enter an area unprotected.

- Your safety is of first importance! No longer can responders rush in to save lives without first thoroughly assessing the scene and the potential dangers. Self-protection is essential for you to perform your duties.

- Have body armor *available* and *wear it* if there is any danger of being attacked.

- The sudden appearance of multiple patients with similar complaints should alert you to the possibility of a terrorist event.

- When called to the scene of a multicasualty incident that involves suspicious symptoms (especially respiratory), do not enter the scene, except to save lives, until it has been cleared by the HazMat team.

- Survey the scene, observing for threats and any persons, vehicles, or containers that appear out of place or out of the ordinary.

- Do not become a victim! If you make an unplanned arrival at a suspicious multicasualty incident, you should immediately retreat to a safe area (upwind, upstream, uphill, and away from smoke, fogs, or liquids) and call the HazMat team and law enforcement.

- If the situation is critical, you may have to don your available PPE and rescue victims. Have appropriate PPE in your vehicle!

- Before leaving your vehicle, call dispatch to notify all other responders, the fire service, EMS, medical control, receiving hospitals, law enforcement, the bomb squad, and hazardous materials assistance.

- Be aware that there could be a second bomb or ambush awaiting responders.

- The senior initial responder to a multicasualty event should establish the incident command system and identify areas for triage, segregation, decontamination/treatment, and staging.

- Direct those fleeing the scene to safe segregation areas.

- To prevent cross-contamination, avoid direct contact with victims unless you are wearing proper PPE.

- Patients who need decontamination should be decontaminated before they are placed in your ambulance.

Want to Know More?

Bibliography

DeLorenzo, R.A. and Porter, R.S., *Weapons of Mass Destruction: Emergency Care,* Brady, Prentice Hall, 2000.

McVey, P.M. *Terrorism and Local Law Enforcement: A Multidimensional Challenge for the Twenty-First Century,* Charles C Thomas, 1997.

Mullins, W.C., *A Sourcebook on Domestic and International Terrorism,* 2nd ed., Charles C Thomas, 1997.

Ronczkowski, M.R., *Terrorism and Organized Hate Crime.* CRC Press, 2004.

Internet Sources

Chemical Protective Clothing
www.Tasco-Safety.com/clothing/standards.html

NIMS Training:
www.fema.gov/nims/nims_training.shtm

Basic Incident Command System
http://training.fema.gov/EMIWeb/IS/is195.asp

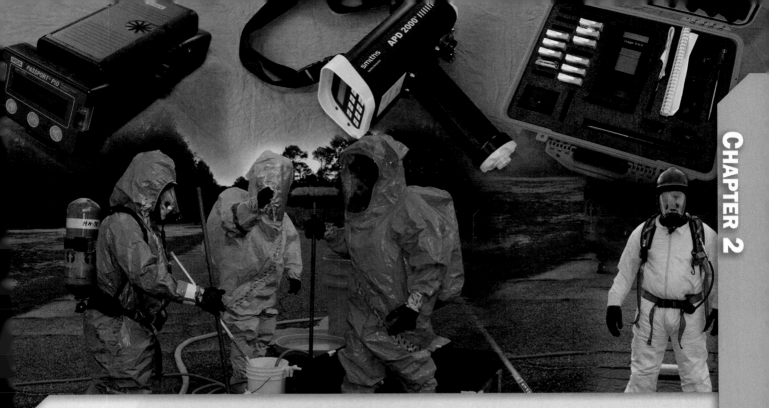

CHAPTER 2

Chemical Agents Used in Terrorist Attacks

Chapter Objectives

Upon completion of this chapter you should be able to:

1. List the methods for dispersing the agent in a chemical weapons attack.
2. Discuss the four methods of decontamination of victims.
3. List the classes of agents used in chemical weapons attacks and differentiate them by clinical presentation.
4. Discuss specific decontamination and treatment of victims of a nerve agent attack.
5. Discuss specific decontamination and treatment of victims of a cyanide agent attack.
6. Discuss why Level C PPE should not be used when working at the scene of a cyanide chemical attack.
7. Discuss specific decontamination and treatment of victims of a blister agent attack.
8. Discuss why hypochlorite solution should not be used to clean equipment that has been contaminated by blister agent.
9. Discuss specific decontamination and treatment of victims of a pulmonary agent attack.
10. Discuss specific decontamination and treatment of victims of a tear gas or pepper spray attack.
11. Discuss basic principles of EMS response to a possible chemical weapons attack.

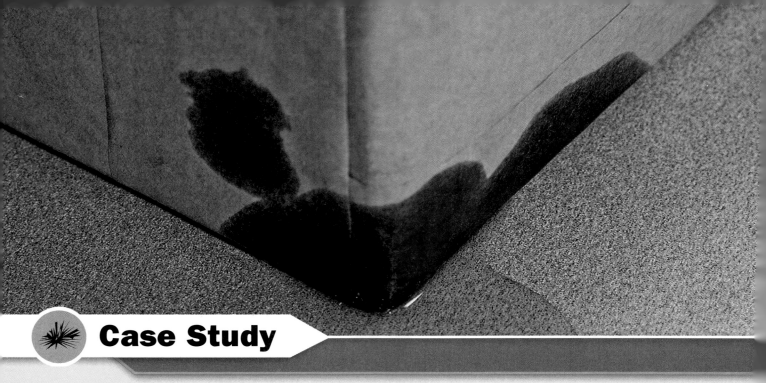

Case Study

You respond with fire, EMS, and law enforcement to a multinational company that has reported a suspicious package leaking a yellow colored liquid. You have responded to this facility on several occasions for bomb threats and demonstrations by radical environmental groups. The two employees handling the mail are experiencing severe eye pain, tearing, and profuse nasal secretions. They are also coughing and report being short of breath. Because the employees cannot see well, safety security personnel have to take them by the hand and lead them to safety. Security has isolated the area and shut down the ventilation system. The personnel in the building are being evacuated in an upwind direction. However, the two security personnel who entered the area to perform these tasks and who led the contaminated workers out of the building are now reporting similar symptoms. The first arriving EMS and fire personnel (not wearing protective clothing or respiratory protection) are now also experiencing tearing, eye pain, coughing, and shortness of breath following their assessment of the four patients. All patients are ambulatory and standing outside and upwind of the facility.

- What has happened?
- Is a toxic material involved?
- How would you control contamination?
- What are the decontamination steps?
- What treatment is indicated?
- Are the EMTs and firefighters on scene in danger?
- What protective clothing is required?

The Case Study will continue at the end of the chapter.

Although bombs are by far the most common method of terrorist attack, the threat of a chemical agent attack is very real. The term *chemical agents* refers to those chemicals that may be released by terrorists in an attempt to produce mass casualties. These chemicals include not only those agents that have been developed by military organizations (chemical warfare agents), but also extremely toxic chemicals that are routinely used in industrial processes. Large tanker trucks and train cars loaded with toxic chemicals pass through our cities every day. There have been several incidents involving chemical agents in the last several years. It is known that during the 1980s Iraq used cyanide gas and nerve agents against Iranian soldiers and Iraqi citizens (Figure 2.1).

Chemical agents are excellent for terror purposes as they have the *potential* to kill or injure thousands of people. The media have referred to chemical and biological agents as the "poor man's atomic bomb." However, these agents are somewhat difficult to manufacture in a clandestine environment (the Aum Shinrikyo cult spent millions to make sarin), so great concern exists about international theft of military agents. There are also concerns that rogue nations could provide terrorists with such weapons. Of even more concern is the vast amount of toxic industrial chemicals that are transported on our highways and railways every day. A tanker truck containing a toxic chemical could be hijacked and the chemical released in a populated area, causing as many casualties as the Bhopal disaster.

It Happens...

On the night of December 2, 1984, an accident at the Union Carbide plant in downtown Bhopal, India, caused the release of 40 metric tons of the deadly gas *methyl isocyanate*. The cloud of gas spread throughout the city of Bhopal, exposing at least half a million people. The number of people killed is still disputed. Union Carbide admits only to 3,800 deaths, but sources in India claiming at least 20,000 people have died over the years from the exposure.

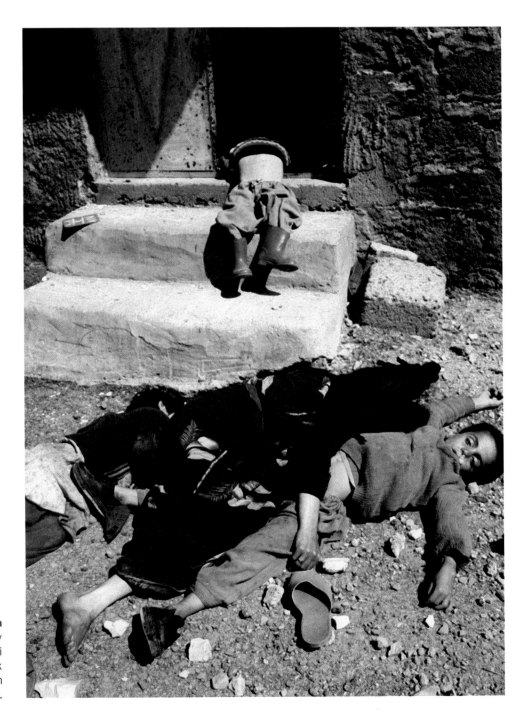

Figure 2.1a
Some of the approximately 5,000 victims of an Iraqi chemical weapons attack against the Kurdish town of Hallabja in 1988.

It Happens...

In Matsumoto, Japan, in June 1994, people complaining of eye pain, numbness of their hands, and difficulty breathing began showing up at a local hospital. Two died soon after arrival. All of the people were from the same residential area. The next day, dead fish were found floating in a pond in the community where these people lived. Around the pond the grass had turned brown, and there were carcasses of dead dogs and birds. Within 150 meters of the pond were found five people dead in their apartments. A total of 274 people were treated for complaints of eye pain and decreased vision, nausea, and difficulty breathing; 58 required hospitalization. The cause was found to be nerve agent poisoning. The perpetrators were not found at that time.

Almost a year later (March 20, 1995) in Tokyo during the morning rush hour, thousands of subway passengers began having the same symptoms as the Matsumoto victims. Five thousand people fled the subways and overwhelmed the unprepared local hospitals, contaminating many of the treating staff. Twelve people died. The Tokyo police suspected the doomsday cult Aum Shinrikyo, and two days after the attack they raided the facilities of this group. The police were astounded to find stockpiles of sarin nerve agent as well as hundreds of tons of chemicals, enough to make sufficient sarin nerve agent to kill millions of people. They also found a Russian military helicopter that had been purchased to use to spray the gas over the city of Tokyo. It was found that the cult had used a modified refrigerator truck to disperse sarin gas in Matsumoto and had carried containers of liquid sarin into the subways, where umbrellas were used to puncture the containers, allowing the sarin to leak out.

According to data from the media reports and FBI's Bomb Data Center, 80 to 85% of terrorist attacks will use conventional explosives in the form of homemade bombs. *However, bombs can also be used to disperse toxic chemicals.* The psychological warfare value produced following the mass hysteria from the use of a chemical agent cannot be underestimated. Unfortunately the vast majority of public safety agencies and medical facilities are not well equipped to handle such an event.

Chemical attacks will usually present suddenly, with many casualties displaying similar symptoms. Such an attack will require an EMS response, but if the attack occurs in a public setting, many patients may bypass the EMS system and transport themselves to the nearest emergency department. In the sarin nerve gas attacks in Tokyo, most of the 5,000 victims arrived by private vehicle or by simply walking to the nearest hospital. When this happens the emergency department can become overwhelmed with both "walking wounded" and the "worried well" (nervous individuals who are not injured but are worried that they might be). The danger in

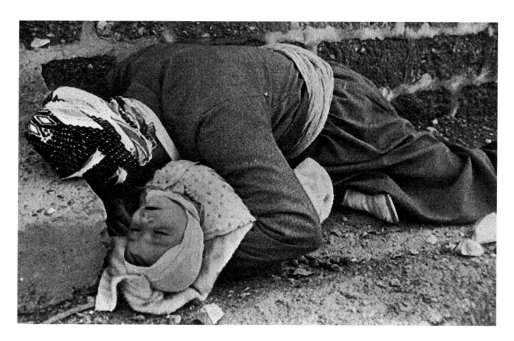

Figure 2.1b
Mother and child killed by
Iraqi nerve gas attack.

Figure 2.2
Unprepared and unprotected emergency personnel caring for sarin nerve agent victims.

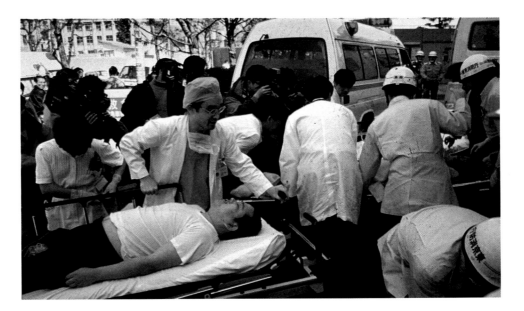

this situation is that the least injured arrive first and the sickest and critically injured will arrive later after the hospital is overwhelmed with victims, further delaying medical care for those most in need. The medical facility also may become contaminated before the nature of the event is realized.

The issue of responder safety is also important. Public safety agencies must adequately train their personnel in the proper methods to protect themselves so that they can respond appropriately to these threats. The sarin attacks in Japan injured a number of public safety and health care providers, demonstrating that chemical attacks present a danger for responders as well as those originally targeted (Figure 2.2). You must also keep in mind that terrorists have used secondary bombs to target public safety responders (Bali, Indonesia) and have even stolen ambulances, placed explosives inside, and detonated them among the rescuers (Israel).

Methods of Attack with Chemical Weapons

While terrorists could deliver chemical agents in liquid form and wait for them to evaporate (as in the Tokyo attack), the most efficient delivery method is aerosol. Aerosols are small droplets suspended in the air. Delivery methods include simple hand sprayers, planes (crop dusters), helicopters, or by a small explosive charge. Both chemical agents and biological agents can be dispersed in this manner. Chemical weapons are not popular with soldiers because it is difficult to control them. The aerosol is carried by the wind, and if the wind changes direction the agent could be carried onto their own forces.

There are several properties of chemical warfare agents:

- Most are liquids and must be converted to an aerosol or vapor for maximum effect.
- If there is no device to disperse the chemical (sprayer, explosion), the hot zone (Chapter 1) will be smaller.
- Sunlight will cause liquids to evaporate into the atmosphere more quickly, so the best time to attack is in the early morning or at night.
- Wind conditions affect a chemical or biological attack. Slow, steady winds will give greater concentration of the chemical over a larger area, while gusty winds will rapidly disperse the chemical, making it less effective or ineffective.
- Attacks in enclosed spaces (buildings, tunnels, or subways) are always going to have higher concentrations of chemicals than outdoor attacks.

Responding to a Chemical Attack

- When responding to an outdoor attack, try to keep the wind at your back so that the wind blows the chemical away from you.

- When responding to an attack in a building, (if you do not have a reason to contain the chemical in the building), immediately have the ventilation system shut down, open doors and windows, and set up fans for ventilation as soon as possible. This is not practical in large buildings.

- Any time chemicals are involved, consider having fans blowing in the decontamination area.

Principles of Decontamination of Victims

Physical decontamination of victims is the removal of hazardous substances from victims to prevent or reduce toxicity. Decontamination reduces the amount of toxic material to which the victim is exposed and also reduces the risk of secondary contamination (cross-contamination) of rescuers and others at the scene or the hospital.

There are four methods of decontamination: dilution, absorption, neutralization, and isolation/disposal.

- *Dilution.* Dilution involves the application of large volumes of water to the contaminated patient. This is called wet decontamination. If possible it should be used with soap to make it more effective. If performed soon enough and well enough, this will reduce the concentration of the material on the skin by 99%. If water is not available, dry decontamination can be performed using a combination of absorption, isolation/disposal, and standing in front of a fan. Wet decontamination will then have to be done upon arrival at the emergency department at the hospital.

- *Absorption.* Absorption involves the use of some substance (fuller's earth, flour, M291 kit, towels, etc.) to blot up the liquid material. This would usually be done when water is not available (dry decontamination) or if there is persistent oily liquid on the skin after showering. It is more commonly used for decontamination of equipment.

- *Neutralization.* Neutralization involves the elimination of a chemical's toxicity by applying another chemical that reacts with it, such as neutralizing an acid with an alkali. These reactions can produce heat, which is potentially as damaging as the original chemical. This method is almost never used on contaminated victims. This is more applicable to decontaminating environmental surfaces than victims.

- *Isolation/Disposal.* Isolation involves the separation of the patient from the hazardous substance. This means first removing the patient from the hot zone and then removing the patient's clothing and jewelry. All contaminated items should be properly stored in hazardous material bags.

Combinations of these methods may be used in any particular situation.

Decontamination equipment (such as tents, pumps, heaters, soap, towels, disposable clothing) is usually stored in a "decon trailer" so that, when needed, everything is ready and available and can be taken directly to the scene of the exposure (Figure 2.3). It can take an hour or more for this equipment to arrive and be set up, so first responders may have to use expedient methods until this is done. This can involve initial dry decontamination or the use of hoses or showers that may be available near the scene. For this initial emergency decontamination to take place, the first responders must wear PPE of at least Level C or they will become cross-contaminated by the victims. Unfortunately most responders don't carry PPE in their vehicles. Hopefully this will change as more receive homeland security training.

Water is the cornerstone of decontamination of victims, but tap, hydrant, and tanker-truck water is usually colder than the ambient temperature so hypothermia can be a problem, especially in winter. There are products on the market to warm

Figure 2.3
A truck used for HazMat response and decontamination.

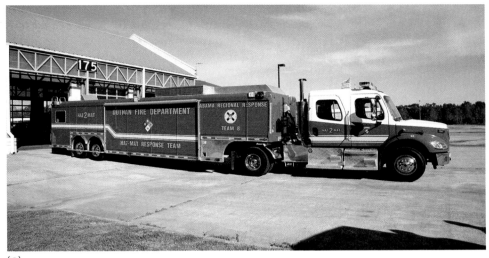

(a)

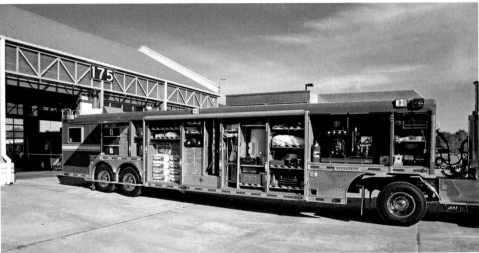

(b)

the water from a tanker truck or hydrant. If such water heaters are not available on-scene, the decision about wet versus dry decontamination depends on the toxicity of the exposure, the danger of hypothermia, and the availability of existing showers with heated water (in private homes, schools, office buildings, barracks, dormitories, etc.).

Many patients who have field decontamination (especially those with only dry decontamination) will require further decontamination at the hospital. If the scene is close to the hospital, many victims may transport themselves directly to the hospital and arrive having had no decontamination at all (as in the Tokyo sarin attacks). Hospitals usually have little in the way of decontamination equipment other than wading pools, water hoses, and soap. Most emergency departments have no PPE available and no training in the use of PPE. Thus, if contaminated victims arrived at the emergency department, the staff would become cross-contaminated while trying to perform decontamination of the patients. Most hospitals depend on the fire service, EMS, or EMA to provide a decon trailer in an emergency situation. The problem with this is the decon trailer may be in use at the scene of the incident and not be available.

Management of contaminated victims can be a problem. Most U.S. citizens (except those who have been indoctrinated by air travel) resent being herded and ordered about, and when told that they must remove and leave their clothes, jewelry (especially those with expensive jewelry or watches), and wallets or purses, they might refuse. Law enforcement help may be needed. It is wise to have available "Doff-it" kits that contain a plastic poncho for privacy, hazardous material bags for their clothes, and sealable hazardous material bags for their jewelry and identification. They can take the sealed bag of personal items with them but the contents will have to be decontaminated or disposed of at some point. Wet decontamination can be performed while the victim is wearing the plastic poncho if the victim is ambulatory.

Generally only lifesaving care is performed (by personnel in appropriate PPE) before the victim is decontaminated. Lifesaving care includes opening the airway, control of serious bleeding, and use of the Nerve Agent Antidote Kit, which can be injected through the victim's clothes. If at all possible, don't let the victim die while awaiting decontamination. See "Practical Skills: 2" for more specific information on decontamination.

Chemical Warfare Agents That May Be Used by Terrorists

We will not try to cover toxic industrial chemicals, because there are far too many of them to cover in a basic course. Chemical warfare agents are generally divided into these categories: nerve agents, cyanide, vesicants, pulmonary agents, and riot control agents.

Nerve Agents

A German scientist (Dr. Gerhard Schrader) developed the first nerve agent (Tabun, or GB) while trying to develop an improved insecticide. He found that the organo-phosphate insecticide he developed not only killed insects; it killed just about everything else as well. Because the nerve agents were developed in Germany, they were called "G" agents (GA, GB, GD, and GF). Germany recognized their value as chemical weapons and had large stockpiles of these agents during WWII but for reasons unclear never used them. The United States has stockpiles of the nerve agents GB and VX. These agents are considered major chemical weapons for military use, but the only known use of them on the battlefield was in the Iran-Iraq war (1980s). These agents are believed to be stockpiled by many countries, and they could be obtained or synthesized by terrorists.

Physical Properties and Mechanism of Action

Nerve agents exist in liquid form (colorless to brown) and evaporate to form vapors. They are also rapidly absorbed through the skin. This makes them ideal for delivery in an aerosol form that can be absorbed through either the lungs or the skin. Nerve agent vapors are denser than air, so they will accumulate along the ground and tend to pool in low spots, such as drainage ditches. How long a particular nerve agent will persist on environmental surfaces depends on how rapidly it evaporates into the atmosphere (volatility). The more volatile the agent is, the less persistent it will be on environmental surfaces. Nonpersistent agents are those that are not a threat after 24 hours. Agents that stay on surfaces for more than 24 hours are considered persistent. VX and many agents improvised from organophosphate insecticides are persistent. Of the G-series of nerve agents, GA and GF are persistent while GB and GD are nonpersistent.

Nerve agents are lethal chemicals originally developed from organophosphate insecticides (such as Malathion or Parathion) that are commonly used in agriculture (Figure 2.4). Nerve agents exert their deadly action by inhibiting the critical enzyme acetylcholinesterase. The proper functioning of the human nervous system depends on the nerve transmitter acetylcholine, which is released from the nerve endings when a nerve impulse is transmitted. The acetylcholine is immediately broken down by the enzyme acetylcholinesterase. This prevents continual firing of the nerve. Nerve agents inhibit acetylcholinesterase, allowing the excessive

Figure 2.4
Malathion insecticide, from which the nerve agents were developed.

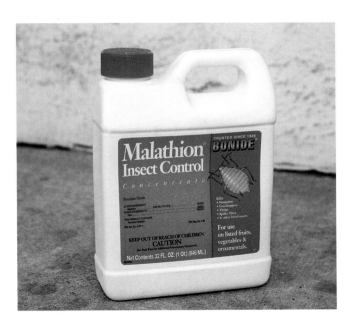

accumulation of acetylcholine, which results in the continuous stimulation of nerve endings. In the proper dose these agents will cause death within minutes.

Clinical Effects

The clinical effects (signs and symptoms) of the nerve agents are upon the parasympathetic nervous system, which tends to regulate "vegetative" functions of the body such as digestion, slowing of heart rate, urination, and defecation. The following are signs (things the examiner can see) and symptoms (things the patient feels) of exposure to a vapor nerve agent: anxiety, salivation (drooling), lacrimation (tearing), urination, defecation/diarrhea, emesis (vomiting), miosis (pinpoint pupils) (Figure 2.5), rhinorrhea (runny nose), dyspnea (difficulty breathing), muscle fasciculation (twitching, jerking). The acronyms **SLUDGEM** and **DUMBELS** can be used to remember these signs and symptoms:

SLUDGEM	**DUMBELS**
S—salivation	**D**—diarrhea
L—lacrimation	**U**—urination
U—urination	**M**—miosis
D—diarrhea	**B**—bronchoconstriction
G—gastric upset	**E**—emesis
E—emesis (vomiting)	**L**—lacrimation
M—miosis	**S**—salivation

These symptoms progress to loss of consciousness, seizures, apnea (cessation of breathing), and death. It is important to remember an acronym, SLUDGEM or DUMBELS, but even more important to know the very early symptoms of exposure. Soon after exposure to nerve agent vapors, most victims complain of *eye pain, decreased vision, and difficulty breathing*. The more rapidly the symptoms

Figure 2.5
Dilated (left) versus pinpoint (right) pupils.

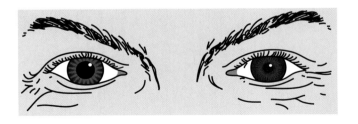

Box 2-1	LD50 of "G" Agents
GA—Tabun	1,000 mg (1 gram)
GB—Sarin	1,700 mg (derived from the insecticide parathion)
GD—Soman	50 mg
GF—(no common name)	30 mg

develop, the greater the probability that the dose was lethal. A victim will usually develop symptoms rapidly after inhalation of a nerve agent vapor but may not develop symptoms for up to 18 hours after exposure to a liquid nerve agent.

"G" Series Nerve Agents

"G" agents are potent acetylcholinesterase inhibitors. They are all more volatile than VX, but GA and GF are considered persistent (will not evaporate for over 24 hours). Box 2-1 lists the LD50 (amount it takes to kill 50% of those exposed) of victims with skin exposure to "G" agents.

"VX" Nerve Agent (Venom Agent)

This agent is oily and does not evaporate quickly, thus it is primarily a skin or eye absorption agent. When sprayed on environmental surfaces, it will last longer than 24 hours (persistent). However, under certain conditions it may be inhaled. VX is very potent. The LD50 of victims with skin exposure to VX is only 10 mg (1 drop).

Specific Decontamination of Nerve Agent Victims

When performing decontamination, you must wear protective clothing and respiratory protection of at least Level C. Removing the victim's clothes should be enough for exposure to vapor only. CROSS-CONTAMINATION POTENTIAL IS HIGH—DOUBLE-BAG CLOTHES (in hazardous waste bags—not garbage bags) THAT YOU REMOVE FROM PATIENTS.

If the victims have liquid on their clothes or skin, you must perform wet decontamination. Use soap and lots of water for victims. Up to 10 to 15 minutes of irrigation with soap and water may be needed. Use 5% hypochlorite solution for contaminated equipment (Figure 2.6). Equipment may require up to 30 minutes

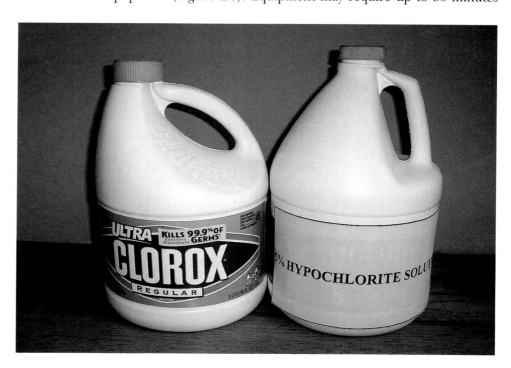

Figure 2.6
5% hypochlorite solution and household bleach (6% hypochlorite solution).

Figure 2.7
M291 decontamination kit.

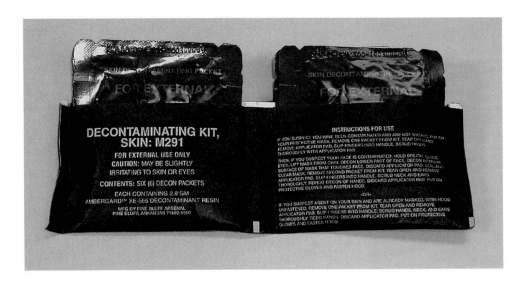

of cleaning with this solution. A 5% hypochlorite solution is for decontaminating equipment, not patients. Hypochlorite solutions should be fresh and alkaline with a pH of 10, but commercial or household chlorine bleach will suffice in emergency circumstances. If there is not enough water for the victims to wash, the 5% hypochlorite solution should be diluted 1:10 (to 0.5%) with water and used to clean liquid agent from the skin and wounds. Control water runoff if possible. Be mindful that exposure to liquids, including water, may diminish the effectiveness of your PPE. Prevent further contact of the agent with the body during irrigation and cleaning. The following can be used to remove liquid nerve agent from the skin but are unlikely to be available when needed:

- Fuller's earth (diatomaceous earth) can be used effectively to blot the oily liquid of nerve agents and also is an excellent indicator of the agents present, as it adheres to the agent on the skin and environmental surfaces.
- Common flour can be used in the same way and is almost equally effective. Both fuller's earth and flour must be wiped off with a tissue once they stick to the liquid.
- The M291 military resin kit may be used for skin decontamination (avoid the eyes) (Figure 2.7). The resin, which both removes the agent and also neutralizes it, leaves a black marking when it absorbs the chemical agent.

All discarded contaminated material should be soaked in a 5% solution of hypochlorite or placed in a hazardous material bag, double bagged, and sealed.

Treatment of Nerve Agent Exposure Victims

Because of the danger of nerve agent attack on U.S. soldiers, the military developed the Mark I Nerve Agent Antidote Kit (NAAK) (Figure 2.8). The NAAK contains two autoinjectors. One injector contains 2 mg of atropine and the other contains 600 mg of pralidoxime (2-PAM). These are the preferred antidotes for nerve agent exposure. They are for intramuscular (IM) use in the field and can be given through two layers of clothes. The military has since developed a new single autoinjector that delivers both the atropine and the 2-PAM through one needle. It will replace the two-injector NAAKs when present stores are used up. At this time the single injector (DuoDote) is available for civilian use.

The atropine works quickly to block the receptor site for the nerve transmitter acetylcholine. This helps prevent the constant firing of the nerves and gives relief of the symptoms. The 2-PAM is a true antidote and it breaks the bond that has formed between the nerve agent and the enzyme acetylcholinesterase. This allows the enzyme to break down the acetylcholine. Some kits also include a CANA (convulsants antidote for nerve agent) injector for treatment of seizures. CANA injectors

Figure 2.8
The NAAK (*left*) contains two injectors (atropine and 2-PAM), while the ATNAA (*right*) contains both antidotes in the same injector.

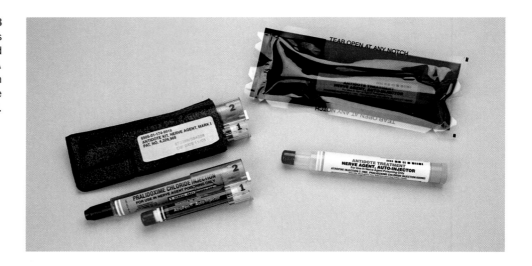

contain 10 mg of diazepam (Valium) and are for IM use (Figure 2.9). Paramedics usually treat seizures by the more effective intravenous (IV) injection of diazepam or lorazepam (Ativan), but in the mass casualty situation these IM injectors can be used to prevent seizures in patients who have not yet been decontaminated.

If there is a potential threat from a nerve agent attack, public safety responders should carry the NAAK and hospitals should stock the kits. Those areas most likely to be threatened are metropolitan areas, areas near military storage sites for nerve agents, and areas near chemical weapons transportation routes. Each rescuer should be issued three MARK I kits (NAAK) with the atropine and pralidoxime injectors and with the consideration of issuing one CANA diazepam injector.

If an area decides to stock the antidote kits, they must train responders and hospital staff on when and how to use them. The Chemical Stockpile Emergency Preparedness Program (CSEPP) provides nerve agent kits to most emergency agencies and hospitals near the military stockpiles of nerve agents. In other areas, emergency agencies and hospitals have used local, state, or federal money to purchase the kits. The kits have a shelf life of approximately 5 years but are probably effective for a much longer period. Atropine stored since World War II has been found to still have 90% effectiveness. Expired kits should be stockpiled for use in case of a massive incident.

Using the NAAK is very simple ("Practical Skills: 3"). Knowing when to use it takes a little more training. Depending upon class size and background, it takes approximately 2 to 4 hours to train public safety personnel in the recognition of symptoms and when to use the kit. First responders (who usually don't administer medications) should carry the NAAKs and be included in the training, because in the event of an attack they are likely to be exposed to nerve agents and will need

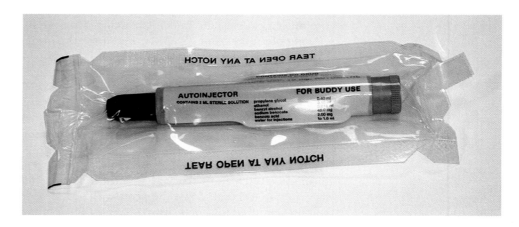

Figure 2.9
An autoinjector of diazepam, to be used to prevent or treat seizures.

immediate self- or partner treatment. The NAAK training program is designed for treatment of mass casualties and also to treat injured responders. Even law enforcement officers with a limited background in EMS pick up the material quickly. Local and state requirements for carrying the NAAK will need to be checked.

Before using the kit it is important to be sure that you are treating a nerve agent exposure. See Table 2.1 for a chart of differences in the presentations of the various chemical agents. Administering atropine when there has been no nerve agent exposure can be dangerous. Atropine can produce dilated pupils, loss of ability to sweat, rapid heart rate, delirium, and hallucinations.

Normally patients are not treated until they have been decontaminated, but use of the Nerve Agent Antidote Kit is an exception. Victims who have eye pain, runny nose, and shortness of breath should get one NAAK immediately injected through their clothes. They may require more, depending on their response. Victims with a history of liquid exposure and having localized fasciculation and sweating should get one NAAK immediately and more depending on symptoms. Victims with more severe symptoms (weakness, shortness of breath, nausea, or vomiting) should get two NAAKs immediately plus one CANA injector to prevent seizures. Those who are even worse (seizing, not breathing, unconscious) should get three NAAKs plus one CANA injector. Seizing patients will need IV diazepam, but the IM CANA injector may have to suffice until the patient can be decontaminated and an IV started (Table 2.1).

Table 2.1	Nerve Agent Exposure Treatment Chart	
Exposure Symptoms	**Number of Mark I Kits to Administer**	**Follow-up Treatment**
Ambulatory patients with history of exposure to vapor or liquid and no symptoms	None	Observe for up to 18 hours for liquid exposure and 1 hour for vapor.
Ambulatory patients with rhinorrhea and miosis and history of exposure to vapor	None	Observe for increasing dyspnea; if improved no treatment required.
Ambulatory patients with a history of liquid exposure with localized fasciculation and sweating	One	Continue to observe and give additional atropine as needed to control symptoms.
Moderate exposure to vapor with continuing dyspnea and/or nausea and vomiting, muscle weakness	One to two. (If two NAAKs are given, the victim should also receive one CANA injector of 10 mg diazepam.)	Continue to observe and give additional atropine to control dyspnea, administer oxygen, and control airway.
Seizing, apnea, post ictal collapse, or effects in two or more body systems	Three. Repeat atropine in 2 mg increments as needed. If seizing or post ictal, administer one CANA injector IM. Consider 2–5 mg of diazepam IV for seizures. **Children with severe symptoms: 2–7 years old—1 NAAK 8–14 years old—2 NAAKs**	Intubate and ventilate as need; large amounts of atropine may be needed.

Cyanide Agents

The cyanide agents were originally called "blood agents," but that antiquated term is no longer used. During World War I there were only three classifications of chemical agents: blister agents (mustard), lung agents (phosgene), and blood agents (cyanides). Since then nerve agents have been developed, and also it has been discovered that cyanide is active at the tissue level, not in the blood, so the term was dropped. The French used cyanide during World War I, but it was not very successful because the two-pound shells used to deliver it were too small to get a high enough local concentration of the gas. Cyanide is so volatile that it quickly evaporated and was carried off by the wind. Japan is thought to have used cyanide against China in World War II. Germany used the cyanide pesticide Zyklon B to murder millions of Jews during the Holocaust. Iraq used cyanide against the Kurds in the 1980s. The United States does not stockpile cyanide, but it is commonly used in U.S. industries (mining, metal processing, and as pesticide fumigant) and large amounts are often stored in poorly guarded tanks (Figure 2.10). Even with the drawbacks to its use outdoors, it would serve well as a terrorist weapon in an attack on victims in an enclosed space like a building, tunnel, or subway.

Cyanide in solid form (sodium or potassium cyanide) can be used to poison food or drinks.

Mechanism of Action and Physical Characteristics

Cyanide is a colorless gas or liquid and comes in two forms: AC (hydrogen cyanide), which is lighter than air, and CK (cyanogen chloride), which is denser than air.

An aerosol would be the best delivery method, but is difficult to use cyanide gas outdoors because of the high concentration required and the high volatility of cyanide. Respiratory exposure gives very rapid onset of symptoms when inhaled. Cyanide is very volatile and is not persistent. Cyanide agents are the least potent of all lethal chemical agents. The LD50 is 100 to 200 mg/kg, or about 7 to 14 grams for an average-size man.

Solid potassium or sodium cyanide, when ingested, is acted upon by stomach acid to liberate the toxic cyanide gas. Cyanogen chloride (CK) is also an irritant to the skin and mucous membranes.

The cyanide chemical warfare agents, when inhaled or ingested, bind cellular enzymes and prevent the cells of the body from using oxygen. The victims "smother" to death even though they have oxygen in their blood. Many toxic industrial chemicals contain cyanide compounds and can cause the same effect. Hydrogen cyanide gas can be made by mixing sodium or potassium cyanide and an acid.

These agents require a fairly high concentration of cyanide to be effective. Their effect is more of an "all or none" phenomenon—they either cause minimal symptoms or are lethal.

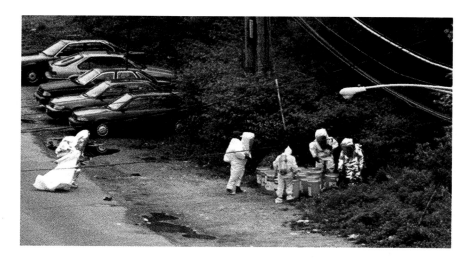

Figure 2.10
Recovery of stolen drums of cyanide. Notice that the members of the recovery team are wearing Level A PPE except for one in Level B.

It Happens...

In 1978 in Jonestown, Guyana, 913 men, women, and children of the Peoples Temple cult died when the cult leader, Jim Jones, ordered them to drink Kool-Aid laced with cyanide.

In 1982 someone tampered with bottles of Tylenol by placing potassium cyanide into Tylenol capsules. The bottles containing poisoned capsules were then placed onto the shelves of stores in Chicago. There were fewer than ten poisoned capsules in each bottle and only one or two tampered bottles in each store. Seven people died from ingesting the poisoned capsules. The person or persons responsible have never been found. In 1986 a copycat killer (Stella Nickell of Washington State) killed her husband with cyanide-poisoned Excedrin in order to collect his life insurance. To try to cover her tracks she also put three packages of cyanide-laced Anacin and Excedrin in three stores,

causing the death of another person. She is currently serving a 90-year sentence.

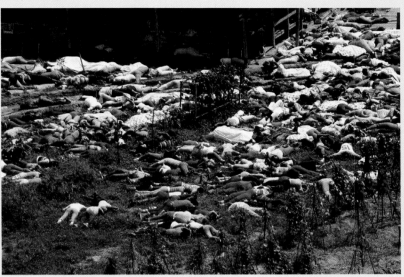

Clinical Effects

The signs and symptoms of aerosol cyanide exposure are initial hyperventilation progressing quickly to loss of consciousness, seizures, apnea, and death. This is somewhat similar to the nerve agents except that *cyanide does not cause pinpoint pupils*. Though the victims are dying of lack of oxygen, their skin or mucous membranes will be pink because there is oxygen in their blood. Cyanogen chloride (CK) is also similar to the incapacitating agents (see page 49), causing immediate burning and itching of skin, nasal passages, nose, lungs, and eyes. Cyanides usually either kill within 6 to 8 minutes or have little effect. This makes the cyanide treatment kit fairly useless because most of those who are significantly exposed are dead before they can be treated. Victims exposed to continuing low levels of cyanide develop headache, nausea, vomiting, and varying neurological symptoms with progressive deterioration and development of metabolic acidosis.

Specific Decontamination of Cyanide Exposure Victims

If cyanide is suspected, you should not enter the scene unless wearing at least Level B protection. Level C PPE cannot be used because *gas mask filters deteriorate rapidly upon exposure to cyanide gas*.

Cyanide is not a persistent agent. You should remove the victims' clothes and place them in HazMat bags. Wash the victims with soap and water.

Treatment of Cyanide Exposure Victims

Support the airway. This may require intubation. All cyanide exposure patients should get 100% oxygen and support of ventilation if needed. Obtain IV access. Use a cyanide antidote kit if you are equipped (Figure 2.11). The cyanide antidote kit is itself toxic, and you should have special training if you are to use it. Most EMS units do not carry the kit, and most hospitals stock only one or two kits. There is an easier and safer treatment being used in Europe (IV hydroxycobalamin) and it has recently been accepted by the FDA for use in the United States.

Figure 2.11
Cyanide treatment kit.

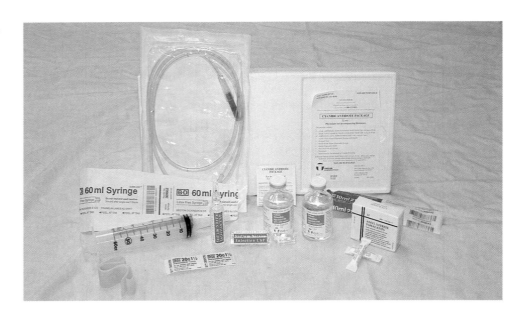

Vesicants or Blister Agents

Sulfur mustard (H or HD) is the prototype blister agent. It was developed in the early 1800s and was first used by Germany during World War I. During World War I mustard gas produced more chemical casualties than all other chemical agents. Most of those casualties survived, though often with severe disabilities (Figure 2.12). Since the First World War mustard has been used militarily by several countries, including Italy, Egypt, and Iraq, and is still considered a major chemical warfare threat. Many countries maintain stockpiles of mustard, and there is always the danger that terrorists may obtain enough to attack.

Mechanism of Action and Physical Characteristics

Sulfur mustard is a very reactive compound and, once in contact with the skin or absorbed into the body, it quickly (within minutes) binds to the tissue enzymes and proteins. Like cancer chemotherapeutic agents (nitrogen mustard was one of the first cancer treatment drugs), sulfur mustard has an affinity for rapidly dividing cells, especially of the skin, mucous membranes, and bone marrow. Sulfur mustard and related compounds are usually delivered by the aerosol route, so their main effects are on the skin, eyes, or respiratory system. Sulfur mustard is a yellow to brown oily liquid with an odor of mustard or garlic. It is not very volatile and so it is dispersed as a liquid aerosol. It will become a vapor at greater than 100 degrees Fahrenheit, but a problem in dispersal is that it becomes a solid below 57 degrees Fahrenheit. For this reason it is often mixed with another similar agent

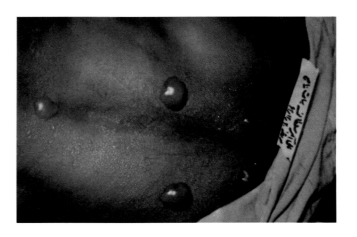

Figure 2.12
A victim of blister agent attack.

such as Lewisite (the mixture is HL) or agent T (the mixture is HT) so that it remains a liquid at lower temperatures.

Clinical Effects

The vesicant agents have a latent period of 1 to 12 hours until symptoms develop. After the latent period, the eyes and nose will be affected first. Signs and symptoms of vesicant poisoning include irritation and red eyes; red skin; severe itching and burning of skin; blisters; sore throat and hoarseness; cough; nausea and vomiting. The eyes are the organs most sensitive to mustard vapor injury; 90% of victims will have eye injury. Experience from military use has shown that most victims will have only mild conjunctivitis with recovery in 1 to 2 weeks. Less than 0.1% had severe damage and long-term vision loss. Inhalation of the vesicant vapor causes long-term lung injury with bronchitis, fibrosis, and chronic obstructive pulmonary disease (COPD). In the first day or two after exposure to sulfur mustard deaths are usually from respiratory failure. However, moderate exposure can cause deaths in the weeks following, usually due to massive infection from the agent's effects on the immune system. After skin exposure the skin will develop erythema like sunburn within 2 to 12 hours, and this may go on to form large thin-walled blisters that are prone to infection. Though the agent reacts with the tissue within minutes and must be removed immediately to prevent injury, the symptoms may be delayed for several hours. Thus, if a victim does not realize he has been exposed to a vesicant agent it will be too late to prevent injury once symptoms develop. Vesicant exposure can also cause nausea and miosis (pinpoint pupils), causing initial responders to mistake it for a nerve agent exposure. The latent period of up to several hours as well as the skin, eye, and respiratory irritation should help differentiate vesicant agent exposure from nerve agent exposure.

Specific Decontamination of Vesicant Exposure Victims

Mustards or vesicant agents react violently with flame, and they also produce poisonous smoke if mixed with bleach. Therefore, *do not try to decontaminate equipment with hypochlorite!* If you suspect a vesicant agent attack, you should wear full chemical protective clothing and respiratory protection in the form of an SCBA or APR (Level B or C) to enter the area. Vapors are heavier than air and so tend to remain along the ground for prolonged times.

Decontamination must be done immediately after exposure to prevent injury. Remove victims from exposure before attempting decontamination. Irrigate all skin with copious amounts of water. Be careful not to wash the agent onto nonexposed body parts. Even after the patients develop symptoms, you should perform wet decontamination to prevent continued absorption of the agent and limit cross-contamination. **Remember that you must decontaminate your equipment with soap and water, not bleach or hypochlorite.**

Treatment of Vesicant Exposure Victims

The first symptoms are likely to be eye irritation, and you should irrigate the eyes with normal saline for 15 minutes. Because the agent causes irritation of the respiratory tract, the patients will likely have airway problems. Severe cases may require intubation and assisted respiration. If they develop bronchospasm, treat like an asthma attack. All patients with respiratory symptoms should get oxygen to maintain a pulse oximeter reading of greater than 95%. Once skin symptoms develop, the patients should be treated much like a burn victim. Fluid loss is not as significant as you see in thermal burns of the same body surface area. Use less IV fluids when treating fluid loss. Victims with a significant exposure will require narcotics for pain relief.

Lewisite and phosgene oxime (CX) are also vesicants but are different from sulfur mustard and have never been used militarily. In liquid or vapor form they produce *immediate* pain and injury. Because of the immediate pain, the victims tend to run away from the exposure and immediately begin self-decontamination.

Thus these agents tend to cause less damage than mustard. Decontamination should be with large amounts of water or soap and water. Lewisite (L) contains arsenic and may respond to British Anti-Lewisite (BAL) injection.

Pulmonary Agents

Certain chemicals, when inhaled, cause damage to the alveolar-capillary membrane of the lungs, causing them to leak and the lungs to fill with fluid. Death comes from literally drowning in these fluids. The prototype agent of this type is phosgene (not the same as phosgene oxime). Phosgene was synthesized in 1812, and it was used as a chemical warfare agent by Germany during World War I. It was dispersed by way of artillery shells. During the same war both sides used it alone or in combination with chlorine. Phosgene was stockpiled during World War II but was not used in the conflict. It has not been used since then, and the United States no longer stockpiles it. It may be available in other countries and possibly could be obtained by terrorists.

Mechanism of Action and Physical Characteristics

There are many chemicals that have toxic effects on the lung membranes. Phosgene (CG), phosphine, chlorine (Cl), anhydrous ammonia, hydrochloric acid (HCl), oxides of nitrogen (NOx) (not the same as nitrous oxide used for pain relief), and smoke from the burning of some plastics (PFIB) all have similar effects on the lung (Figure 2.13). Phosgene is a vapor at room temperature but is heavier than air so it remains close to the ground until it is dispersed by the wind. It smells like newly mown hay. Though only slightly soluble in water, once dissolved, phosgene breaks down into carbon dioxide and hydrochloric acid. The hydrochloric acid causes irritation of the eyes and respiratory passages, but other reactions directly on the alveolar capillary membrane account for the leaking of fluid into the lungs.

Clinical Effects

After exposure to phosgene gas there is usually an asymptomatic period of 20 minutes to up to 24 hours (depending on concentration of the gas) and then the development of persistent cough, burning in the throat and chest, and increasingly severe shortness of breath (SOB). Agents of this type usually must be inhaled to cause death, but topically they can cause eye injury and skin irritation. The usual signs and symptoms are irritation of the eyes and respiratory tract, burning in the chest, coughing, and increasingly severe dyspnea. Fatalities are from pulmonary edema and hypoxia.

Specific Decontamination of Pulmonary Agent Exposure Victims

If you suspect an attack by a pulmonary agent, you should not enter the scene unless you are wearing at least Level C PPE. Removal of the victims from additional exposure is critical. Those exposed must be decontaminated prior to treatment and transport. Their clothing should be removed as soon as they are out of the area of exposure. Clothing will absorb the agent and off-gas. The patient should

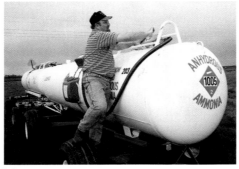

Figure 2.13
(a) Anhydrous ammonia storage tank. (b) Chlorine gas storage tank.

(a)   (b)

be decontaminated with a soap and water bath or shower. Irrigation of the eyes with several liters of normal saline (use water if saline is not available) is needed in exposures to phosgene as well as many toxic industrial chemicals such as chlorine, anhydrous ammonia, hydrochloric acid, and similar caustic or acidic agents.

Treatment of Pulmonary Agent Exposure Victims

Once respiratory symptoms develop, treatment is supportive. All patients with respiratory symptoms should receive oxygen and be put at strict rest. Many will need positive-pressure ventilation. Patients with dyspnea will require hospital treatment. If the patient survives 48 hours, then long-term survival is probable.

Riot Control Agents (Incapacitating Agents)

These agents will generally render the victim incapable of fighting or resisting. Agents of this type were first used by Paris police to break up riots that occurred just before World War I. DM (vomiting agent) was the first incapacitating agent developed but is very uncommon now. During WWI, the Germans used DM along with phosgene. The DM would make the soldiers vomit so they could not wear their gas masks and they would get a worse exposure to phosgene. The gas masks of that day did not filter out DM.

Though many agents have been used over the years, only a few are commonly used today. Each group of agents will be discussed separately.

CN and CS (Tear Gas, Mace)

Mechanism of Action and Physical Characteristics

CN and CS are white, tan, or yellow crystals or dust. They are solids that vaporize easily. They are dispersed as fine particles or in solution. These agents are frequently dispersed using a flammable propellant such as isopropyl alcohol. They may ignite if there is an open flame. They may be dispersed by small spray cans, large spray tanks, or by explosive devices (tear gas grenades or shells) (Figure 2.14).

The mechanism of action is not well understood for these agents, but they cause pain and irritation on contact with the skin or mucous membranes without causing actual tissue injury. Though incapacitating, these agents have a high safety margin and rarely cause death or serious injury. However, they can be lethal for persons who are debilitated or have severe lung disease or allergic reaction.

Clinical Effects

CS (tear gas) is used by police and military for crowd control or riot control. CN (mace) is less potent than CS and is used by individual citizens for personal protection. Tear agents produce immediate intense stinging, burning,

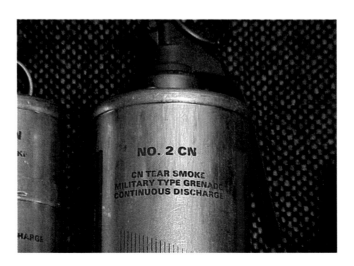

Figure 2.14
Tear gas (CN) grenade.

and itching of the skin. These effects are heightened if the skin is hot and sweaty. They also cause tearing and swollen eyes with blurred vision. When inhaled they cause coughing, difficulty breathing, and tightness in the chest. Most symptoms will disappear within 30 to 60 minutes even without treatment. In rare cases, exposure to CN may produce a severe allergic reaction.

Specific Decontamination of Tear Gas Exposure Victims

If you suspect an attack by any riot control agent, you should wear waterproof outer garments and a full-face or hood-type air-purifying respirator (Level C). Patients should be decontaminated before they are placed in your ambulance or taken into the emergency department. Flush the skin with large amounts of water (showering is best). Irrigate the eyes with saline or water for 10 to 15 minutes. DO NOT RUB THE AFFECTED AREAS, particularly the eyes. You may use soap and water on affected skin, but avoid bleach and oils. Be aware that initial contact with water may temporarily increase symptoms.

Treatment of Tear Gas Exposure Victims

For most victims, decontamination is all the treatment that is needed. If there is substantial pulmonary exposure and the patient complains of severe dyspnea, treat like an asthma attack (oxygen and bronchodilators).

Pepper Spray (OC)

Mechanism of Action and Physical Characteristics

OC is a yellowish to orange oily liquid that contains oil from cayenne pepper (oleoresin capsicum), dissolved in a propellant. It is usually dispersed by an aerosol canister or as a liquid delivered as a launched munitions or explosive device. Like tear gas, it is a skin irritant. This is nontoxic food product and not a lethal agent. It has a large safety margin.

Clinical Effects

Pepper spray is commonly used by police because of its effectiveness on both humans and dogs (CS and CN don't have much effect on dogs). Pepper spray causes an intense irritation of the skin and mucous membranes. It has a latent effect period, when no effects are felt or observed, that varies from a few seconds to up 30 seconds. OC is very effective, causing temporary incapacitation of more than 95% of persons exposed. OC has a distinctive smell and taste that some persons describe as a "pepper smell," "metallic taste," or "copper taste." The first effects are intense burning of the eyes resulting in blepharospasm (involuntary closing of eyelids), and irritation of the mucous membranes of the nose, mouth, and throat. The irritation also causes swelling of the airways, resulting in difficulty breathing with runny nose and excessive saliva production. The sensitive skin of the face, neck, and ears is reddened (erythema). Much of the rapidity of the effect and total effect of OC spray depends upon whether the person sprayed is inhaling when the aerosol reaches them. If so, the effects usually are significant and more rapid than in those who do not initially inhale the aerosol.

Specific Decontamination of Pepper Spray Exposure Victims

As with all riot control agents, you should wear Level C attire. Gloves and normal clothing will afford significant protection from this agent, but it is prudent to wear waterproof outer garments. Immediately remove victims from the source and then remove contaminated clothing. Victims should be decontaminated before placing them in your ambulance or taking them into the emergency department. Gentle washing is needed. Be aware that washing may temporarily increase symptoms. Showering with water is probably the most practical way to decontaminate a patient who has been exposed to pepper spray. A dishwashing detergent with agents to encapsulate and disperse oils is an effective aid in removing the OC from the skin, but avoid the eyes. Contaminated clothes can be decontaminated by normal washing.

It Happens...

On October 23, 2002, forty Chechen terrorists took about 700 people hostage in a Moscow theater. The terrorists demanded the withdrawal of Russian forces from Chechnya. The terrorists had bombs strapped to their bodies and threatened to detonate them if the Russians attacked the theater. After two and a half days of negotiations, forces from Russia's elite Spetsnaz commando unit of the Federal Security Service (FSB) pumped an incapacitating agent into the theater through a hole in the wall before storming the building from the roof and from all entrances. All of the terrorists were killed, along with 130 of the hostages. All of the terrorists were shot in the head to prevent them from detonating their explosive belts. Almost all of the 130 hostage fatalities were from the "knock-out gas." Russian authorities have never disclosed the identity of the gas (even to the doctors treating the hostages). It is speculated that BZ may have been a component of this gas.

Avoid contaminated environmental surfaces. Contaminated items and surfaces will off-gas the vapor for several hours, and this should be a consideration in an attack inside a building. Ventilation will help disperse the product. Persons exposed should be advised to not rub the areas affected, as this will drive the oily OC into the skin, prolonging it effects.

Treatment of Pepper Spray Exposure Victims

For most victims, decontamination is all the treatment needed. Some persons with preexisting reactive airway disease or allergies to OC products may show an exaggerated response. Treat these as you would an asthma attack.

BZ, CS2, Persistent Agent

Mechanism of Action and Physical Characteristics

BZ is a white or grayish solid. These agents are anticholinergics (like atropine), and they cause confusion, hallucinations, loss of coordination, and depression. They can cause heat stroke and seizures. These agents are more dangerous than the other riot control agents.

Clinical Effects

Effects may be rapid and immediate, or delayed for up to 90 minutes, and they can last for hours. Victims will have confusion, dry skin, delirium, hallucinations, memory loss, and loss of coordination. They will also have dry mouth, inability to speak, and anxiety. They may lose their ability to control their body temperature and develop heat stroke. They may have seizures, tachycardia, fever, and flushing of the skin. Some may develop cardiac dysrhythmias.

Specific Decontamination of Persistent Agent Exposure Victims

Responders entering the scene should wear chemical-resistant clothing and full respiratory protection of at least Level C. Immediately remove victims from the source and then remove their contaminated clothing. Victims should be decontaminated before they are placed in your ambulance or taken into the emergency department. Flush skin and eyes with water.

Treatment of Persistent Agent Exposure Victims

Patients may require oxygen, airway control, and temperature control. Diazepam or lorazepam may be used for seizures and excitability.

DM—Vomit Agent

Common names for this agent include vomit agent, DM, and Adamsite.

Mechanism of Action and Physical Characteristics

DM is a solid that appears yellow to green. DM stimulates the vomiting center in the brain. It is also a mild irritant.

Clinical Effects

DM causes rapid nausea, vomiting, and incapacitation. Symptoms are immediate but of short duration. It has a peppery sensation when inhaled. Because it is a mild irritant, it also causes tearing and sneezing. DM was the first incapacitating agent developed but has never been used in the United States.

Specific Decontamination of Vomit Agent Exposure Victims

Responders entering the scene should wear PPE of at least Level B. Gas masks may not filter out the DM. Caution: DM produces very toxic fumes if burned. Immediately remove victims from the source and then remove their contaminated clothing. Victims should be decontaminated before they are placed in your ambulance or taken into the emergency department. Flush the skin with large amounts of water and the eyes with several liters of normal saline (use water if normal saline is not available). Use soap and water on affected skin, but avoid bleach and oils.

Treatment of Vomit Agent Exposure Victims

Patients will need injectable antiemetics and may require fluid replacement.

Smoke HC, FM, FS, WP, PWP, SGF

Common names for this agent include smoke, white phosphorus (WP), and "Willie Pete." Smoke-producing agents are not used for riot control but rather for concealment of troops on the battlefield. They might be used as chemical weapons by terrorists, so they are included in this section.

Mechanism of Action and Physical Characteristics

The active contents of smoke grenades or shells are various colored solids, powders, or liquids. They produce various colors of smoke. The liquids are acid and can cause burns of the skin. Some solids are potent irritants. White phosphorus burns on exposure to air. Burning white phosphorous also produces toxic fumes.

Clinical Effects

The smoke produced by these agents causes irritation of the eyes, bronchi, and lungs. It may also cause dyspnea and decreased oxygenation. The liquids may also cause acid burns to the skin. Chemical pneumonia is common, and symptoms may be delayed for several hours. Pulmonary edema may be a significant problem. Many smoke grenades produce phosgene gas, hydrochloric acid gas, and other acid gases that would put them in the pulmonary agent category (see above). Like the pulmonary agents, they produce dyspnea, coughing, and irritation of the skin and eyes.

Specific Decontamination of Smoke Grenade Exposure Victims

Responders who enter the scene should wear flame-resistant clothing and full respiratory protection in the form of an SCBA (Level B). Immediately remove victims from the source of the smoke and then remove their contaminated clothing. Victims should be decontaminated before they are placed in your ambulance or taken into the emergency department. Wash the skin with large amounts of water and irrigate the eyes with large amounts of normal saline (or water if saline is not available). Wash the liquid smoke agent off with lots of water followed by a dilute sodium bicarbonate solution.

Treatment of Smoke Grenade Exposure Victims

If the patient has pieces of white phosphorus (WP) stuck to or embedded in his skin, keep the WP covered with a wet dressing or submerge the extremity in water. Use fresh 2 to 4% copper sulfate solution to inactivate and remove particles of WP. Once removed, WP particles must be kept underwater or in a copper sulfate solution or they may spontaneously burn. All embedded WP must be removed to avoid chemical poisoning of victim. Use care to avoid cross-contamination. Treat thermal burns in the usual manner. If the patient is having respiratory problems, give oxygen, bronchodilators, and respiratory support.

Detection and Identification of Chemical Agents

Detection can come from a variety of sources and methods. Obviously if there are casualties having similar signs and symptoms consistent with a chemical agent, this will be a strong indication of a hazardous material spill or a chemical attack. You may be able to establish the type of agent by the clinical signs and symptoms produced (see Table 2.2); however, electronic detectors should be used to confirm the type of agent. Electronic chemical detectors use photoelectric ionization detectors to detect and categorize chemical warfare agents, toxic industrial agents, halogen gases such as chlorine and bromine, and OC (Figure 2.15). Some instruments will give the strength of the agent, usually in parts per million (PPM). False positives are infrequent but do occur. There are also colorimetric test strips that can provide qualitative indicators of exposure to a particular chemical agent (Figure 2.16). These are fairly reliable but sometimes slow to react to the agent.

Colorimetric testing tubes may be used if a specific chemical agent is suspected (Figure 2.17). These tubes with their indicator will usually reveal the nature of the chemical agent and its level. It should be remembered that cross-reactions are common among chemical agents measured in this manner (see "Practical Skills: 5" for use of these detection devices).

The best method of agent identification is for a fully protected HazMat team to move into the incident area to make an assessment of the nature, extent, and quality of a chemical agent attack. This team *should* be able to deploy within 15 to 20 minutes of arrival and report via radio to the incident commander.

Table 2.2 Comparison of Clinical Effects of Chemical Agents

Agent	Eye Pain/Pupils	Breathing	Rhinorrhea	Seizures	Skin	Time to Symptoms
Nerve	Pain, **pinpoint pupils,** dim vision, tearing	SOB or absent, bronchorrhea	Present	Likely	Muscle fasciculation from liquid agent exposure	Symptoms immediate for vapor, delayed for liquid
Pulmonary	Burning, tearing	SOB, delayed pulmonary edema	Possible	Not likely	Burning	Immediate
Vesicant	Delayed eye pain	Normal	None	None	Delayed blisters	Delayed
Cyanide vapor	Normal	Hyperventilation, or apnea	None	Likely	Normal	Immediate
Anhydrous ammonia	Eye pain, tearing	SOB, pulmonary edema likely	Possible	Not likely	Burning sensation	Immediate
Chlorine	Eye pain, tearing	SOB, pulmonary edema likely	Possible	Not likely	Burning sensation	Immediate
Phosgene	Delayed irritation	Normal, delayed pulmonary edema	Delayed	Not likely	Normal	Delayed
OC, CS/CN	Eye pain, cannot open eyelids, tearing	SOB, rapidly passes when removed to fresh air	Present	Not likely	Burning sensation, initially increases, then stops when flushed with water	Immediate

Figure 2.15
Photoionization chemical
detector.

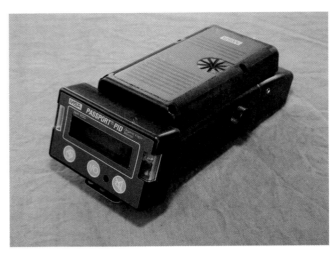

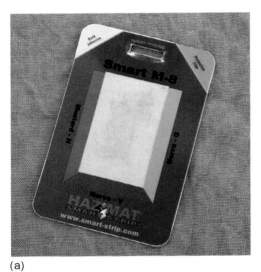

(a)

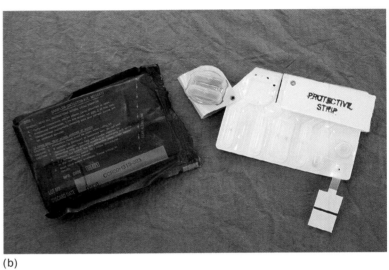

(b)

Figure 2.16
Military M8 and M256 colorimetric test strip kits.

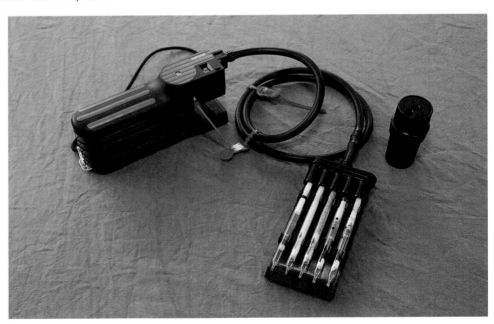

Figure 2.17
Commercial colorimetric
chemical detector.

Responding to a Chemical Attack Scene
Before You Arrive at the Scene

Because public safety responders are likely to be first on the scene of a chemical attack, your recognition of the incident as a chemical attack can prevent the contamination of responders, including yourself. In a chemical attack there are usually reports of a number of persons reported to be "sick" or down. If dispatch states that you are responding to a scene of multiple people down, you know you are responding to a high-risk call. Keep in mind that in addition to the chemical attack, there may be other hazards, such as additional explosive or chemical devices designed to attack responders, terrorists lying in ambush to shoot responders, or contamination of the scene by radiation or biological agents.

When responding to the call, you should shut down emergency equipment (turn off lights and siren, turn radio down) before the scene comes into view. You should slowly approach the scene using your through-the-windshield survey (binoculars are recommended), looking for any indicators of hazards, such as:

- Persons fleeing
- Persons concealing themselves
- Armed persons
- Disorderly crowds
- The demeanor of persons present (angry, scowling)
- Lack of anyone present

You should listen for shouts, altercations, gunshots, or other audible information as you observe the scene. If there is any doubt as to scene safety, you should stop and wait for law enforcement to clear the scene. If the incident is known to be a HazMat or chemical attack, the scene needs assessment by hazardous materials technicians. You should stage in a safe place uphill and upwind until they have finished their mission and give you the OK to enter. While you continue your observation of the scene, you should communicate with dispatch and with other responders to obtain any additional information.

When You Depart Your Vehicle at the Scene

When you begin your on-the-ground scene size-up, evidence that you are dealing with a chemical attack includes the presence of mists, smoke, fogs, or liquids at the scene. The victims may exhibit signs and symptoms of a chemical agent (Box 2-2).

Box 2-2   Signs and Symptoms of a Chemical Agent

- **Nerve agents** initially cause eye pain, dimness of vision, and shortness of breath. Constricted pupils are extremely suspicious for nerve agent poisoning (vesicants can also cause this, but most other symptoms are different). Patients will soon exhibit the "DUMBELS" or "SLUDGEM" signs.
- **Cyanide** causes gasping for air; red eyes, skin, and lips; seizures; unconsciousness; and death.
- **Blister (vesicant) agents** cause burning of eyes, cough, and burning, then blistering, of skin. The symptoms can be delayed for several hours.
- **Pulmonary agents** (phosgene, phosphine, chlorine, anhydrous ammonia, etc.) cause immediate irritation of eyes and throat and then coughing, tightness in chest, and difficulty breathing.
- **Incapacitating agents** generally cause the same signs and symptoms as the pulmonary agents, but may be more severe. However, they wear off quickly.

Box 2-3   When There Are Critical Victims

If there are obvious critical victims needing immediate treatment, you should have the senior responder select a place for decontamination and triage while the other responders don at least Level C PPE (unless it is a cyanide attack, which requires Level B) and begin rescuing critical patients and directing ambulatory patients to the decontamination area. You should spend the absolute shortest time possible in the hot zone.

As soon as you suspect that you are dealing with a terrorist attack, you should immediately notify dispatch and have them notify all appropriate agencies and local hospitals. Resist the urge to *immediately* rush into the scene and rescue the victims (Box 2-3). You should immediately withdraw to a safe place and wait for the HazMat team to enter and size up the scene. They will test for chemical and radiological hazards as well as search for bombs and booby traps.

While HazMat is performing the scene size-up, you should establish the Incident Command System and find a safe place for the command post and for decontamination, evaluation, and treatment of patients. Remember to choose a **good** place upwind, upstream, and uphill, but not the **best** place. Terrorists are clever, and they may have already scouted the best place and targeted it.

Depending on wind conditions, consider evacuation of nearby areas using the North American Emergency Response Guide (NAERG) section on evacuations. Ambulatory victims may see you and approach you. They are likely contaminated with the chemical agent, so you should direct them to a safe place for decontamination but do not approach them or let them approach you until you are in at least Level C PPE. A bullhorn (loudspeaker) can be used to direct these patients to the decontamination area.

When You Enter the Scene

Once the HazMat team has identified the chemical agent, you should don the appropriate PPE (see Chapter 1). If you are using Level C attire, you must also use a full-face shield or hood to protect you from liquid splashes. Keeping the number of responders to a minimum, enter the scene from upwind, uphill, and upstream. Continually scan the area for hazards while on scene (see above). Have a planned escape route.

Ambulatory patients should be directed to the decontamination area. They should have a thorough wet decontamination as soon as possible. Alive but non-ambulatory patients should be removed rapidly from the scene using "load and go" principles. They should have a thorough wet decontamination as soon as possible. If it is a nerve agent attack, some critical patients may need the nerve agent antidote kit before they are moved. Leave the dead in place until law enforcement has investigated the crime scene.

While on scene, avoid contact with any contaminated areas and avoid liquids or powdered materials. Persons fleeing from the event may be contaminated and should be isolated until they can be examined and cleared (Table 2.3). This should be the responsibility of law enforcement (in proper PPE), because terrified victims may refuse to obey EMS orders and may try to transport themselves to the hospital before decontamination. Preserve the crime scene as described in Chapter 1.

Table 2.3   Cross-Contamination Potential for Chemical Agents

Cross-Contamination Potential	Potential for Off-Gassing from Clothing	Potential Harm from Off-Gassing Vapors	Liquid Exposure from Clothing or Skin	Potential Harm from Liquid Exposure
Nerve agent vapor	High, with immediate effects	Moderate	Not applicable	Not applicable
Nerve agent liquid	Low	Low	Very high	Lethal, may be delayed
Pulmonary	Moderate	Low	Not likely	Not likely
Vesicant	Low	Low	Very high, delayed effects	Very high, delayed effects
Cyanide vapor	Moderate	Low	Not likely	Not likely
Anhydrous ammonia	Moderate	Low	Not likely	Not likely
Chlorine	Moderate	Low	Not likely	Not likely
Phosgene	Low	Low	Not likely	Not likely
OC/CS/CN	High, with immediate effects	Low	Moderate	Not likely

When You Leave the Scene

When you leave the scene, proceed to decontamination and perform wet decontamination if possible. Report to your supervisor and to incident command. Box 2-4 lists actions for civilians to take if they think they have been exposed to a chemical.

Box 2-4   Advice to Citizens (or Off-Duty Public Safety Personnel) from the Department of Homeland Security

Possible Signs of Chemical Threat

- Many people suffering from watery eyes, twitching, choking, having trouble breathing, or losing coordination is a sign of chemical threat.
- Many sick or dead birds, fish, or small animals are also cause for suspicion.

If You See Signs of Chemical Attack: Find Clean Air Quickly

- Quickly try to define the impacted area or where the chemical is coming from, if possible.
- Take immediate action to get away.
- If the chemical is inside a building where you are, get out of the building without passing through the contaminated area, if possible.
- If you can't get out of the building or find clean air without passing through the area where you see signs of a chemical attack, it may be better to move as far away as possible and "shelter in place."
- If you are outside, quickly decide what is the fastest way to find clean air. Consider if you can get out of the area or if you should go inside the closest building and "shelter in place."

If You Think You Have Been Exposed to a Chemical

If your eyes are watering, your skin is stinging, and you are having trouble breathing, you may have been exposed to a chemical.

- If you think you may have been exposed **to a chemical,** strip immediately and wash.
- Look for a hose, fountain, or any source of water, and wash with soap if possible, being sure not to scrub the chemical into your skin.
- Seek emergency **medical attention.**

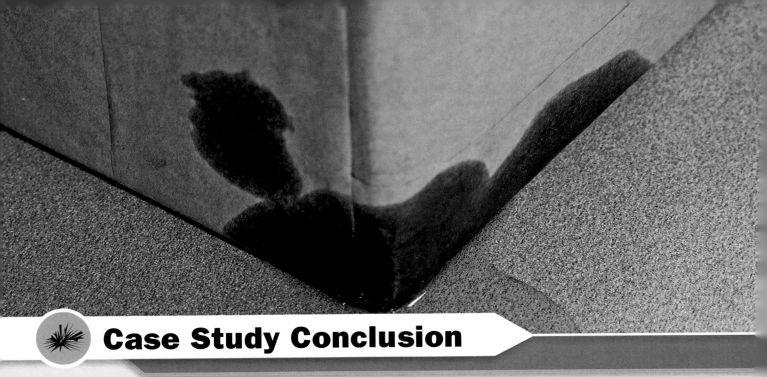

Case Study Conclusion

You immediately recognize that some form of toxic material is involved and the initial responders are being contaminated by a chemical agent being off-gassed from the victims' clothing. You temporarily retreat from the victims until you can put on your Level C PPE. The reports of immediate eye pain, tearing, shortness of breath, and runny nose are all consistent with nerve agent, vesicant agent, some toxic industrial chemicals, or OC exposure. Several patients have reported dimness of vision, which would be consistent with nerve agent vapor exposure. Because all patients are ambulatory, you have them disrobe and wet decontamination is performed using a shower in a nearby building. The patients report little relief on contact with water, and their symptoms do not improve dramatically. You note they all have pinpoint pupils and continued nasal discharge, and one patient has difficulty breathing. You hear rales in his lungs when you examine him. After 5 minutes of high-flow oxygen by nonrebreather mask, this patient continues to have profuse runny nose, and his shortness of breath is worsening. Based upon your clinical exam you presume these symptoms are due to nerve agent exposure. You administer one NAAK with 2 mg atropine and 600 mg pralidoxime IM to the distressed patient. You continue to monitor the other patients and prepare them for transport. At this point the HazMat team and the police bomb squad arrive. They enter the area in Level A or Level B chemical suits and report their electronic detector readings are positive for nerve agents, negative for halogen gases such as chlorine, and negative for anhydrous ammonia. You transport all patients to the local hospital, where those patients who are ambulatory undergo additional decontamination with a shower and washing with soap. Within 30 minutes three patients are symptom free and the distressed patient has improved. Emergency department personnel administer an additional 2 mg atropine and the distressed patient is admitted. Within 8 hours all but the distressed patient are released.

The bomb squad's X-ray of the suspicious package reveals that the package contains what appear to be several plastic containers but no items consistent with an explosive. The area is evacuated and isolated. The FBI is notified, and agents respond and assume incident command. The media responds in force, and this story is the lead story on all the news networks. A joint information center is established at a nearby school. The county emergency operations center becomes the joint operations command post. Federal assets begin to arrive. A technical team from the U.S. Army flies to the site, and in concert with local and federal officials a plan to remove the suspect item is developed over a 72-hour period. Initial laboratory tests reveal that the item contains a crude form of sarin nerve agent. The package is placed in a leak-proof box and removed to a secure location under guard by members of the U.S. Army Technical Escort Group. The structure and involved areas are decontaminated, and the building is certified safe for occupancy by a hazardous material cleanup vendor. The cleanup cost is in excess of $1 million and takes more than 90 days. The sarin is destroyed using heat and a chemical process. Evidence is recovered from the package and containers by FBI agents and turned over to the FBI forensic personnel. An intense federal investigation ensues and, based upon fingerprints obtained from the package and other corroborative evidence, several members of a radical environmental group are arrested. Following a search of their remote compound by the FBI Hostage Rescue Team and Hazardous Materials Response Unit, a sophisticated chemistry laboratory is found. Agents find the instructions and apparatus for the manufacture of sarin, ricin, and cyanide gas devices. They also locate the raw materials for the manufacture of these items and directions obtained from the Internet to make sarin nerve agent. They also find numerous firearms, incendiary devices, and pipe bombs. The federal prosecution of several members of the group for possession of weapons of mass destruction, firearms, and illegal explosives is successful.

Case Study Discussion

This is an example of a terrorist attack by use of a chemical (sarin nerve agent) weapon sent through the mail. The security personnel were correct in shutting down the ventilation system of the building to limit spread of the agent, but they were contaminated as they rescued the workers in the mailroom. The initial responders were not alert and allowed themselves to become contaminated by the nerve agent that off-gassed from the victims' clothes. They should have retreated and put on Level C PPE before examining the patients. The second responders followed this protocol and saved the day. The victims were decontaminated by having them remove their contaminated clothes and shower before being transported to the emergency department. Law enforcement is responsible for keeping the victims together on-scene until they are decontaminated and transported. In many cases, such as the Tokyo subway sarin attack, this is impossible because people leave the scene before law enforcement arrives. One victim had symptoms of a dangerous exposure to a nerve agent and required treatment with the Mark I nerve agent antidote kit before transport. This patient required a second kit before symptoms were controlled. If not for the quick thinking of the security guards, everyone in the building could have been exposed and a major disaster might have occurred.

Pearls

- Approach all emergency calls as if they are dangerous calls.

- To avoid becoming a victim, survey the scene from your vehicle before rushing in.

- Stage in a safe location upwind and uphill. Avoid fumes, smoke, mists, and liquids. Look for other attackers or hazards.

- Identify the scope and extent of the event. A chemical weapons attack will usually present with victims reporting the same signs and symptoms, or a large number of persons reporting ill. Be especially suspicious of a large number of persons with respiratory complaints and eye pain.

- Notify supervisory personnel and dispatch of your intentions. Have dispatch notify all other responders and request fire service, EMS, medical control, receiving hospitals, law enforcement, bomb squad, and hazardous materials assistance.

- If there are multiple casualties, the first arriving responders should establish incident command.

- Choose triage and segregation/decontamination areas.

- Put on protective clothing, especially respiratory protection of at least Level C. Be sure your gas mask canister is fresh (seals not broken) and appropriate for the incident.

- Continue to be alert for threats and any persons, vehicles, or containers that appear out of place or out of the ordinary.

- Direct those fleeing the scene to segregation areas. Communicate to all in the hot zone to exit to the same segregation area. Do not allow them to carry anything with them that might hide a dispersal device.

- Remember that terrorist attack scenes are crime scenes.

- To prevent becoming contaminated, you should avoid contact with victims (as much as possible) until you have put on the proper PPE.

- If possible, identify the chemical agent using symptoms of victims and/or electronic or other test means. You will probably have to depend on the HazMat team detection by electronic or colorimetric tests.

- Treat patients only after decontamination to prevent cross-contaminating yourself and your co-workers.

- Initial decontamination should include removing clothing and rinsing the patients with water. A shower with soap and water is best.

- When adequate resources are available, enter the affected area, if possible and reasonably safe, to rescue those who are nonambulatory.

- Use "load and go" tactics to remove nonambulatory victims from the hot zone. Leave the dead.

- Treat symptoms until definitive identification of the agent is made.

- Remember that multiple agents may be involved.

- Remember that there may be a second attack (bomb or ambush) on the responding personnel.

Want to Know More?

Bibliography

Copenhaver, R.C., *Agent Characteristics and Toxicology First Aid and Special Treatment,* Oak Ridge National Laboratories, 1997.

DeLorenzo, R.A. and Porter, R.S., *Weapons of Mass Destruction: Emergency Care,* Upper Saddle River, NJ., Brady, Prentice Hall, 2000.

Horton, D.K., P. Burgess, S. Rossiter, and W. Kaye, "Secondary Contamination of Emergency Department Personnel from o-Chlorobenzylidene Malononitrile Exposure, 2002." *Annals of Emergency Medicine,* 45 (2005): 655–657.

Marrs, T.C., *Chemical Warfare Agents: Toxicology and Treatment,* John Wiley and Sons, 1996.

Medical Management of Chemical Casualties, U.S. Army Medical Research Institute of Chemical Defense, Aberdeen Proving Ground, 1995.

Textbook of Military Medicine: Medical Aspects of Chemical and Biological Warfare. Office of the Surgeon General at TMM Publications, Borden Institute, Walter Reed Army Medical Center 1997.

U.S. Army *Chemical and Biological Countermeasures Course,* 1997.

U.S. Army Field Manual (FM)

FM 3-3 *Nuclear, Biological, and Chemical (NBC) Contamination Avoidance*

FM 3-4 *NBC Protection*

FM 3-4-1 *Fixed Site Protection*

FM 3-5 *NBC Decontamination*

FM 3-6 *Field Behavior of NBC Agents*

FM 3-100 *NBC Operations*

Internet Sources

Decontamination of Chemical Casualties
www.vnh.org/CHEMCASU/08Decontamination.html

The Guide for the Selection of Chemical Agent and Toxic Industrial Material Detection Equipment for Emergency First Responders, DHS, March 2005. The guide, produced for the Department of Homeland Security (DHS), does not make recommendations. It provides you with ways to compare and contrast commercially available Chemical Agent and Toxic Industrial Material detection equipment. After registration, type in "DHS AND guide" in the search box. The link to the Chemical Agent and Toxic Industrial Material Detector Guide will be seen.
www.rkb.mipt.org.

Textbook of Military Medicine: Chemical and Biological Warfare
www.vnh.org/MedAspChemBioWar/

Advice for Citizens from Department of Homeland Security
www.ready.gov/america/chemical.html

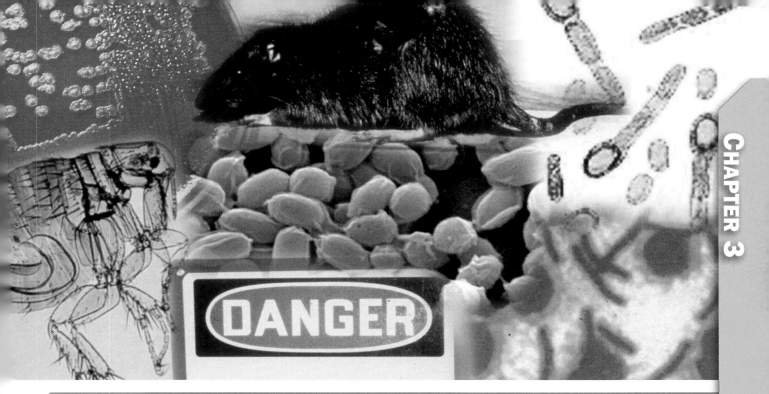

CHAPTER 3

Biological Weapons I

Chapter Objectives

Upon completion of this chapter you should be able to:

1. Discuss the methods terrorists might use to expose people to biological agents.
2. Explain the categories of threats from biological agents.
3. Discuss the prehospital presentations of the common biological agents that generally produce respiratory symptoms.

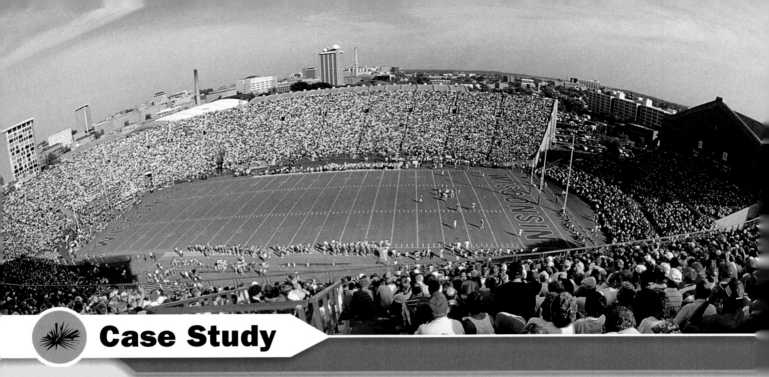

Case Study

At a hospital in a university town, the prehospital EMS service reports to their medical direction physician that they have transported, from multiple locations, patients with fever, muscle aches, nonproductive cough, and midchest pain. They have taken these patients to several hospitals. The local emergency physician recalls that today he has seen six patients complaining of similar symptoms. Their exams were unremarkable and he ordered no laboratory tests or X-rays. He had diagnosed them with viral syndrome and sent them home with cough syrup and analgesics. It is not the influenza season and none of the patients were related. The emergency department contacts the patients and finds that the only common factor is that each had attended the local university football game the past weekend. Nobody recalls anything out of the ordinary, other than that the home team lost.

Because of the concern of the paramedics, the emergency physician notifies the local public health officer of the patients with similar symptoms and asks if there is a new kind of flu going around. The health officer checks his health department's online disease surveillance system for information on the latest communicable diseases in the area. He quickly finds that there have been multiple patients with similar symptoms over the entire state. The health officer immediately alerts state health officials by email about a possible statewide outbreak. The state health officer alerts the epidemiology team and the state EMS department. After a rapid statewide investigation, it is discovered that almost all of the patients with flu-like symptoms had attended the football game the past weekend. Those ill include many of the players on both teams. The number of patients is rising into the hundreds already. When specifically asked about possible aerosol sprays during the game, some people remember that there were the usual planes flying around the stadium pulling banners and there was a shower of mist that they assumed was spray from someone's drink being thrown into the air.

By the morning of the next day there are thousands more people with flu-like symptoms but nobody has become seriously ill.

- Is this an influenza epidemic or a terrorist attack with a biological agent?

- If this is a bioweapon attack, what is the probable agent?

- What should be done now?

The Case Study will continue at the end of the chapter.

Disease has always been associated with war. Until the twentieth century, most casualties of war (soldiers and civilians) were due to disease rather than combat. In the Middle Ages, bubonic plague wiped out a third of the population of Europe (40 million deaths), and in modern times influenza outbreaks and the recent SARS epidemic have caused deaths worldwide. Biological agents are well suited for terrorism because they not only kill and disable but also cause fear out of proportion to their actual potential killing power.

Biological agents were used as far back as the sixth century BC when the Assyrians poisoned wells using rye contaminated with ergot. In 1346 during the siege of Kaffa in the Crimea, the attacking army, using siege catapults, hurled the corpses of plague victims into the city. An outbreak of plague developed that caused the surrender of the city. People from Kaffa fled to Italy and carried the plague with them. This incident is thought to have started the bubonic plague (Black Death) pandemic that spread across Europe and the known world.

In South America, Pizzaro used smallpox-contaminated clothing to cause an epidemic among the natives in the fifteenth century. In North America, during the French and Indian War, the English provided smallpox-contaminated blankets to Indians loyal to the French.

During World War II, the Japanese experimented with biological weapons at their secret facility "Unit 731" in Manchuria, China. These agents (mainly aerosolized anthrax) were tested on prisoners of war and caused an estimated 3,000 deaths. In 1940, Japan reportedly dropped plague-infected fleas on cities in Mainland China, causing plague epidemics. To this day, some cities in China have endemic plague because of this. By 1945 Japan had a stockpile of 400 kilograms of anthrax to be dispersed in specially designed bombs. Japanese troops burned Unit 731 in 1945, before the advancing Americans could capture it.

The United States began studying the offensive use of biological weapons in 1943 in response to perceived threats of German use of similar agents. Japanese use of such weapons was unsuspected at that time. By executive order in 1969, President Nixon stopped all research into biological and toxin weapons. All U.S. stockpiles of those weapons were destroyed by 1972. The United States began a defensive program for biological weapons in 1953 that continues to this day.

In 1972 the United States and many other countries, including Iraq and the Soviet Union, agreed to a treaty prohibiting the development, production, and stockpiling of biological agents for offensive purposes. Evidence suggests that many countries have ignored this treaty. In Laos and Kampuchea during the late 1970s, sickness and death followed the spraying of toxic material by unidentified planes. These attacks were labeled "yellow rain" and are thought to have been T2 mycotoxin. In 1979 there was an accidental release of anthrax from a biological weapons facility in the former Soviet Union. Ninety-four people downwind of the facility became sick, and at least sixty-four died.

After the Gulf War in 1991, UN inspectors found multiple facilities in Iraq that were working on weapons programs for anthrax and botulinum toxins. By 1995 investigations revealed that Iraq had tested these biological agents in rockets, bombs, and spray apparatus. Iraq produced 19,000 liters of concentrated botulinum toxin, 8,500 liters of concentrated anthrax, and 2,200 liters of aflatoxin. Over half of the toxins produced were placed in munitions. It is unknown what percentage of the biologicals and weapons were actually destroyed.

It Happens...

In two separate attacks in September and October 2001, letters containing anthrax spores were mailed to several news media offices and two U.S. senators. All of these letters had a Trenton, New Jersey, postmark. Five people died as a result of these mailings, and over $220,000,000 was spent in cleanup. In late 2003 and early 2004, several letters containing the toxin ricin were mailed to government addresses, including the White House and Senator Bill Frist. There were no injuries associated with the ricin mailings. No arrests have been made in either case.

Biological warfare remains a threat, with many countries still developing offensive weapons. An awareness of the dangers and general principles of management is necessary for emergency personnel as well as law enforcement and even the general public.

Methods of Exposure

To be useful as a weapon, a biological agent must have certain characteristics. One of the best dispersal methods for infectious agents or toxins is by aerosol. Dispersal by aerosol requires that the substance be produced in a particle size of no larger than 5 microns. In certain weather conditions, such small particles will stay suspended in the air for hours. If they are inhaled by humans, the particles will penetrate down to the terminal alveoli, where they can be absorbed into the blood. Particles larger than 5 microns will be filtered out by the upper airway.

Liquids or powders made up of 5-micron (or smaller) particles could be aerosolized by simple sprayer equipment that can be purchased at any hardware or home supply store. Individuals, boats, planes, helicopters, or low-power bombs could be used to deliver this spray. In the right place (a highly populated area), with the right wind conditions, these agents could travel up to 12 miles and impact hundreds of thousands of people.

The second most efficient way to expose many people to a bioweapon is by highly contagious infectious agents that are introduced into a community by infected individuals, vectors (such as fleas or mosquitoes), or fomites (clothing, blankets, pillows, etc.). It has been estimated that if one person infected with smallpox were to arrive in a busy airport, there would be 40,000 victims within a week.

Direct contamination of food, water, or individuals is also possible but is difficult and not generally an efficient way to infect large numbers of people. However, a terrorist can be successful by harming small numbers of victims, as this can still cause large-scale fear, if not terror. The cyanide-contaminated Tylenol in 1982 (see Chapter 2) and mailed anthrax spores in 2001 are past examples of terrorist attacks that killed a small number of people but caused nationwide fear and disproportionately large economic losses.

Recognition and Response to Biological Attack

Individual response to biological attack depends on the agent and whether immunization or prophylaxis has been provided prior to the attack. Active immunization is available for several biological agents, such as smallpox and anthrax. Immunization is the best protection against such agents. Most bacterial infections can be treated or prevented with antibiotics, but this may not be effective if there is an overwhelming exposure. In a biological attack, those first exposed may die before the diagnosis is made and an organized medical response is mounted. Viruses and toxins cannot be treated with antibiotics, and generally resistance must be obtained by immunization (when available).

It is likely that a major biological attack would quickly overwhelm the local medical care infrastructure. In some instances, medical facilities and personnel might become contaminated early and thus immediately become off-limits for the rest of the population. Even in the best situations it is likely that both victims and the "worried well" (healthy individuals who are not infected but are worried that they might be) will inundate emergency departments. The local EMS system would most likely be overwhelmed and break down rapidly. It is also likely that stocks of medication and vaccines would soon be exhausted and might not be immediately replaceable, even from national stores.

Response to any recognized terrorist attack probably would immediately be federalized and perhaps even militarized (see the section "National Incident Management System" in Chapter 1). In today's world it is not a question of whether such an attack will happen but only where, when, and by what method?

Biological Agents

Biological weapons can be made using bacteria, viruses, rickettsia, or toxins. Bacteria are one-celled, microscopic organisms. Bacteria capable of injuring humans do so either by actively invading the tissue or by producing toxins that poison tissue. In some cases, such as staphylococcal food poisoning, the bacteria may live and die without coming in contact with humans but the toxin they produce can then cause disease when ingested by humans.

Viruses are much smaller than bacteria and have no metabolism of their own. They are composed of DNA or RNA, and they reproduce by entering the nucleus of a cell and causing the cell to manufacture more virus. This process eventually kills the cell. Viruses can infect plants, animals, humans, and even bacteria. Because viruses reproduce only inside living cells, they are difficult and expensive to culture.

Rickettsia are infectious organisms that have some of the qualities of both viruses and bacteria.

Toxins are natural substances that are poisonous. Animals (snake venom), plants (ricin from castor beans), bacteria (botulism toxin), and fungi (trichothecene mycotoxin T2) produce toxins. A man-made chemical substance that is poisonous is called a poison, not a toxin. To be useful as a weapon, a toxin has to be stable enough to be stored and must be producible in sufficient quantities. Some very potent toxins do not lend themselves to weapons use because they cannot be produced in more than minute quantities.

Categories of Biological Agents

The U.S. Centers for Disease Control and Prevention (CDC) rates biological agents with the greatest potential for harming public health as "Category A." Current Category A agents include anthrax, botulism, plague, smallpox, tularemia, and viral hemorrhagic fevers.

Category B agents are those agents that are more difficult to disseminate and/or would result in moderate morbidity and low mortality rates. Current Category B agents include ricin, Q fever, staphylococcal enterotoxin B, Venezuelan equine encephalitis, cholera, and T2 mycotoxin.

Category C agents are agents that could be engineered for mass dissemination in the future. Category C agents include various viruses that cause encephalitis and influenza.

These lists are dynamic and more diseases continue to be added. In this text we will cover the listed Category A and B agents.

Recognition and Identification of Biological Agents

Unless announced by the terrorists, attacks using infectious agents will usually go unrecognized until the incubation period is over and patients begin to flood the medical facilities. In these cases the diagnosis must be made by examination of the patients combined with epidemiological investigation. The original attack scene is usually unknown or is too cold for detection to be useful.

Biological toxins (ricin, staphylococcal enterotoxin B, T2 mycotoxin, and botulinum toxin) are not infectious agents and they manifest symptoms much faster (in minutes to hours rather than days), so the attack scene may be recognized and tested.

Although this is still an evolving technology, there are biological detectors that can be used in the field to screen for biological agents. The Department of Homeland Security's *Guide for the Selection of Biological Agent Detection Equipment for Emergency First Responders* is available on the Internet (see "Internet Sources" at the end of this chapter). In the field setting, biological agent detectors would be most useful for testing a suspicious powder for anthrax or for testing for an aerosol attack for ricin or staphylococcal enterotoxin B. All such screening tests will need laboratory confirmation. At this point, field screening tests for biological agents are still evolving and most are very expensive, but they hold promise for the future.

Because the recognition of a biological attack and the diagnosis of the offending agent will usually depend on the victims' presenting symptoms and signs, the various agents will be discussed in terms of their main presenting symptoms.

Biological Agents That Generally Produce Respiratory Symptoms
Influenza and SARS

Because most of the following biological agents present with flu-like symptoms, you should be familiar with influenza (flu) and SARS (severe acute respiratory syndrome). Influenza is a contagious respiratory illness caused by various influenza viruses. It is spread by aerosol droplets during coughing. Flu presents with sudden onset of fever, aching, sore throat, dry cough, and weakness. In the United States, 5 to 20% of the population gets flu every year; more than 200,000 are hospitalized, and about 36,000 die. Many people develop complications of flu, such as bacterial pneumonia, or worsening of other chronic conditions, such as congestive heart failure or asthma. Flu can be prevented by taking the flu vaccine (flu shot) each year. Flu can also be treated with certain antiviral medications. Influenza is not known to have been used as a biological weapon, but it might be in the future and so is rated a Category C threat.

Severe acute respiratory syndrome (SARS) is a relatively new respiratory illness that has had only one known major outbreak. It first appeared in southern China in November 2002 and caused a global outbreak in 2003. SARS presents much like flu: fever, aching, weakness, and dry cough. Unlike the flu, though, it usually causes pneumonia and often severe dyspnea (shortness of breath). It is caused by a family of viruses (coronaviruses) that are usually associated with mild upper respiratory infections like the common cold. Like flu, SARS is spread by coughing. At this time the only treatment for SARS is supportive care. During the global outbreak in 2003, a total of 8,098 people became sick and about 10% (774) died. Only eight people in the United States became sick (all were exposed to the virus in other countries) and none died. In the three years since the outbreak in 2003 there have been only two cases of SARS and these were associated with laboratory exposures. SARS is not rated as a bioweapon threat at this time.

Anthrax
Overview and History
Anthrax is a spore-forming bacterium (*Bacillus anthracis*) that usually causes infection by inhalation, ingestion, or skin contamination by the spores. The spores are very stable and will resist heat, disinfectants, and sunlight. Under favorable

It Happens...

In 1972 the United States terminated its offensive biological warfare program and destroyed all stocks of biological weapons. It is known that Russia has weaponized anthrax because an accidental release of spores in 1979 caused at least 64 deaths downwind of the facility. In 1995 Iraq was found to have produced 8,500 liters of concentrated anthrax spores.

conditions the spores will remain infectious for years. The disease is most often seen in animals, with cattle, sheep, and horses most commonly infected. Humans can contract the disease by handling hair, wool, hides, meat, or by-products from infected animals. The disease can be transmitted by inhalation of the spores or by contamination of skin wounds (abrasions, scratches, lacerations) by the spores. Flies are a common carrier. Ingesting undercooked meat of infected animals can also transmit the disease. Recovery from the disease usually confers immunity to further infection by the anthrax bacterium.

Because of their stability under many adverse conditions, anthrax spores are ideal for use as a biological weapon. Many countries, including the United States, have developed anthrax weapons, and in spite of treaties eliminating such programs, such weapons are believed to still exist.

Anthrax spores are stable in both wet or dry form and can be delivered to large groups of victims by either an aerosol spray (ground or air sprayers) or by airbursts from missiles, bombs, or artillery shells. They can also be sent in the mail in packages or letters, as the five deaths in 2001 attest. There is an inexpensive test available for field screening to see if a suspicious powder is anthrax (see "Practical Skills: 4"). There are also newer, more specific field tests available for screening, but all field tests must be confirmed by laboratory testing.

The CDC rates anthrax as a Category A threat.

Clinical Presentation

In humans, infection by anthrax appears in three forms: cutaneous (skin), pulmonary (lung), or gastrointestinal. The skin form, called malignant pustule (a misnomer, because it does not form pus and is usually not fatal), is seen most frequently in persons who handle infected livestock. The victim develops skin ulcers that form coal-black scabs (Figure 3.1). *Anthrax* is a Greek word meaning "coal." There is usually extensive edema (swelling from edema toxin) around the infected area, and bullae (large blisters) are also common early. Though cutaneous anthrax usually spreads locally, it may become a systemic (generalized) infection. Untreated, cutaneous anthrax has a mortality rate of up to 25% (<1% if treated).

The inhalation (lung) form of anthrax, called woolsorter's disease, is caused by inhalation of the spores. Historically this was seen among people who handled wool, hides, or fur of infected animals. Interestingly, in workers who were frequently exposed to contaminated hides, inhalation anthrax was rare. The inhalation infection would be the expected presentation of the weaponized form of anthrax. After inhalation of the spores there is an incubation period of 1 to 6 days, and then the signs (what the physician finds during examination of the patient) and symptoms (what the patient feels—symptoms can be described over the phone) begin as a flu-like illness. The patient will complain of fever, weakness, and aching and may have a nonproductive cough (a cough that does not produce sputum) and mild chest pain. Occasionally the cough may produce blood-tinged sputum. These symptoms are often followed by a short period of improvement and then the sudden onset of severe respiratory symptoms. The patient will develop severe dyspnea (shortness of breath), diaphoresis (sweating), stridor (high-pitched, labored respiration), and cyanosis (bluish skin color). Death follows within about 24 to 36 hours of onset of the severe respiratory symptoms. The sudden worsening of the disease

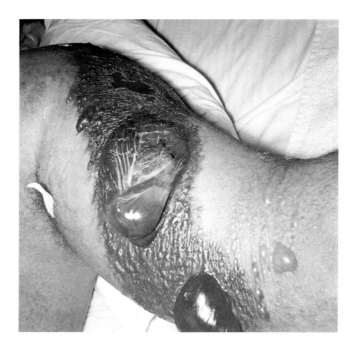

is from the production of a deadly toxin by the anthrax bacteria. Unless treatment is begun early, the mortality rate for inhalation anthrax approaches 100%.

The intestinal form of anthrax is caused by the ingestion of undercooked meat from infected animals and is very rare. This is not a likely route for weaponized anthrax.

Prehospital Presentation

It is unlikely that EMS would be called for the flu-like symptoms, but if you begin to transport multiple patients with a history of flu-like symptoms who have suddenly developed severe respiratory signs and symptoms, you should consider that this may be an epidemic of influenza or SARS but also could be a mass casualty incident involving anthrax infection or pneumonic plague. Though the patients may have all been exposed to the spores at the same location, because of the incubation period the patients would likely have become sick after leaving that location. The anthrax bacterium does not form spores during human infection, and person-to-person transmission is highly unlikely unless the patient is still wearing clothes or fomites that are contaminated by anthrax spores. However, you will not know for certain that the patient is infected with anthrax, so you must protect yourself from other contagious diseases that present in the same way. Practice respiratory as well as standard precautions against infection (gloves, handwashing). The severely dyspneic patient will require oxygen by nonrebreather mask (or even endotracheal intubation) and so you will have to wear a face mask (N-95 mask) to prevent inhaling any infectious material. Carefully disinfect your equipment after delivering the patient. Notify the emergency department personnel of your suspicions. They may be slower to notice the trend of patients with severe respiratory symptoms, especially if the patients are spread among multiple hospitals.

You might be called upon to determine whether a suspicious powder is anthrax. A screening test for anthrax can be performed at the scene. Screening tests are usually performed by a designated HazMat team, but in certain areas law enforcement or EMS may be designated to do this.

Treatment

Historically, parenteral penicillin (2 million units of pen. G IV every 2 hours) has been the treatment of choice, with tetracycline or erythromycin used for those patients allergic to penicillin. However, the weaponized anthrax made by the former Soviet Union countries was selected and produced to be resistant to many of the antibiotics used in the United States. Because of this, until culture and antibiotic sensitivity results are available, the suggested treatment regimen is ciprofloxin (400 mg q 8–12 hours IV or PO) or doxycycline (200 mg IV followed by 100 mg IV q 12 hours).

Prophylaxis

There is a vaccine available to protect against anthrax infections, but it requires a primary series of six doses at 0, 2, and 4 weeks, then at 6, 12, and 18 months. A yearly booster is required. There is limited data, but the first three doses are thought to give good protection against the skin form of anthrax but little is known about protection against the respiratory form. It is thought that protection would depend on the amount of exposure. A heavy dose of spores would probably overwhelm the protective effect. Obviously a mass vaccination program will offer no protection to those already exposed to anthrax, but vaccination should be started and those who have been, or might be, exposed should begin taking oral ciprofloxin (500 mg PO bid) or doxycycline (100 mg PO bid).

Pneumonic Plague

Overview and history

Pneumonic or bubonic plague is a disease caused by a non-spore-forming, gram-negative coccobacillus bacteria (*Yersinia pestis*). The bacteria will live for several weeks in water or moist grain and will last months to years if kept at near-freezing temperatures. It will also live for some time in dried sputum, flea feces, or dead bodies. The bacterium is rapidly killed by heat (boiling water) or sunlight. Plague is normally a disease of rats, mice, and ground squirrels. It can be passed on to humans by the bite of fleas that live on the infected animals.

The first recorded incidence of a bubonic plague epidemic occurred around 1000 BC and is found in the Bible (1st Samuel 5:6–6:6). It is thought that use of plague as a biological weapon (siege of Kaffa in 1346) was the event that precipitated the Black Death plague pandemic that killed a third of the population of Europe. Several countries have been, or are suspected of, developing programs for offensive use of *Y. pestis*. The United States studied its use before the offensive program was terminated. During World War II, to release plague-infected fleas Japan developed a special clay "bomb" that simply shattered when it struck the ground (explosive devices would have killed the fleas). The bombs also contained grain to attract rats. These bombs are believed responsible for WWII plague epidemics in several Chinese cities that caused over 200,000 deaths (plague is still endemic in many of those cities today). The most efficient weaponized form would be an aerosol spray of the bacteria, and it could be delivered in much the same way as *B. anthracis*.

The CDC rates plague as a Category A threat.

Clinical Presentation

Plague appears in three forms in humans: bubonic, primary septicemic, and pneumonic. *Buboes* means inflamed, swollen lymph nodes. Bubonic plague is usually seen after fleabites. Fleas usually bite on the legs of humans, so the affected lymph nodes are usually in the inguinal region (Figure 3.2). Up to 80% of untreated bubonic plague proceeds on to septicemia, though primary septicemia may occur without seeing lymph node enlargement. There is an incubation period of 2 to 10 days, but then the onset of symptoms is acute and the disease often takes a rapid, fulminant course. The patient presents with malaise, high fever, and at least one swollen, tender lymph node (usually in the groin) that may appear to be an abscess. Up to 25% of patients have skin lesions such as vesicles or papules around the swollen nodes. Black or purple necrotic skin lesions caused by bacterial toxins may be present (Figure 3.3). The black skin lesions were the origin of the name "Black Death." The majority of patients with bubonic plague, if untreated, will proceed to septicemia or

Figure 3.2
Draining inguinal
buboes in bubonic
plague victim.

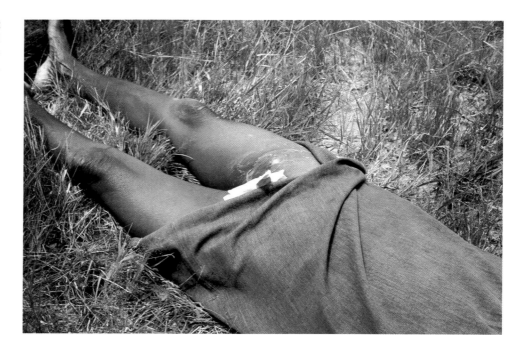

pneumonic plague. There is a 50% mortality rate for untreated bubonic plague. A naturally occurring bubonic plague epidemic in humans would be preceded by the death of animal vectors, especially cats, which have little natural resistance to the disease. However, during World War II the Chinese cities attacked by Japan with infected fleas saw no animal deaths until after the human infections started.

The pneumonic form of plague is usually caused by inhalation of the organism but may spread to the lungs from septicemia. The incubation period of pneumonic plague is only 1 to 6 days (depending on the amount of inhaled bacteria)

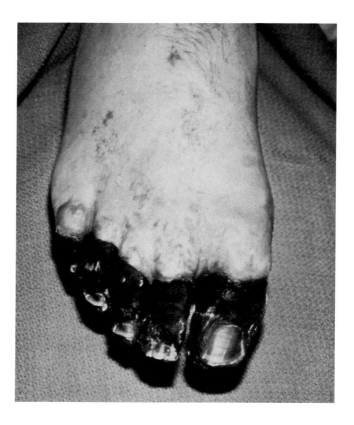

Figure 3.3
Black, gangrenous skin
lesions gave plague the
name "Black Death."

and then symptom development is rapid and frequently fulminant. The patient complains of fever, weakness, aching, headache, chest pain, and cough producing bloody or watery sputum. Occasionally gastrointestinal symptoms (nausea, vomiting, diarrhea, and abdominal pain) may be present. The patient usually appears acutely toxic. The patient usually dies of respiratory failure, circulatory collapse, and generalized bleeding. In humans, the pneumonic form is universally fatal if untreated. The time between respiratory exposure and death averages 2 to 4 days. Generally all patients with pneumonic plague die if treatment is not started within 18 to 24 hours of onset of symptoms.

Prehospital Presentation

Because the disease has a sudden and often severe presentation, you are likely to be called to transport the patient to the hospital. Because of the incubation period, you would likely be called not to the scene of the exposure but rather to patients' homes. You should become suspicious for something unnatural occurring if you suddenly begin to be called for multiple patients with sudden onset of severe flu-like symptoms, especially if they are having bloody sputum and appear extremely ill. The plague bacterium is in the blood and respiratory secretions and is very contagious, so you must practice careful respiratory precautions as well as standard precautions against infection (barrier face mask, gloves, eye protection, and disposable gown). The severely dyspneic patient will require oxygen by non-rebreather mask (or even endotracheal intubation) and so will probably not tolerate wearing a barrier face mask. Carefully disinfect your equipment after delivering the patient. Notify the emergency department personnel of your suspicions. They may be slower to notice the trend of patients with severe respiratory symptoms, especially if the patients are spread among multiple hospitals.

Once it is determined there is a multicasualty incident involving pneumonic plague, the receiving hospital may become quarantined and you may have to take all patients (except those with symptoms of plague) to hospitals that have not been contaminated by the plague. Such hospitals may have to set up triage outside the hospital to determine which patients will be allowed into the hospital. Federal laws that specify guidelines regarding patient treatment and transfer (COBRA) may have to be suspended during such an emergency. Anytime a bioweapon attack is confirmed or strongly suspected, law enforcement (to include FBI) as well as the local public health department should be notified.

Treatment

Plague is sensitive to streptomycin, tetracycline, chloramphenicol, and gentamicin, but weaponized plague bacteria may be genetically engineered to be resistant to these antibiotics. Aggressive antibiotic treatment must be started within 18 to 24 hours of onset of symptoms if the patient is to be saved. If there is a plague epidemic, you will need to take oral doxycycline or ciprofloxin to prevent contracting the disease.

Prophylaxis

At this time there is not a U.S. vaccine available for those at risk for exposure to plague. The old vaccine was discontinued in 1999. This is no great loss as it only protected against bubonic plague and did not protect against the aerosolized bacteria. Doxycycline (100 mg BID) is effective for prophylaxis for those who are known contacts of patients with plague (including pneumonic). Fluoroquinolones are known to be effective in animals and can also be used for prophylaxis.

Tularemia
Overview and History
Tularemia (rabbit fever or deer fly fever) is a disease caused by *Francisella tularensis*, a gram-negative coccobacillus that does not form spores. It is normally a disease of animals, and the disease is transmitted to humans by the bite of infected biting

Figure 3.4
Typical hand ulcer
from tularemia.

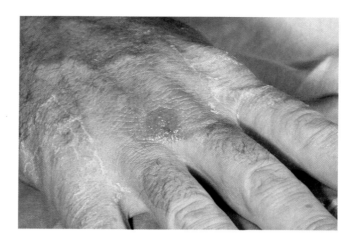

flies, mosquitoes, or ticks. The disease was first described in Tulare County, California, and thus was named tularemia. The bacterium is very infective and it only takes a few organisms to cause disease in humans. The organism can remain viable for weeks in water, soil, and animal tissue. It is resistant to cold and freezing but is rapidly killed by heat and common disinfectants. The United States weaponized this organism in the 1950s before the offensive program was terminated. It is suspected that other countries have also developed a weaponized form of *F. tularensis*. The agent is stable enough to be delivered by spray or explosive devise.

The CDC rates tularemia as a Category A threat.

Clinical Presentation

Depending on the route of inoculation, tularemia can appear in three different forms in humans. If the bacteria enter the body through the skin or mucous membranes, the disease usually presents with swollen tender lymph glands and flu-like symptoms. There is usually a skin ulcer. This is called ulceroglandular tularemia (Figure 3.4). If the bacteria are inhaled, the presentation is of nonproductive cough and substernal chest pain along with the flu-like symptoms but no swollen glands or skin ulcers. This is called typhoidal tularemia. The incubation period can vary from a few days to several weeks, depending on the number of bacteria inhaled. Some people don't present with the cough or swollen glands but have only fever, weakness, and weight loss. This is called septicemic tularemia. The weaponized form of tularemia would be spread by aerosol and so should present with the typhoidal or septicemic picture. Diagnosis is difficult because the symptoms are so nonspecific. Untreated, the disease has about a 5% mortality rate. Recovery confers permanent immunity.

Prehospital Presentation

Because of the incubation period, the patients would not all be from the exposure site but would more likely come from other locations. The incubation period varies, and patients might trickle in over several days, eluding suspicion until you notice a trend for patients with flu-like symptoms. Because the disease is so nonspecific, initially the patients are likely to be misdiagnosed as having a viral infection. You may be well into a mass casualty incident before anyone recognizes that the patients have tularemia and not influenza. As with any patient with flu-like symptoms, you should practice standard precautions plus place a face mask on the patient or on yourself. If you notice that you are having excessive calls for flu-like symptoms at the wrong time of year for influenza, you should voice your concerns to the emergency department staff. You can easily decontaminate your equipment by the usual methods.

Figure 3.5 Castor beans are used to produce the deadly toxin ricin.

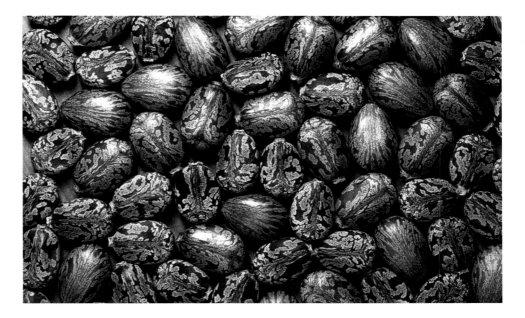

Treatment

Once the diagnosis is made, the treatment of choice is streptomycin or gentamicin. Tularemia is usually not spread by human-to-human contact, so isolation is not necessary.

Prophylaxis

Patients known to have been exposed to the bacterial aerosol should be treated with oral doxycycline 100 mg BID for 2 weeks. EMS and emergency department personnel should not have to take this because caring for the patients does not expose them to the disease. There is a vaccination available and it could be used in large exposures.

Ricin

Overview and History

Ricin is not an infectious agent but rather is a potent protein toxin produced from castor beans (Figure 3.5). Castor beans are common worldwide and the toxin is easy to produce. It makes a good bioweapon (better for assassination than for mass exposure) because it is stable and can be administered by several routes (inhalation, oral, or injection). Although ricin is not as deadly as some toxins, the ease of its production makes it attractive as a weapon. It has been especially attractive for small terrorist organizations that lack funds for obtaining more deadly weapons. Aerosol would be the most effective delivery method, but it is difficult to produce ricin particles in the 5-micron range so it is less useful for mass exposures.

Clinical Presentation

The clinical presentation depends on the route of exposure. If inhaled, ricin causes flu-like symptoms (fever, chest tightness, cough, dyspnea, and joint pain) within 4 to 8 hours, and then generalized airway and alveolar inflammation

It Happens...

Ricin has been used for at least one political assassination via injection. In 2003–2004, letters containing ricin were mailed to several U.S. government agencies, including the White House and Senator Bill Frist (no intoxications resulted). It is certain that several countries have weaponized ricin toxin. Quantities of ricin have been found in al Qaeda caves in Afghanistan.

progresses to pulmonary edema and death within 36 to 72 hours. Survival would depend on the amount inhaled. Oral ingestion of ricin causes gastrointestinal hemorrhage with necrosis of the liver, spleen, and kidneys. The patient dies of vascular collapse. If ricin is given IV, the patient will die of multiple organ failure. If given IM there will be local necrosis of muscle tissue and eventually multiple organ involvement. Patients living longer than 5 days usually recover.

The CDC rates ricin as a Category B threat.

Prehospital Presentation

Inhalation

Because symptoms develop rapidly from inhalation of ricin, you may get multiple calls to the same address or close geographical area. Although the initial symptoms are flu-like, they would occur simultaneously in multiple victims in close proximity, so your suspicion should be immediately aroused. You would be in no danger from the patients you treat, but if you respond to the area of attack you might be exposed to any residual aerosolized ricin.

Anytime you are called to a mass casualty event in which all patients have pulmonary symptoms, you should not enter the scene or approach victims until the HazMat team has made an investigation. This approach may have to be modified if HazMat is not available within minutes. If you must respond to save lives, you should wear Level B or C PPE, and the patients should be decontaminated before being transported. This toxin will not be detected by chemical agent detectors, so you would suspect either a chemical that is not detectable by current detectors or one of the biological toxins (ricin, staphylococcal enterotoxin B, or mycotoxin T2).

Table 3.1		Summary of Biological Weapons		
Disease Agent	**Incubation period**	**Common Presentation**	**Less Common Signs and Symptoms**	**Diagnostic Tests**
Inhalation anthrax (bacterial spore)	1–6 days, may be longer	Fever, weakness, aching, non-productive cough, chest pain. Usually a short period of improvement followed by seveve dyspnea, diaphoresis, and cyanosis. Death occurs within 36 hours of onset of severe symptoms.		Chest X-ray may show widened mediastinum and bilateral pleural effusions. Rarely pneumonia. Consult public health about other tests.
Pneumonic plague (bacteria)	1–6 days	Fever, weakness, aching, chest pain, cough producing bloody or watery sputum. Symptoms progress rapidly to respiratory failure, shock, and generalized bleeding.	May have abdominal pain with nausea, voimting, and, diarrhea.	Chest X-ray may show bilateral infiltrates and consolidation. CBC shows high WBC with most cells being PMNs. Liver enzymes usually elevated, tests for DIC positive. Gram stain shows gram-negative coccobacillus with bipolar staining. Immunoassay available.
Typhoidal tularemia (bacteria)	A few days to several weeks	Nonproductive cough, fever, chest pain, aching, weakness.	Fever, weakness, and weight loss but no cough.	Chest X-ray may show pneumonia or mediastinal adenopathy. Serology test available. Consult with public health.
Ricin (toxin)	4–8 hours	Fever, chest tightness, cough, dyspnea, arthralgias. Symptoms progress rapidly to pulmonary edema and death within 72 hours.	Oral ingestion causes gastrointestinal hemorrhage, with necrosis of liver, spleen and kidneys. Death from vascular collapse.	Chest X-ray may show bilateral infiltrates. CBC suggests bacterial infection. Consult public health for other tests.
Staphylococcal entero-toxin B	3–12 hours	Ingested: fever, abdominal cramping, diarrhea, vomiting. Inhaled: flu-like symptoms that can lead to septic shock.		Lab is of little value. Consult public health for tests. Urine test available. Patients who inhale the toxin will have cough but normal chest X-ray.

Treatment   Unfortunately, supportive treatment is all that is available for inhalational ricin exposure. Clean your equipment in the usual way, but do not use compressed air when cleaning the vehicle as it may re-aerosolize any ricin particles present.

Gastrointestinal

If a food or water source were contaminated by ricin, the picture would be much like a staphylococcal food poisoning incident. There would be multiple patients with sudden onset of vomiting, diarrhea, abdominal pain, and gastrointestinal bleeding. Unless you were expecting a terrorist attack, it is unlikely you would initially consider ricin as the cause. You should treat these patients with IV fluids, antiemetics, and analgesics, just as you would the victims of staphylococcal food poisoning. You would not be in danger from the patients because you would have to ingest the contaminated food or water to be affected.

Treatment   Treatment is supportive only.

Prophylaxis   You are not in danger from contamination by your patients, and a simple fitted face mask will provide protection from aerosolized ricin. There is currently no vaccine available.

Staphylococcal Enterotoxin B
Overview and History
Staphylococcal enterotoxin B (SEB) is one of several toxins produced by the bacteria *Staphylococcus aureus*. SEB commonly causes food poisoning in humans. If

Differential Diagnosis	Treatment	Prophylaxis	Mortality	Transmission
Dissecting aortic aneurysm, mediastinitis, influenza, mediatinal tumor, pneumonia	Fluoroquinolones or doxycycline.	Vaccine available	100% if untreated. About 50% if treated early.	Pulmonary form not transmitted from person to person.
Tularemia, community-aquired pneumonia, meningococcemia, tuberculosis, influenza	Streptomycin, tetracycline, chloramphenicol, gentamycin. If buboes are present, do not drain.	Doxycycline or fluoroquinolone	Very high unless treated within 24 hours of onset of symptoms.	Very contagious. Isolate for first 48 hours of treatment.
Q fever, brucellosis, anthrax, community-aquired pneumonia, pneumonic plague, influenza	Streptomycin, gentamycin.	Doxycycline	Low, 5% if untreated.	No patient-to-patient transmission for the pulmonary form.
Anthrax, pneumonic plague, pulmonary irritant gas exposure, Q fever, tularemia, staphylococcal enterotoxin B, influenza	Supportive.	None	High.	No patient-to-patient transmission.
Staphylococcal food poisoining, influenza	Supportive.	None	Low.	No patient-to-patient transmission.

certain foodstuffs are contaminated by *Staph. aureus*, the bacteria will grow, reproduce, and form multiple toxins, including SEB. When the contaminated food is ingested, the toxin produces, fever, abdominal cramping, and severe vomiting and diarrhea. This is not an infection but rather an intoxication. This is the classic case of "food poisoning." Although victims of food poisoning are very sick, they rarely die. As with most diseases, the very young, the very old, and those with underlying medical illnesses are most at risk for death. If the toxin is inhaled, it produces flu-like symptoms that can lead to septic shock and death. SEB could not be used to cause widespread death, but it could overwhelm the medical system with mass numbers of significantly ill patients and the worried well. SEB could be an effective weapon of terror because it can be delivered by aerosol or through contamination of food or limited water supplies.

Clinical Presentation

Ingestion of the toxin produces fever, severe stomach cramps, vomiting, and diarrhea. There is marked fluid loss that can lead to death from dehydration and hypovolemic shock. Within 3 to 12 hours of inhalation of SEB, patients will develop high fever, headache, myalgias, and nonproductive cough. The more severe cases will develop midsternal chest pain and dyspnea.

Exam of the patient is often unremarkable with normal chest exam (except in rare cases of pulmonary edema). Those who ingest the toxin are frequently dehydrated and thus have postural hypotension. The fever lasts up to 5 days, the cough up to 4 weeks, and GI symptoms several days. Patients are likely to be sick for at least a week, though almost all will recover with only supportive therapy.

The CDC rates SEB as a category B threat.

Prehospital Presentation

A biological attack using SEB could present in two ways, depending on the route of ingestion. The key would be that there would be multiple patients with similar symptoms presenting over a short period of time (probably not greater than 24 hours). They will all have been in a common small geographical area within the past few hours.

If the SEB was delivered by aerosol, the victims will complain of flu-like symptoms including nonproductive cough. If they are all still in the same area, there may be residual SEB aerosol and you may be exposed. Anytime you are called to a mass casualty event in which all patients have pulmonary symptoms, you should not enter the scene or approach victims until the HazMat team has investigated. This approach may have to be modified if HazMat is not available within minutes. If you must respond to save lives, you should wear Level B or C PPE and the patients should be decontaminated before being transported.

If the SEB is delivered by contamination of food or water, the victims will have shared a common meal or water source and within a few hours all will develop severe abdominal cramping along with profuse vomiting and diarrhea. This will be the same presentation as (and in fact is) staphylococcal food poisoning. These patients may require IV fluids for their dehydration. You will be unlikely to think of a bioweapon attack in this situation.

Your equipment can be decontaminated by the usual methods.

Treatment

There is no treatment other than supportive care, and fortunately most patients, though ill and uncomfortable, will recover.

Prophylaxis

At this point there is no vaccine available to protect against SEB. Table 3.1 provides a summary of bioweapons discussed in this chapter.

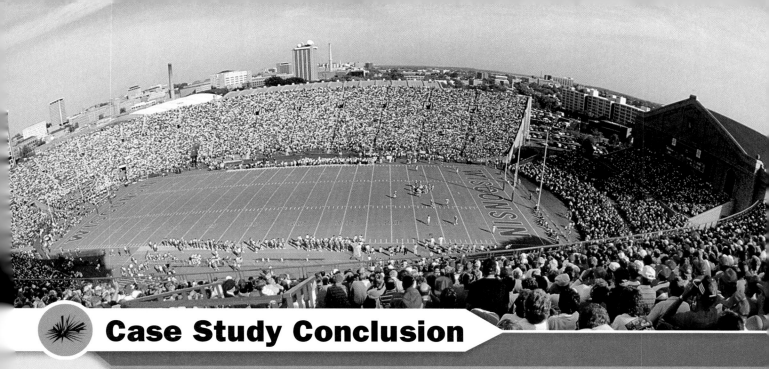

Case Study Conclusion

Tests done on the blood of affected patients are positive for anthrax bacteria and anthrax toxin. The CDC, the medical community, and law enforcement are notified immediately. Screening and treatment protocols are sent out and a press release is issued to the media to inform the public and to ask anyone who was at the football game to go to the nearest emergency department and have them contact the public health department. The national media are immediately notified, not only because of the attack itself but because many football fans were from out of state and so the warning must go out to the entire nation. The FBI assumes control over the investigation of the attack, and the government mobilizes stocks of antibiotics to meet the sudden demand for treatment and prophylaxis for nearly a hundred thousand people.

By the third day, untreated patients are appearing with severe respiratory distress. Most of these patients die in spite of treatment. Most of those who were treated early do well.

Case Study Discussion

This is an example of a biological attack using an aerosol of anthrax spores. This particular attack was a challenge for the public health service because the exposed football fans came from widely different areas (many from other states). Anthrax infection by aerosol has an incubation period of a few days and then presents with flu-like symptoms that may improve for the first couple of days before suddenly worsening to respiratory distress, shock, and death. Most of the early victims will die before the disease is diagnosed and an effective medical response is mounted. Early detection of the disease is the key to saving lives. The public health service is extremely important in the diagnosis and management of any biological attacks.

Pearls

- If you find yourself transporting multiple patients with similar complaints, you should consider the possibility of bioterrorism.

- When called to the scene of a multicasualty incident involving suspicious symptoms (especially respiratory), do not enter the scene until it has been cleared by the HazMat team or until you put on proper personal protective equipment.

- If called to a scene where there are multiple patients with similar complaints, patients should be decontaminated before they are allowed to enter your ambulance.

- The public health department has resources to help you with any potential terrorist event.

- Try to approach any suspicious multicasualty event from uphill, upstream, and upwind.

- Do not become a victim! If you make an unplanned arrival at a suspicious multicasualty event, you should immediately retreat and call the HazMat team and law enforcement.

- Patients with respiratory symptoms (especially cough) should wear a face mask while in the ambulance. If the patient is too short of breath to wear a face mask, then you and your team should wear mask.

- Most biological agents (95%) can be effectively blocked by wearing an appropriately fitted N-95 mask, along with simple universal precautions and PPE that protects your skin.

Want to Know More?

Bibliography

DeLorenzo, R.A. and Porter, R.S., *Weapons of Mass Destruction: Emergency Care.* Brady, Prentice Hall, 2000.

Gilbert, D.N., R.C. Moellering, G.M. Eliopoulos, and M.A. Sande. *The Sanford Guide to Antimicrobial Therapy.* Antimicrobial Therapy, Inc., 2004, 34:39, 46.

Inglesby, T.V., et al. "Anthrax as a Biological Weapon: Medical and Public Health Management," *JAMA,* 281(1999): 1735–45.

Inglesby, T.V., et al. "Plague as a Biological Weapon." *JAMA,* 283(2000): 2281–2290.

Medical Management of Biological Casualties Handbook, 2nd ed. U.S. Army Medical Research Institute of Infectious Diseases, 1996.

Medical Management of Chemical Casualties Handbook. Chemical Casualty Care Office, Medical Research Institute of Chemical Defense, 1995.

Internet Sources

Centers for Disease Control and Prevention
www.cdc.gov/agent

Occupational Health and Safety Administration
www.osha.gov/SLTC/emergencypreparedness/index.html

U.S. Army Medical Research Institute of Infectious Diseases
www.usamriid.army.mil/education/bluebook.html

E-medicine articles on biological warfare agents. Go to the website and type in "CBRNE" in the search module.
www.emedicine.com/emerg/

The Guide for the Selection of Biological Agent Detection Equipment for Emergency First Responders, DHS, March 2005. The guide, produced for the Department of Homeland Security (DHS), does not make recommendations. It provides you with ways to compare and contrast commercially available biological detection equipment. After registration, type in "DHS AND guide" in the search box. The link to the Bioagent Detector Guide will be seen.
www.rkb.mipt.org.

Advice to citizens from the Department of Homeland Security
www.ready.gov/america/biological.html

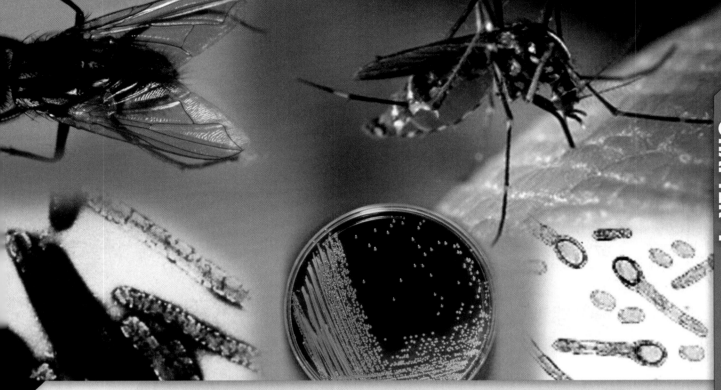

CHAPTER 4

Biological Weapons II

Chapter Objectives

Upon completion of this chapter you should be able to:

1. Discuss biological agents that commonly produce fever and generalized symptoms but not primarily respiratory symptoms.
2. Discuss the biological agent that primarily produces gastrointestinal symptoms.
3. Discuss the biological agent that primarily produces skin lesions.
4. Discuss the biological agent that primarily produces weakness and paralysis.

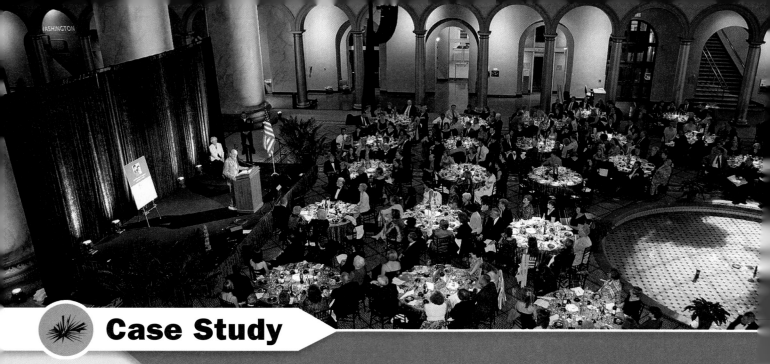

Case Study

At 8:00 a.m. your ambulance has been called to a local hotel where there are multiple cases of people complaining of severe weakness. The hotel manager meets you and tells you that they are hosting a scientific convention for medical research physicians and this morning multiple guests have complained of severe weakness. You call for more ambulances and then examine the first patient. She tells you that last night she was nauseated and her vision was blurry so she went to bed early. This morning she had a sore throat and difficulty speaking and swallowing. Her vision was worse. She had difficulty lifting her arms but was able to call the front desk for help. The manager called 911. When you examine the patient, you find that she cannot fully open her eyes and her pupils are dilated and fixed. She states that light hurts her eyes. She is able to stand but cannot raise her head or lift her arms. You consider Guillain-Barre syndrome but can't explain the other cases in the same hotel. You briefly consider nerve agent exposure, but the patient has dry mucous membranes and her pupils are dilated, not constricted. At this time your dispatcher calls to tell you that they have had 33 more calls from the same hotel, all complaining of weakness.

- What is going on here?
- Is this a natural event or a terrorist attack with a chemical or biological agent?
- If a bioweapon attack, what is the probable agent?
- What should be done now?

The Case Study will continue at the end of the chapter.

Chapter 3 covered biological agents that primarily produce respiratory symptoms. In this chapter we will cover biological agents that produce other symptoms.

Biological Agents That Produce Fever and Generalized Symptoms

Smallpox

Overview and History

Smallpox is a disease caused by the variola virus. The disease is transmitted from person to person but is not transmitted by animals or insects. In the past, smallpox caused major epidemics worldwide, but (except for laboratory specimens) the virus was eradicated by 1980. There have been no reported cases of smallpox in the world since 1977 (Somalia). The last case in the United States was in 1949. There is a vaccine that is very effective, but immunization of civilians and the military was stopped in the 1980s because, out of millions vaccinated, there would

It Happens...

be a few deaths from adverse complications each year (about 1 to 2 deaths per million persons vaccinated).

Smallpox has been effectively used as a biological weapon since the 1500s when Pizzaro used contaminated clothing to infect South American natives. During the French and Indian War (1754–1757) the British used contaminated blankets to infect Indians loyal to the French (50% of some Indian tribes died). Japan experimented with smallpox as a bioweapon in World War II, and many other countries are thought to have developed offensive bioweapons using smallpox.

The CDC rates smallpox as a Category A threat.

Clinical Presentation

After the patient is exposed to the variola virus, the disease incubates for an average of 12 days and then the patient develops fever, aching, and weakness. Many patients will also have vomiting; some will have a mild cough. Two or 3 days later a rash develops on the mucosa of the mouth, face, hands, and forearms (a few patients develop the rash along with the original symptoms). The lesions that first appear in the mouth quickly ulcerate, releasing large amounts of virus into the saliva. The patient is most contagious at this time. The rash then spreads to the trunk over a week's time. The original rash is macular (flat like a freckle) but quickly progresses to papules and then pustules (Figure 4.1). Most lesions are on

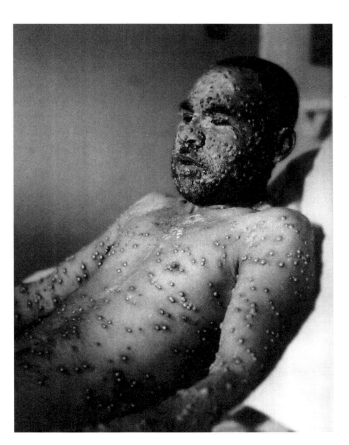

Figure 4.1
Person with severe smallpox. Though the lesions are all over his body, they are worse on the head and distal extremities. Note that the lesions are all in the same stage of development.
Photo: CDC Public Health Image Library.

Figure 4.2
Smallpox rash tends to be
worse on the face and
extremities, whereas
chickenpox rash tends to
be worse on the trunk and
proximal extremities.

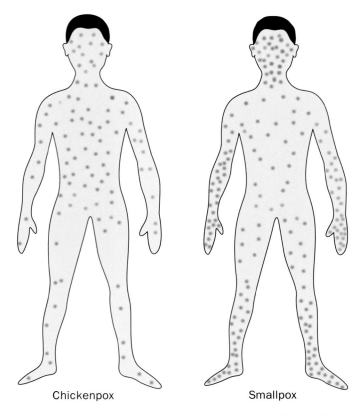

Chickenpox   Smallpox

the face and extremities (centrifugal), and this distinguishes early smallpox from varicella (chickenpox), which tends to be on the trunk (centripetal) (Figure 4.2). The smallpox pustules tend to be synchronized in their stage of development, whereas the lesions of chickenpox will be in various stages of development. Eight to 14 days after appearing, the pustules form scabs that separate leaving depressed, depigmented scars. The patient remains infective until all scabs are gone. The mortality rate for smallpox is 30% in unvaccinated patients but only 3% in patients previously vaccinated.

There is another pox virus of which we must be aware. Monkeypox is a rare viral illness that occurs mostly in central and western Africa. It belongs to the same group of viruses that cause smallpox, cowpox, and chickenpox. The disease is usually found in rats, mice, rabbits, squirrels, and monkeys. It got its name because it was first discovered in laboratory monkeys (1958). In humans the virus causes a disease similar to smallpox but milder (1–10% mortality). The virus entered the United States by way of an infected Gambian giant rat that was imported for sale as a pet. While still at a pet wholesaler, the rat infected prairie dogs. People who bought the prairie dogs for pets developed monkeypox (1970). So far the only known infections among humans have been in Indiana, Wisconsin, and Illinois. The western U.S. wild prairie dog population has not been infected with the virus. A person infected with monkeypox would have a rash similar to smallpox but would also have swollen lymph nodes. The smallpox vaccine is effective against monkeypox. Your local public health officer can arrange for tests to differentiate monkeypox from chickenpox or smallpox.

Prehospital Presentation

Because of the incubation period you would not likely be called to the site of the exposure, but would rather be called to transport most patients from their homes. Most patients will transport themselves to medical care by private vehicle. The presenting symptoms will be flu-like except for a lack of cough or dyspnea. The patient may or may not have a macular, erythematous rash on the face and extremities. You would be likely to think of some viral process, but unlikely to think of smallpox at this stage, and yet the patients are all contagious. This underlines the importance of strict standard precautions against becoming contaminated. If you begin to see many patients like this, you should notify the emergency department of your suspicions. Decontaminate your equipment in the usual way.

Treatment

The only proven treatment is vaccinia-immune globulin (VIG) and supportive care. The antiviral drug cidofovir may be helpful but can cause renal toxicity. The patient and all persons who have been in direct contact with the patient must be quarantined with respiratory isolation for 17 days. Spread of the disease is much more likely if the patient has a cough. Immediate vaccination or revaccination (if vaccinated many years previously) should be performed on all personnel who have been exposed.

Prophylaxis

Smallpox vaccine is very effective, and everyone in the area should be vaccinated except those who:

- Are immunosuppressed
- Have HIV infection
- Have a history of eczema
- Have a current household, sexual, or other close physical contact with persons that have one of these conditions.

The vaccine is given by intradermal inoculation. A vesicle develops in 5 to 7 days and forms a scab that falls off in another 1 to 2 weeks. For healthcare workers who have been exposed to the virus, it is important to remember that if not immunized previously, you have about 3 to 4 days to obtain the smallpox vaccination. If given after that time, you will have the same 30% mortality rate as unvaccinated victims. Those patients who are known contacts should get VIG (0.6 mg/kg IM) within the first week of exposure. Those receiving this within 24 hours of exposure get the highest level of protection.

Venezuelan Equine Encephalitis
Overview and History

Venezuelan equine encephalitis (VEE) is caused by an alphavirus that is endemic to northern South America, Central America, Mexico, and Florida. The virus causes disease in horses, mules, burros, and donkeys (Equidae), and the disease is transmitted to humans by the bite of infected mosquitoes that have previously bitten an infected animal. Many kinds of mosquitoes can transmit the virus. In natural VEE epidemics, human disease is always preceded by disease in the equine population. The disease is deadly in horses (80% mortality) but causes death in only about 1% of infected humans. However, in those who actually develop encephalitis the mortality rate goes up to 20%. In a bioweapon attack, human and equine populations would develop the disease at the same time.

The United States weaponized VEE before the offensive program was terminated. Other countries are also thought to have developed weaponized VEE. The virus could be produced in a wet or dry form and delivered by aerosol. Secondary spread from human to human is possible but rare. It would require mosquito transmission or exposure to blood or body fluids.

The CDC rates VEE as a Category B threat.

Clinical Presentation

The VEE virus has an incubation period of 1 to 5 days and then presents with sudden onset of spiking fever, weakness, severe headache, photophobia, and muscle aches in the legs and back. The patient may develop nausea, vomiting, cough, sore throat, and diarrhea. Most patients (99%) slowly recover over 3 to 14 days with only supportive treatment. VEE can cause inflammation of the covering of the brain (meninges) and the brain itself (encephalitis). Almost everyone who is infected will develop overt disease, but only 2 to 5% will develop encephalitis. Recovery results in long-term immunity.

Prehospital Presentation

If there were an aerosol bioterrorism attack with VEE, you would begin to get multiple calls to the same geographic area. Because of the incubation period, you would not likely be called to the site of the exposure, but would rather be called to transport most patients from their homes. The patients would complain of severe headache, fever, aching, and weakness, and your assessment might suggest encephalitis or meningitis. Children are more prone to have seizures, coma, or paralysis. Because the number of patients would be out of proportion to what would occur in a natural encephalitis epidemic, you should notify the emergency department personnel of your suspicions. You should practice standard precautions plus gown and mask. Decontaminate your equipment by the usual method.

Treatment

Treatment is supportive only, but most patients will recover within 2 weeks. Some patients (usually children) may require anticonvulsants, and many will need IV fluids. You should practice blood and body substance precautions. If the patient has a cough, you should protect against respiratory transmission, though such transmission has not been proven. The virus is inactivated by the usual disinfectants.

Prophylaxis

At this time there is an experimental vaccine available, but it can cause moderate to severe reactions and almost 20% of people fail to develop detectable neutralizing antibodies.

Viral Hemorrhagic Fevers

Overview and History

The viral hemorrhagic fevers are a diverse group of diseases caused by RNA viruses from several different families. These diseases include yellow fever, dengue fever, Ebola and Marburg viruses, Argentine and Bolivian hemorrhagic fevers, Lassa fever, Congo-Crimean hemorrhagic fever, and Rift Valley fever. They are not known to have been weaponized but are included because they have the potential to be weaponized and delivered by the aerosol route. All of these viruses (except for the mosquito-borne yellow fever and dengue fever) can be spread by aerosol or infected fomites. None of these viruses are endemic to the United States, so any epidemic here would likely be caused by intentional attack.

The CDC rates viral hemorrhagic fevers as a Category A threat.

Clinical Presentation

All of these viruses cause a clinical syndrome referred to as viral hemorrhagic fever (VHF). The incubation period varies with each particular virus. The target organ is the vascular bed, and symptoms reflect damage to the microvascular system with changes in vascular permeability. This results in easy bleeding, bruising, and petechiae (multiple pinpoint hemorrhages in the skin). Common complaints are fever, muscle aching, and extreme weakness. Some may have nausea, vomiting, and diarrhea. Examination may only reveal flushing, mild hypotension, generalized petechial hemorrhages, easy bruising, conjunctival injection, and generalized edema (Figure 4.3). Severe cases will show generalized mucous membrane hemorrhage and shock. Some of these viruses, such as Ebola, have very high mortality rates.

Prehospital Presentation

If there were an aerosol bioterrorism attack with VHF, you would begin to get multiple calls to the same geographic area. Because of the incubation period, these patients will usually come from their homes. The patients would complain

Figure 4.3
The viral hemorrhagic fevers cause bleeding into the skin. This looks like large bruised areas.

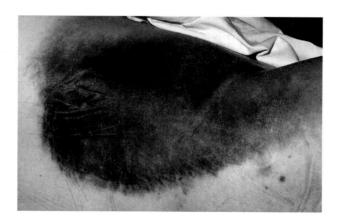

of severe aching, high fever, and weakness. Your assessment would reveal acutely ill patients with fever, multiple petechiae, bruises, and generalized edema. These patients are extremely contagious, and you should wear gloves, gowns, and a face mask. Extreme care must be taken when disposing of gowns and gloves to prevent secondary infection.

Treatment

The treatment is mainly supportive, and many patients will require intensive care to survive. The antiviral drug ribavirin can be used to treat some of these fevers, but its use will depend on a definite diagnosis of the etiology of the disease.

Prophylaxis

Of this group of diseases, a vaccine is available only for yellow fever, though vaccines are under investigation for several others. Public health officials can tell you if any vaccines are available once they have made a diagnosis of the cause of the fever.

Q Fever
Overview and History

Q fever is caused by a rickettsia, *Coxiella burnetii*. The disease naturally occurs in animals (sheep, cattle, and goats), which excrete the organism in their milk, urine, and feces. Humans contract the disease when they inhale aerosols containing the organism. The disease was first described in Australia and was called "Query fever" because the causative agent was unknown. The infective agent was discovered in 1937. *C. burnetii* is very stable and is resistant to heat and drying. It is highly infectious by the aerosol route (one organism can cause illness). These characteristics make it attractive as a biological weapon, and some countries are believed to have weaponized *C. brunetii*. It would most likely be delivered by the aerosol route.

The CDC rates Q fever as a Category B threat.

Clinical Presentation

Q fever has an incubation period of 10 to 20 days, depending on the number of organisms inhaled. The disease presents with flu-like symptoms of fever, myalgias, headache, and weakness. Of infected patients, about half will develop pneumonia but only half of those will have a cough (usually nonproductive) and about 25% will have pleuritic chest pain. Q fever can cause abortion in pregnant patients. The disease is usually self-limiting and lasts from 2 days to 2 weeks. Rarely patients develop chronic hepatitis, culture-negative endocarditis (heart valve infection), aseptic meningitis, encephalitis, or osteomyelitis.

Prehospital Presentation

Because of the incubation period, you would not be called to the exposure site but would usually be called to the patients' homes. If you are called to transport significant numbers of patients with flu-like symptoms (especially if not during flu season), you should consider other causes and express your suspicions to the emergency department personnel. As with all patients with cough, you should use standard precautions and mask the patient or yourself. You can decontaminate your equipment by the usual methods.

Treatment

Most patients will recover without antibiotics, but oral doxycycline (100 mg BID) for 5 to 7 days will shorten the duration of the illness.

Prophylaxis

In the event of a biological attack with *C. burnetii* there is a vaccine available but it causes severe local reactions in individuals who are already immune to the organism. Doxycycline given during the incubation period will prevent the disease but, interestingly, only if it is **not** given **too soon.** If doxycycline is begun the day after exposure, the clinical disease will occur about 3 weeks after treatment, but if the drug is begun a week after exposure, the disease is prevented.

Biological Agents That Produce Primarily Gastrointestinal Symptoms

Cholera

Overview and History

Cholera is a disease caused by the bacterium *Vibrio cholerae,* a curved (vibrio), motile, gram-negative rod that does not form spores. Cholera exerts it effect on the intestinal mucosa, which it adheres to but does not invade. All strains of cholera produce an enterotoxin that causes a toxigenic diarrhea. Natural transmission is through direct or indirect fecal contamination of food or water. The bacterium will not survive in pure water but will survive up to 24 hours in sewage and as long as 6 weeks in contaminated water that contains organic matter. It is resistant to freezing but is easily killed by heat or ordinary disinfectants.

There have been multiple natural epidemics of cholera. Without treatment, the mortality rate approaches 50%. Although cholera is almost unknown in the United States, it continues to cause epidemics in developing countries. The agent has been investigated as a bioweapon, but effective use would require contaminating major drinking water supplies.

The CDC rates cholera as a Category B threat.

Clinical Presentation

After an incubation period of 12 to 72 hours, the disease suddenly presents with abdominal cramping and then painless, profuse "rice water" diarrhea (5–10 liters per day). Some patients may also have vomiting, weakness, and headache. Fever, if present, is low-grade. The response to infection varies greatly. Many patients have few or no symptoms (400:1 ratio of asymptomatic to symptomatic); others lose massive amounts of fluids and develop hypovolemic shock. As with other diseases, cholera is worse in the very young and very old. Deaths are from fluid loss and electrolyte abnormalities.

Prehospital Presentation

If there were a bioterrorism attack with cholera, you would begin to get multiple calls to the same geographic area for patients complaining of severe painless diarrhea. Because of the incubation period, you would likely be called not to the site of the exposure but rather to the victims' homes. The patients would likely share the same water supply or have shared a common meal in the last 3 days. Many will require IV fluid replacement for hypovolemia. Weakness and watery diarrhea will be the common complaint. Standard precautions are adequate to protect against infection, and your equipment can be disinfected in the usual manner.

Treatment

The disease usually lasts from 2 to 7 days. The mainstay of treatment is fluid and electrolyte replacement. This can be done orally for those patients who are not vomiting (3.5 g NaCl, 2.5 g $NaHCO_3$, 1.5 g KCl, 20 g glucose per liter). Some patients will lose fluid so rapidly that they require oral and IV replacement. Antibiotics (doxycycline 100 mg BID for 3 days or ciprofloxin 500 mg BID for 3 days) shorten the diarrhea and thus decrease fluid loss.

Prophylaxis

Oral cholera vaccines are available and can be used in those at risk for exposure. Public health officials will have the latest protocols for use of such vaccines. The most important method to stop an epidemic is to find the contaminated water or food supply and quarantine it. The public health department is tasked and trained to do this sort of investigation. Careful safeguarding of our water supply is the best way to prevent the use of cholera as a bioweapon.

Ricin, staphylococcal enterotoxin B, and trichothecene mycotoxins T2 can also present with vomiting and diarrhea if ingested. See descriptions of these diseases under the respiratory and skin sections.

Biological Agents That Primarily Produce Skin Lesions

Trichothecene Mycotoxins T2

Overview and History

The trichothecene mycotoxins are low-molecular-weight nonvolatile compounds produced by certain molds. They are not water soluble but are soluble in alcohols. They are very stable to heat and ultraviolet light but are inactivated by alkaline solutions.

The communists used aerosolized mycotoxins ("yellow rain") in Laos (1975–1981), Kampuchea (1979–1981), and Afghanistan (1979–1981), causing over 10,000 deaths. It is almost certain that weaponized mycotoxins are still available in some countries.

The CDC rates trichothecene mycotoxins as a Category B threat.

Clinical Presentation

T2 and other mycotoxins are rapid-acting, potent inhibitors of protein and nucleic acid synthesis. They can be absorbed through the skin, inhaled, or ingested. Victims may be contaminated by all three methods if the mycotoxin is aerosolized and contaminates their clothing and skin and is also inhaled and swallowed. Signs and symptoms depend on the route of exposure. If the skin is contaminated, symptoms of burning pain develop within minutes and progress to erythema, blistering, and then skin necrosis with formation of a leathery eschar and sloughing of skin. If inhaled, there will be burning pain in the nose, pharynx, and tracheobronchial tree along with cough, sneezing, epistaxis (nosebleed), bloody sputum, and wheezing. If ingested, there will be nausea, vomiting, and watery or bloody diarrhea with abdominal cramps. Mycotoxin in the eye causes intense burning pain, tearing, redness, and blurred vision. Skin, eye, and pulmonary symptoms usually occur within minutes, but GI symptoms may take several hours to develop. As the toxin is absorbed, the victim may develop ataxia, weakness, and loss of coordination. Severe cases will develop shock and die.

Prehospital Presentation

Because the effect is immediate, you are likely to get a call for a multicasualty incident involving an aerosol spray (yellow fluid droplets). If you know you are responding to a multicasualty incident with symptoms of skin irritation, you should not enter the scene or approach victims until the HazMat team has done an evaluation. This approach may have to be modified if Hazmat is not immediately available. You will likely have to wear chemical protective clothing (including hood) and an SCBA (Level A or B) to care for the victims. The victims will complain of burning of their eyes and skin and will likely have erythema and blistering of the skin and erythema and watering of their eyes. They may have cough, dyspnea, and wheezing. Remember, their clothes and skin are probably contaminated by the mycotoxin and you can become cross-contaminated by touching either. You may initially consider an attack by one of the riot control chemical agents or sulfur mustard (aerosol) as the cause. Riot control agents manifest quickly and would cause erythema of the skin but not blistering. Sulfur mustard has a latent period of several hours and has a distinct garlic or onion odor. Mycotoxin has a much shorter latent period (just minutes) and no odor. The HazMat chemical agent detectors will be negative for a chemical agent, and this should make you think that a mycotoxin is the likely agent.

You should decontaminate the victims in the field before taking them to the emergency department. Remove and double-bag all clothing and have the patients wash with soap and uncontaminated water. Patients who have inhaled the toxin may require endotracheal intubation and ventilation. The patients' eyes should be thoroughly irrigated with saline. The runoff water should be captured for secure disposal if possible, but *do not delay decontamination of patients*. Patients should be given activated charcoal if they have ingested any of the toxin. Public health officials should be notified immediately.

Treatment

Treatment consists of removal of the mycotoxin from the skin and eyes and then supportive and symptomatic treatment. Death can occur in minutes to days, and it is expected that the mortality rate will be very high for those exposed to this bioagent.

Prophylaxis

There is currently no prophylaxis other than preventing exposure to the toxin.

Biological Agents That Primarily Produce Weakness and Paralysis

Botulinum Toxins

Overview and History

Botulinum toxins are a group of seven related neurotoxins produced by the bacterium *Clostridium botulinum*. As a group these are the most potent toxins known to man. The bacterium is an anaerobic, gram-positive, spore-forming rod. The disease caused by theses toxins is called "botulism." Botulism occurs naturally when food contaminated by the botulism spores or bacteria is improperly canned, allowing the bacteria to grow and produce toxins. Botulism was first described in Germany after the ingestion of spoiled sausage (*botulus* is Latin for sausage).

Botulinum toxins have been isolated and have been weaponized by several countries. During World War II, the British furnished a grenade containing botulinum toxin to Czech patriots who used it to assassinate Reinhard Heydrich, deputy chief of the Nazi Gestapo. He survived the grenade explosion but died from botulism. In 1995, Iraq admitted to have weaponized botulinum toxin and possessed over 100 bombs containing the toxin. It is unknown how many more might still be hidden. The toxins can be delivered by aerosol or by contamination of food.

The CDC rates botulism as a Category A threat.

Clinical Presentation

The symptoms of botulism are the same whether ingested or inhaled. The latent period varies from 24 hours to several days, depending on the amount of exposure. The toxin has a longer latent period when inhaled than when ingested orally. Early, patients complain of blurred vision and double vision and often have difficulty speaking and swallowing. Examination reveals drooping of the eyelids (ptosis) with photophobia (light hurts the eyes) and dilated, often fixed pupils (pupils may be normal). The patients then develop a progressive, symmetrical, descending weakness and then paralysis. Death results from respiratory failure. The patient will be alert, awake, and afebrile. Mucous membranes will be dry and the patient may complain of sore throat. The patient will have difficulty speaking and swallowing and may not have a gag reflex. Nausea and vomiting are seen with some of the toxins.

Prehospital Presentation

Because of the latent period you are not likely to be called to the scene of the exposure but rather will usually be called to pick up victims at their homes. You would notice an epidemic of cases of weakness, difficulty speaking, and difficulty swallowing. The patients will be alert and afebrile with ptosis, dilated pupils (usual), dry mucous membranes, and profound weakness that begins with the eyes and works downward. They may require ventilatory assistance. With a single patient, you may think of Guillain-Barre syndrome, myasthenia gravis, or tick paralysis. With many patients you will immediately suspect a biological attack. The patients will not likely remember an attack, but they will have been at some common area or shared a common meal within the last couple of days. You are likely to think of organophosphate nerve agents, but these cause copious secretions and small pupils (miosis). You should immediately notify the emergency department of your suspicions.

Decontaminate your equipment in the usual manner. Botulinum toxins are not absorbed through the skin, and the patients do not transmit the disease.

Treatment

Treatment is supportive and may require prolonged intensive care (weeks to months). The severe cases may require intubation and ventilatory support. Respiratory failure is the usual cause of death, but with good care the mortality rate should be less than 5%. There is an antitoxin available for use in certain circumstances.

Prophylaxis

There is an investigational pentavalent toxoid available for special cases, but because the disease is not contagious and the toxoid would not help those already exposed, there are few indications for its use unless repeated attacks are feared.

Table 4.1 provides a summary of the bioweapons discussed in this chapter. Box 4-1 discusses what to do if you suspect that you have been exposed to a biological threat.

Table 4.1	Summary of Biological Weapons			
Disease Agent	**Incubation Period**	**Common Presentation**	**Less Common Signs and Symptoms**	**Diagnostic Tests**
Smallpox (virus)	7–17 days	Fever, aching, headache, weakness, centripetal rash that progessess to pustules in the same stage of development.	Rarely, nonproductive cough.	Consult public health for tests.
Venezuelan equine encephalitis (virus)	1–5 days	Fever, aching, headache, weakness, photophobia. Children may have convulsions, coma, or paralysis.	May develop sore throat, nausea, vomiting, diarrhea, nonproductive cough.	CBC reveals low WBC and low lymphocyte count. Lumbar puncture reveals high pressure and high white cell count, usually mononuclear cells. Consult public health for other tests.
Viral hemorrhagic fevers	Varies with agent	Fever, aching, weakness, petechiae, bruising, edema.	Nausea, vomiting, diarrhea.	CBC reveals low WBC and low platelets, liver enzymes elevated. U/A reveals protein and blood. Consult public health for specific viral tests.
Q fever (rickettsia)	10–20 days	High fever, aching, weakness, sore throat, severe headache.	Chest pain or cough (25%), hepatitis, endocarditis, encephalitis, pneumonia, aseptic meningitis, osteomyelitis, nausea, vomiting, abdominal pain.	Usually are not as toxic as plague or anthrax. Chest X-ray may show patchy infiltrates like mycoplasma or viral pneumonia.
Cholera (bacterium)	12–72 hours	Abdominal cramping and then painless "rice water" diarrhea, dehydration, weakness.	Low-grade fever, vomiting, headache.	Motile, curved rods seen on gram stain of stool. No WBC in stool. Consult public health for confirmation.
Trichothecene mycotoxin T2 (yellow rain) (toxin)	Inhaled or skin: symptoms develop in minutes. Ingested: 2–4 hours.	Skin contamination: almost immediate burning and redness progressing to blisters and necrosis. Inhaled: immediate burning pain in respiratory tree with cough, wheezing, epistaxis, bloody sputum. Ingested: nausea, vomiting, watery or bloody diarrhea. Patients may develop ataxia and weakness, then shock.		Consult public health.
Botulinum toxins (toxin)	1–5 days (Incubation period longer for inhaled toxin than for ingested toxin)	Blurred or double vision, ptosis, generallized weakness, difficulty speaking and swallowing, photophobia, descending paralysis.	Sore throat, nausea, vomiting.	Consult public health.

Differential Diagnosis	Treatment	Prophylaxis	Mortality	Transmission
Influenza, varicella, vaccinia, disseminated herpes zoster.	Supportive. Vaccine-immune globulin.	Vaccine available.	30% in those who are not vaccinated, 1% in vaccinated.	Very contagious. Patients must be isolated until scabs have healed.
Influenza, West Nile virus, western equine encephalitis, St. Louis encephalitis, eastern equine encephalitis.	Supportive.	None for humans.	Low, 1%. But patients who develop encephalitis (2–4%) will have a 20% mortality.	Spread is by mosquitoes. Patient-to-patient transmission very rare.
Malaria, meningococcemia, acute leukemia, typhoid fever, thrombocytopenic purpura.	Supportive. Possibly Ribavirin.	Consult public health for possible vaccines.	Varies, can be very high.	Very contagious via aerosol or on fomites.
Influenza, tularemia, mycoplasma, or viral pheumonia.	Oral doxycycline, fluoroquinolone. Most recover without treatment.	Doxycycline started a week after exposure.	Low, 1–2% if untreated.	Patient-to-patient transmission rare.
Viral diarrhea, typhoid fever.	Supportive plus doxycycline or fluoroquinalone orally.	Vaccine available.	50% without treatment.	Usually transmitted by contaminated food or water. Patient-to-patient transmission rare.
Vessicant gas or liquid exposure.	Decontamination, supportive.	None.	High.	Can get patient-to-patient contamination with the toxin on skin or clothes.
Guillan-Barre syndrome, organophosphate poisoning, myasthenia gravis, magnesium intoxication, tick paralysis, atropine poisoning.	Antitoxin, supportive.	None.	High if untreated.	No patient-to-patient transmission.

Box 4-1   What to Do If You Are Exposed to a Biological Attack

A biological attack is the deliberate release of germs or other biological substances that can make you sick. Many agents must be inhaled, enter through a cut in the skin, or be eaten to make you sick. Some biological agents, such as anthrax, do not cause contagious diseases. Others, like the smallpox virus, can result in diseases you can catch from other people.

If There Is a Biological Threat
Unlike an explosion, a biological attack may or may not be immediately obvious. Although it is possible that you will see signs of a biological attack, as was sometimes the case with the anthrax mailings, it is perhaps more likely that local health care workers will report a pattern of unusual illness or there will be a wave of sick people seeking emergency medical attention. You will probably learn of the danger through an emergency radio or TV broadcast, or some other signal used in your community. You might get a telephone call, or emergency response workers may come to your door.

In the event of a biological attack, public health officials may not immediately be able to provide information on what you should do. It will take time to determine exactly what the illness is, how it should be treated, and who is in danger. However, you should watch TV, listen to the radio, or check the Internet for official news, including the following:

- Are you in the group or area authorities consider in danger?
- What are the signs and symptoms of the disease?
- Are medications or vaccines being distributed?
- Where? Who should get them?
- Where should you seek emergency medical care if you become sick?

During a Declared Biological Emergency
1. If a family member becomes sick, it is important to be suspicious.
2. Do not assume, however, that you should go to a hospital emergency room or that any illness is the result of the biological attack. Many common illnesses have similar symptoms.
3. Use common sense, practice good hygiene, and cleanliness to avoid spreading germs, and seek medical advice.
4. Consider if you are in the group or area authorities believe to be in danger.
5. If your symptoms match those described and you are in the group considered at risk, immediately seek emergency medical attention.

If You Are Potentially Exposed
1. Follow the instructions of doctors and other public health officials.
2. If the disease is contagious, expect to receive medical evaluation and treatment. You may be advised to stay away from others or may be quarantined.
3. For noncontagious diseases, expect to receive medical evaluation and treatment.

If You Become Aware of an Unusual and Suspicious Substance Nearby
1. Quickly get away.
2. Protect yourself. Cover your mouth and nose with layers of fabric that can filter the air but still allow breathing. Examples include two to three layers of cotton, such as a T-shirt, handkerchief, or towel. Otherwise, several layers of tissue or paper towels may help.
3. Wash with soap and water.
4. Contact authorities.
5. Watch TV, listen to the radio, or check the Internet for official news and information, including what the signs and symptoms of the disease are, if medications or vaccinations are being distributed, and where you should seek medical attention if you become sick.
6. If you become sick, seek emergency medical attention.

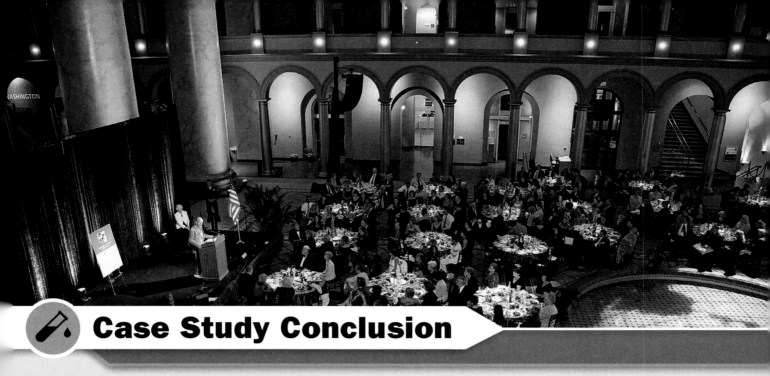

Case Study Conclusion

Eventually 164 patients arrive at local hospitals. They all have weakness that progresses to a descending paralysis. All of the patients are found to have eaten at the same banquet two nights before. The victims include everyone who ate at the banquet, including several waiters and cooks. The local public health officer is consulted, and she initiates an investigation. Laboratory tests determine the patients have botulism. Law enforcement is also notified and, because of the possibility of bioterrorism, the FBI is consulted. The food served at the banquet cannot be tested because it had already been discarded and the contents of the hotel dumpster have been emptied in the city landfill. The hotel food stocks were negative for botulinum toxins. An investigation of the hotel food suppliers was also negative.

An investigation of the hotel workers revealed a temporary cook who was a member of a radical animal rights group, but he denies any involvement. In spite of searches of the group's headquarters, computer files, and several members' homes (including the cook's), no evidence is ever found.

The patients are treated with botulism antitoxin and supportive care. All require endotracheal intubation and mechanical ventilation. Most recover over the next 6 weeks, but seven older patients die.

Case Study Discussion

This is an example of a biological attack using botulism toxin. Because of the incubation period before the victims developed symptoms, the banquet food had already been dumped in the local landfill before an investigation could begin. The medical responders were not affected because the agent was a toxin placed in food and not a contagious agent.

The botulinum antitoxin neutralizes toxin that has not yet bound to nerve terminals but does not reverse toxin that is already attached. If given within the first 24 hours of onset of symptoms, the antitoxin will decrease the severity of the disease and improve survival. Older patients and those who already have chronic diseases are more likely to succumb to the toxin.

It is often very difficult to positively identify the persons responsible for a biological attack because the latent period before symptoms occur usually gives them plenty of time to dispose of evidence.

Pearls

- If you find yourself transporting multiple patients with similar complaints, you should consider the possibility of bioterrorism.

- When called to the scene of a multicasualty incident involving suspicious symptoms (especially respiratory), do not enter the scene until it has been cleared by the HazMat team or until you put on proper personal protective equipment.

- If you are called to a scene where there are multiple patients with similar complaints, the patients should be decontaminated before they are allowed to enter your ambulance.

- The public health department has resources to help you with any potential terrorist event.

- Try to approach any suspicious multicasualty event from uphill, upstream, and upwind.

- Do not become a victim! If you make an unplanned arrival at a suspicious multicasualty event, you should immediately retreat and call the HazMat team and law enforcement.

- If victims have symptoms of a vesicant chemical agent but chemical agent detector tests are negative, consider trichothecene mycotoxin T2.

Want to Know More?

Bibliography

DeLorenzo, R.A. and Porter, R.S., *Weapons of Mass Destruction: Emergency Care,* Brady, Prentice Hall, 2000.

Gilbert, D.N., R.C. Moellering, G.M. Eliopoulos, and M.S. Sande. *The Sanford Guide to Antimicrobial Therapy.* Antimicrobial Therapy, Inc. 2004: 34, 39, 46.

Inglesby, T.V., et al. "Anthrax as a Biological Weapon: Medical and Public Health Management," *JAMA.* 281 (1999): 1735–45.

Inglesby T.V., et al. "Plague as a Biological Weapon," *JAMA.* 283 (2000): 2281–2290.

Medical Management of Biological Casualties Handbook, 2nd ed. U.S. Army Medical Research Institute of Infectious Diseases 1996.

Medical Management of Chemical Casualties Handbook. Chemical Casualty Care Office, Medical Research Institute of Chemical Defense 1995.

Internet Sources

Centers for Disease Control and Prevention
www.cdc.gov/agent

Occupational Health and Safety Administration
www.osha.gov/SLTC/emergencypreparedness/index.html

U.S. Army Medical Research Institute of Infectious Diseases
www.usamriid.army.mil/education/bluebook.html

E-medicine articles on biological warfare agents. Go to the website and type in "CBRNE" in the search module.
www.emedicine.com/emerg/

The Guide for the Selection of Biological Agent Detection Equipment for Emergency First Responders, DHS, March 2005. The guide, produced for the Department of Homeland Security (DHS), does not make recommendations. It provides you with ways to compare and contrast commercially available biological detection equipment. After registration, type in "DHS AND guide" in the search box. The link to the Bioagent Detector Guide will be seen.
www.rkb.mipt.org

Advice to citizens from the Department of Homeland Security
www.ready.gov/america/biological.html

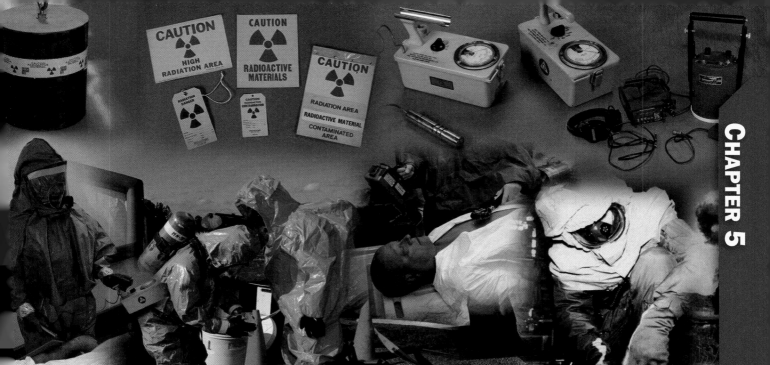

CHAPTER 5

Radiological or Nuclear Incidents

Chapter Objectives

Upon completion of this chapter you should be able to:

1. **Discuss the signs and symptoms of radiation sickness.**
2. **Discuss methods of attack by radioactive or nuclear devices.**
3. **Discuss the response to a nuclear attack.**
4. **Discuss how the detection of radiation at a suspicious event would change your scene response.**
5. **Discuss detection devices available for identifying radioactive contamination.**
6. **Discuss decontamination of victims exposed to radiation.**

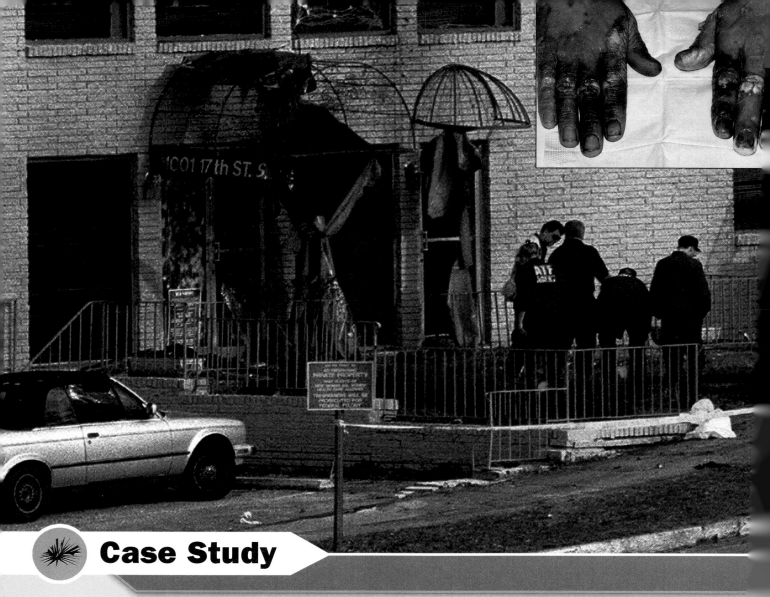

Case Study

Abortion Clinic

EMS, fire service, and law enforcement responders are dispatched to a report of an explosion at an abortion clinic on a Sunday morning. The clinic has been the target of numerous organized protests, picketing, death threats, and harassment of the staff. There have been bomb threat hoaxes, and after business hours shots have been fired into the empty clinic. The clinic is a stand-alone structure and is closed and unoccupied at this time. Upon arrival, responders note debris, dust, and glass in the street in front of the facility. A passing motorist reports he smelled the stench of "vomit" as he drove by the clinic following the explosion.

- What steps should responders take?
- What are the potential hazards?
- Should responders proceed into the scene?
- Has the motorist been exposed to any harmful substance?
- What created the smell?

Emergency Department

Several weeks following the bombing, emergency department personnel treat a middle-aged male farmer who has unusual necrotic ulcers on both hands along with what appears to be healing burns on both hands. The patient says he was burned while working on his farm tractor several weeks before. The emergency department physician has seen many burns in the past but none that would take so long to heal. He is also concerned the patient waited so long to seek medical care. In addition to the burns, the individual complains of malaise, fatigue, nausea, and vomiting. He has a temperature of 39 °C (102.2 °F) and is obviously dehydrated. A CBC (complete blood count) reveals a very low white blood cell count and anemia.

- What is wrong with this person?
- Does he present a threat to the emergency department staff?
- What is the source of his illness and injury?

The Case Study will continue at the end of the chapter.

The use of radioactive material is a true terror weapon because it generates fear far out of proportion to the actual hazard, disrupts society, and creates a great economic impact. Radiation is especially frightening because, though it is deadly, human senses cannot detect it. Radiation cannot be seen, smelled, or felt.

Radioactive material will produce "denial of use" of a contaminated facility or location and can cause long-term health problems to those persons exposed. Contamination by radiation also creates economic issues such as the great costs associated with radiation cleanup, the long-term public health issues of contaminated victims, and the economic impact of loss of use of the affected facilities. The detonation of a nuclear weapon could cause catastrophic damage plus contaminate the surrounding area with radioactive material.

Radiation Primer

Atomic Structure

An atom of an element is made up of protons, neutrons, and electrons. It looks like a miniature solar system. The protons and neutrons make up the nucleus of the atom and they are surrounded by orbiting electrons (Figure 5.1). Most of the atom is empty space. The protons and neutrons make up almost all of the mass. Protons have a positive charge, neutrons have no charge. Electrons have almost no mass but have a negative charge. A neutral atom has the same number of protons as electrons.

Radiation

An atom that has an excess of mass or energy is unstable and will try to become stable by emitting an energetic (radioactive) particle and/or energy in the form of electromagnetic rays. This emission process is called radioactive decay. An element that releases one of these rays or particles is said to be radioactive or a radionuclide.

We are constantly exposed to background radiation from cosmic radiation (interaction of energy from the sun with the earth's atmosphere), terrestrial radiation from breakdown of uranium in the soil, and natural internal radiation in our bodies from carbon-14 that is present at birth. Man-made radiation sources include diagnostic X-rays, nuclear medicine (bone scans, thyroid scans, etc.), radiation therapy for cancer, nuclear power facilities, and nuclear weapons.

Radioactive Emissions

There are four primary forms of radioactive emissions (Figure 5.2): alpha particles, beta particles, gamma rays, and neutrons.

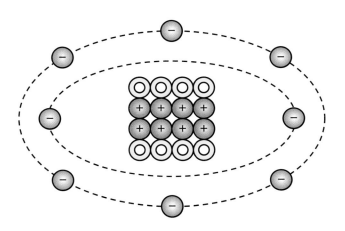

Figure 5.1
Components of an atom. The nucleus is made up of protons and neutrons. Electrons orbit the nucleus like tiny planets.

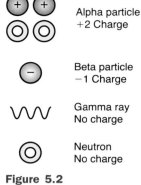

Figure 5.2
Four primary forms of radioactive emissions.

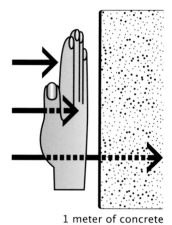

1 meter of concrete

Figure 5.3
Comparison of penetrating powers of alpha and beta particles, and gamma radiation.

- *Alpha Particle:* This particle is emitted from the nucleus of a radioactive atom and has the largest mass of any ionizing particles. It is made up of two protons and two neutrons and has a plus-two (+2) positive charge. These particles can strip negatively charged electrons from atoms that they pass through. Though they have a lot of energy, these particles can travel only a few centimeters in air and have very little penetrating ability. They can be shielded by a sheet of paper. They can't penetrate the skin and generally can't harm the human body except through open wounds, inhalation, or ingestion. They are the most ionizing but least penetrating type of radiation. Polonium-210, an alpha emitter, was used to assassinate Aleksander Litvinenko in November, 2006.

- *Beta Particle:* This is a negatively charged (−1) particle emitted from the nucleus of an atom and has the mass and charge equal to an electron. They will interact electrically with cells they encounter, but because they have only half the charge of an alpha particle, they are less ionizing and cause less damage. They will travel up to several meters in air and a few millimeters in tissue. They are both an internal and an external threat (can burn the skin) but are easily shielded by thin plastic, glass, aluminum, or wood.

- *Gamma Rays:* These are short-wavelength electromagnetic radiations from the nucleus of a radioactive atom. Other than the fact they come from the nucleus rather than the outer shell, they are identical to X-rays. They have no electrical charge and cause cellular damage by directly colliding with the nucleus of an atom in their path. They are the most penetrating form of radiation and travel many meters in the air. Gamma rays can be both an internal and an external threat. X-rays are only an external threat because the X-ray generator cannot be swallowed. Gamma rays require heavy shielding materials, such as 6 inches of lead or 3 feet of concrete (Figure 5.3).

- *Neutron:* Neutrons are man-made and do not occur in nature. They are used in industry and in neutron bombs. They have no charge and cause cellular damage by directly colliding with the nucleus of an atom in their path (like gamma rays). Because of their mass they are 20 times more damaging than gamma rays. Neutrons travel several meters and penetrate skin well, though not as well as gamma rays. They can be shielded with water or plastic. Neutrons require a special detector. If neutrons are detected outside of their industrial use, they are evidence of a terrorist attack and the FBI should be notified immediately.

Radiation Injury

Living cells can be damaged by exposure to ionizing radiation. Radiation can ionize (remove electrons from) atoms in a cell, causing breakage of molecular bonds. When the affected molecules are part of critical cell structures such as chromosomes, cell damage occurs. There are four possible outcomes to a cell's exposure to ionizing radiation:

- There may be no damage.
- The cell may be able to repair itself and continue to function normally.
- The cell may repair itself but no longer function normally (in some cases, become cancerous).
- The cell may die.

The effect of radiation on the skin cells is the same as thermal burns, and *there is no difference in the appearance of burns from thermal and radiation sources.* Unless radioactive material is still present, radiation burns are not radioactive and there are no definitive tests to prove that a burn was caused by radiation. However, radiation burns will heal more slowly than thermal burns and may eventually develop skin cancer. Rapidly dividing (growing) cells are more affected by radiation, and so hair follicles, bone marrow (produces blood cells), and cells of the gastrointestinal tract tend to manifest the effects of radiation poisoning first. Thus a person exposed to toxic levels of radiation to the whole body would, in a few days, develop severe radiation sickness—vomiting and diarrhea, low white and red blood cell counts, and severe hair loss. These are the same symptoms as caused by chemotherapy. Radiation sickness is usually caused by gamma rays, because they penetrate the whole body. Alpha and beta particles cause localized injury. Persons exposed to high levels of radiation frequently die of overwhelming infection because of the damage to their protective white blood cells. However, cells of the nervous system don't grow once they are mature, and they are very resistant to radiation damage.

The amount of radiation to which a person is exposed is measured in RADs or REM. *RAD* stands for "radiation absorbed dose," and it measures the amount of radiation the body has received. One RAD equals 0.01 Joules/kg. *REM* stands for "roentgen equivalent in man." For practical purposes a REM and a RAD are equal. Effects of varying whole-body doses of radiation on humans are listed in Table 5-1.

Table 5-1	Short-Term Effects of Varying Radiation Doses
25 REM	No detectable effect.
50 REM	Slight temporary blood changes.
100 REM	Mild radiation sickness (nausea and fatigue) a couple of days later.
400 REM	Severe radiation sickness. Half of those exposed will die.

The energy transfer of the radioactive waves and particles varies. Alpha particles do not penetrate very deep into tissue but transfer a great deal of energy. A single sheet of paper will shield against alpha particles. Beta particles penetrate farther, but clothing will shield against many beta particles. Once again, the energy transfer is great but the particles do not penetrate deeply. Alpha and beta particles are particularly dangerous when inhaled or ingested, because they irradiate internal tissues directly and impart large amounts of energy to the tissue. Gamma rays are very penetrative but transfer only small amounts of energy. However, gamma rays present a great danger because substantial shielding is required to stop them. Even though the energy transfer is small, the waves travel a long distance and penetration is far greater than for alpha or beta particles. Neutrons penetrate like gamma radiation, and their mass makes them more damaging. Neutrons have the ability to make the irradiated material, including tissue, radioactive. This makes neutron radiation extremely dangerous.

Methods of Exposure to Radiation

Terrorism by way of radioactive materials can come in several forms. If the radioactive isotope is a fissionable material (material that can be used to create a chain reaction that could result in a nuclear explosion), such as some plutonium and uranium isotopes, it is possible that it could be combined into a nuclear weapon. Otherwise the radioactive material might be dispersed by a conventional explosion or by airborne means such as a powder or spray from an aircraft. A building could be contaminated by placing finely ground radioactive particles or powder in the ventilation system. The material could also be spread by hand (more dangerous for the terrorist) or mailed in a package or envelope.

The types of exposure to radiation include simple exposure to the radiation itself, such as from a sealed source in which the radioactive material is securely

Figure 5.4
Examples of medical and industrial X-ray generators.

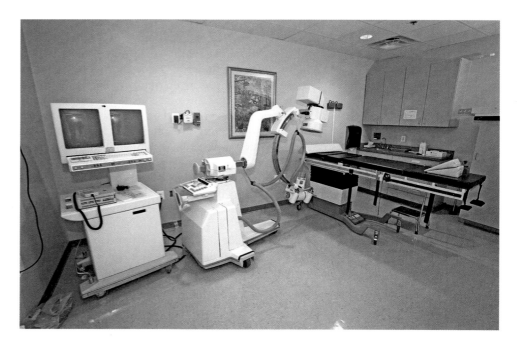

contained, or through electronic means such as an X-ray generator (Figure 5.4). In the case of an X-ray generator no radioactive material is released and the target absorbs the radiation along with the environment. The only hazard is the radiation itself, and the target does not become radioactive. An example is a person who has had an X-ray taken. The person has been exposed to a low dose of radiation (about the same as being out in the sun all day), but is not radioactive or a danger to others.

In other cases where the radioactive material is released, it can be deposited upon environmental surfaces or skin. It could also be inhaled or ingested. The radioactive material on skin and environmental surfaces can usually be washed away, but the close contact with skin may give high doses of radiation to the skin from those isotopes that emit alpha and beta radiation. When radioactive material is inhaled or ingested, it continues to emit radiation and gives the internal areas of the body exposure. If the radioactive material has a chemical affinity for a particular organ of the body, it may accumulate there and selectively irradiate that particular organ. Examples are radioactive iodine (accumulates in the thyroid), radioactive cesium (accumulates in the liver), or radioactive strontium (accumulates in bone).

There is a difference between being exposed to radiation and being contaminated by radioactive material. Persons who have been exposed to radiation are not radioactive and are not dangerous to rescuers or medical personnel. Persons who have radioactive contamination of their skin or clothes will be "radioactive" until the clothes are removed and the material is washed from their skin. A person who has ingested a radioactive material may or may not be dangerous to others, depending on the penetrating power of the particle or wave involved. One way to think of the difference between exposure and contamination is the barnyard example. If you smell a cow pile, you have been exposed. If you step in a cow pile, you have been contaminated.

Nuclear Weapons

A nuclear weapon is a weapon that derives its energy from the nuclear reactions of fission and/or fusion. Even the smallest nuclear detonation would be significantly more powerful than that from the largest conventional explosives.

A simple nuclear weapon derives its energy from nuclear fission. A mass of fissionable material is rapidly assembled into a critical mass, in which a chain reaction develops and releases tremendous amounts of energy. This is known as an atomic bomb. Nuclear fusion can be used to make a more powerful weapon. In such a weapon, the X-ray thermal radiation from a nuclear fission explosion is used to heat and compress a small amount of tritium, deuterium, or lithium, causing nuclear fusion, releasing even more energy. Such a weapon is called a hydrogen bomb and can be hundreds of times more powerful than an atomic bomb.

The nuclear explosion releases four kinds of energy:

- Blast energy—about 50% of the total energy (see Chapter 6).
- Thermal radiation (heat)—about 40% of total energy.
- Ionizing radiation—about 5% of total energy.
- Residual radiation (fallout)—5 to 10% of total energy.

The first three are immediate, whereas radioactive fallout is a delayed release of energy. The total energy release is expressed in equivalent tons of TNT (kilotons or megatons). The heat from the explosion travels farther than the blast wave. The ionizing radiation travels the shortest distance, but the radioactive fallout may be carried great distances by the wind.

Plans for nuclear bombs are public record. The essential component, special fissionable nuclear material, is probably not obtainable except by a nation-state or by a well-funded terrorist group with support from a nation-state. Easier, and more likely, is the theft or purchase of a small nuclear device from a nation with nuclear capability. This could be detonated or used for extortion purposes. Several hoax devices have been located by law enforcement. These devices have been purposely designed to resemble nuclear weapons. Such devices are frightening, because even to qualified personnel, externally they closely resemble small portable nuclear weapons.

It Happens...

The first atomic bomb (only two have ever been used against humans) was dropped on the city of Hiroshima in Japan on August 6, 1945. The bomb detonated 2,000 feet above the city with a blast equivalent to 13,000 tons (13 kilotons) of TNT. The blast leveled the city (Figure 5.5), except for a few very sturdy buildings. Eighty thousand civilians were killed immediately and another 60,000 died of radiation poisoning by the end of the year.

The threat of the use of nuclear devices against the United States by terrorists is not a new threat. There have been threats to use nuclear bombs and radiological devices against the United States since the 1970s. The media reports there are numerous nuclear weapons missing from the former USSR. The media also reports the following countries possess nuclear weapons or are developing the technology: the United States,

former republics of the USSR, France, the U.K., Brazil, Argentina, China, India, Pakistan, Iran, North Korea, South Africa, Israel, Libya, Taiwan, and others.

In the 1970s the city of Orlando, Florida, was the victim of nuclear extortion. It received a viable threat that a nuclear weapon would be detonated if money was not received. A juvenile, who did not really have such a device, committed the crime. Boston, Des Moines, Iowa, and Lincoln, Nebraska, have also been targets of nuclear extortion threats.

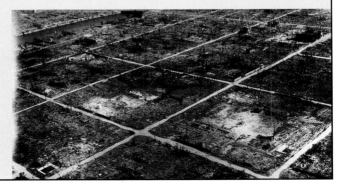

Figure 5.5
An example of the effects of a nuclear blast.

Personal Response to a Nuclear Explosion

If there is advanced warning of a nuclear attack, you should seek shelter as far below ground as possible. This will help protect you from the blast pressure wave and the thermal wave. If a nuclear explosion occurs without warning, you should immediately seek shelter inside a building to reduce your exposure to radioactive material. Go as far below ground as possible, close windows and doors, turn off air conditioners, heaters, or ventilation systems. If possible, use TV, radio, or the Internet to obtain news about the event. Remember to keep as much shielding (earth, concrete, steel) as possible between you and the radioactive material, stay as far away from the nuclear explosion site as possible, and limit the time you are exposed. Public safety personnel will be required to respond to the incident but only after HazMat has evaluated for levels of radiation and other dangers. Once working zones (see Chapter 1) have been defined, you will be able to respond to the surviving victims. This will be covered in more detail later in this chapter.

Radioactive Devices as Weapons

What is more practical, therefore more probable, for a terrorist attack is the use of a radiological dispersion device (RDD), which can either deploy a long-lived radioactive isotope to contaminate a wide area or release a biologically active isotope and affect those exposed more rapidly. Such devices would likely use high explosives to disperse the radioactive material into the atmosphere, causing contamination of a large area. These are referred to as "dirty bombs" (Figure 5.6).

Even if the explosion of a dirty bomb caused few immediate casualties, there is the fear of long-term health risks as well as the astronomical cost of cleanup of a site contaminated by radioactive material.

Other simple methods of attack could involve placing the powdered radioactive material into a ventilation system or sending the radioactive material in an envelope or package via mail.

Long-lived radioactive isotopes such as cobalt-60 (>5-year half-life) or cesium-137 (30-year half-life) can contaminate and render an area uninhabitable for many years. Biologically active isotopes (such as iodine-131) attack specific organs (such as the thyroid) or systems in the human body, causing serious health effects such as cancer. Many radioactive isotopes are not only radiation hazards but are also heavy metals and poisons.

Plutonium is very difficult to obtain but presents a *very* long-lived radiation hazard and is a poisonous heavy metal. In 1986 a nuclear incident at the Russian nuclear power plant at Chernobyl, Belarus, sent 190 tons of radioactive material, including uranium and plutonium, into the atmosphere. Twenty-five percent of the farmland and forests of Belarus were contaminated and will be so for the next 25,000 years! Four hundred thousand people were forced to leave their homes forever, and nine million people were directly or indirectly affected. Exceedingly high rates of certain cancers have been found among those exposed to the radiation. Even to this day,

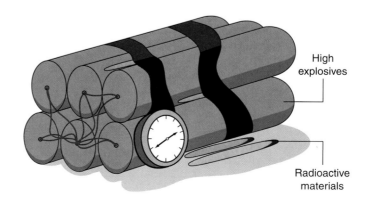

Figure 5.6
A dirty bomb is an explosive device packed with radioactive material that disperses upon detonation.

High explosives

Radioactive materials

It Happens...

The first dirty bomb was found in a park in Moscow after a tip. The bomb had been made by Chechnyan rebels and contained cesium-137 and about 15 pounds of explosives. It was deactivated and removed without harm. Plans for making a dirty bomb were found in al Qaeda caves in Afghanistan, and at least one al Qaeda operative has been arrested for trying to carry out a dirty bomb attack.

25% of the budget of the country of Belarus is spent on cleanup and public health issues related to this radiation accident. Most (97%) of the radioactive material is still within the crumbling power plant structure and may yet be released if the structure collapses. A concrete shelter was erected around the reactor to allow use of other reactors at the plant. This shelter is neither strong nor durable, and a new structure is needed. Though American nuclear power plants are far better built and operated, it is easy to understand why people fear living near them.

There have been many civilian and military nuclear incidents in the past 60 years. The most significant civilian radiation exposures, besides Chernobyl, have been incidents involving cobalt-60 (Co-60) and cesium-137 (Cs-137). Both of these isotopes have long half-lives (30 years for Cs-137), and both are powerful gamma-ray emitters. These radioactive isotopes are used for industrial radiography and food sterilization. In these situations strong gamma rays are needed to penetrate metals to detect imperfections or to kill bacteria (Figure 5.7). In Mexico an incident occurred in which a cobalt-60 source was removed from an abandoned industrial radiography system and placed in a home. The residents become critically ill and several died due to high doses of radiation.

A nuclear accident, second only to Chernobyl, occurred in 1987 in Goiania, Brazil. An abandoned cancer teletherapy (radiation therapy) radiation source containing Cs-137 was stolen and broken open. Many people rubbed the "luminous blue powder" on their bodies. Extensive contamination and radiation exposure occurred. More than 250 persons were known to have been contaminated and irradiated. More than 60 people required hospitalization, and many died. Much of the city was contaminated, and in the ensuing years a significant increase in leukemia has been documented there. It is estimated that the actual number contaminated was in the tens of thousands and that thousands experienced serious health problems.

Federal agencies in the United States report that more than 1,000 sealed radiation sources have been reported stolen, missing, or simply unaccounted for. There are many more sources missing worldwide, and the International Atomic Energy Administration (IAEA) is attempting to recover as many as possible. According to the IAEA, there are thousands of radiation sources (including nuclear weapons) unaccounted for within the former USSR.

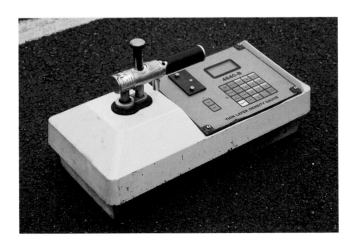

Figure 5.7
An example of an industrial radiological device used in road construction to test the density of road beds.

It Happens...

In 1995 (Operation Sapphire) the United States purchased 600 kilograms of weapons-grade uranium (enough to build 20 to 50 nuclear weapons) from Kazakhstan to prevent Iran from buying it.

The Two-Edged Sword of Radiation

The very nature of radioactive material that makes it suitable as a terrorist weapon also makes it dangerous to the terrorist who must handle it. Persons who improperly handle radioactive materials may receive large whole-body doses of radiation, and can receive skin burns on the hands and arms from close contact with the material. Those handling radioactive material that can become aerosolized (powder or liquid) may also ingest some of the material. This leads to body burdens of the radioactive material, with continuing exposure to the affected tissues. Radiation burns on the hands should at least raise a red flag, suggesting that the patient might be associated with some terrorist event. This would be especially true if the patient gave a false story about the cause of the injuries.

Security of Radiation Sources

Medical and industrial radiographic sources have only minimal security. The Nuclear Regulatory Commission (NRC) reports that most incidents involving theft, loss, or overexposure in the United States are from such sources. This radioactive material is protected only by simple industrial security or, in many instances, no security other than locks. Theft of radioactive material is simple, and purchase on the open market is inexpensive.

There are many sources of radioactive materials in quantity. Some (commercial nuclear power facilities or military facilities) have security to resist theft or attacks. Other sources, such as medical or industrial sites, may have minimal security.

Some sources of radioactive material might include:

- Military facilities where nuclear weapons are housed
- Nuclear weapons construction and maintenance facilities
- Nuclear power plants
- Fuel-reprocessing facilities
- Nuclear waste facilities and transport vehicles
- Medical facilities with medical isotopes, nuclear medicine units, and cancer teletherapy units
- Radiographic (X-ray) sources
- Industrial sites that use radiation to sterilize products
- Highway departments that use radiation devices to test concrete or metal structures

Detection of Radiological Events

The human senses cannot detect radiation and so radiation detectors must be used. Small detectors called "radiation pagers" (Figure 5.8) are readily available and should be worn by responders to any suspicious event. These devices will readily detect even small amounts of gamma radiation. Older, Civil Defense type, (Figure 5.9) units can be utilized to detect energetic gamma-beta emitters such as Cs-137 or Co-60; however, biologically active and medical isotopes such as radioactive

Figure 5.8
An example of a radiation detection pager.

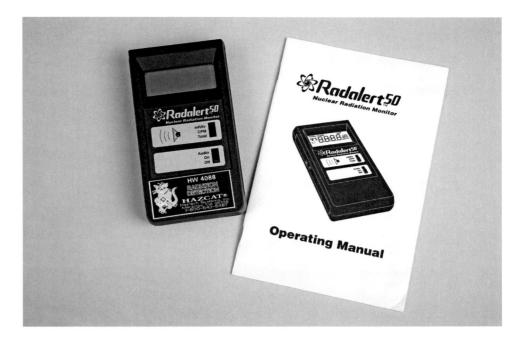

Figure 5.9
Civil Defense radiation detection instruments with "hotdog" probe.

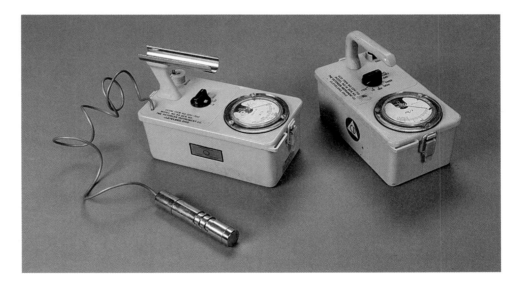

iodine do not give off enough radiation to be detected by this equipment. None of these instruments detect neutron radiation, which is commonly associated with nuclear bombs. Furthermore, shielding with lead or other dense materials (Figure 5.10) may render even strong emitters of gamma rays undetectable by these instruments. Specialized training and equipment such as gamma scintillation and neutron detectors may be required (Figure 5.11). These resources must be identified before you have need of them. In most instances they are available at the local level with hazardous materials teams, bomb squads, and emergency management agencies. At the state level, they are available with radiological health units. Hospital nuclear medicine units can sometimes support emergency department operations involving radioactive materials and usually have the required knowledge and equipment. It is extremely important that emergency responders are well trained in the use of their particular radiation detector.

Emergency responders entering an area where they may be exposed to radiation need to wear radiation dosimeters. A dosimeter records the amount of gamma

Figure 5.10
Shielded medical isotope
container.

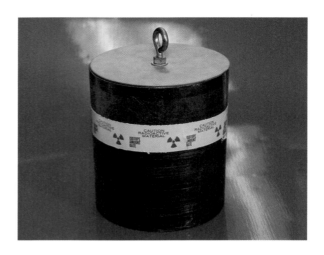

Figure 5.11
Radiation detection
instruments, including a
"pancake probe."
(a) Instrument in fitted
case.

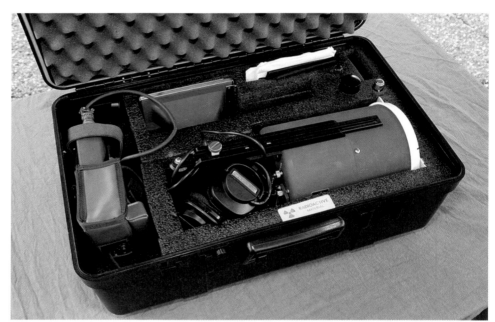

(b) Instrument removed
for use.

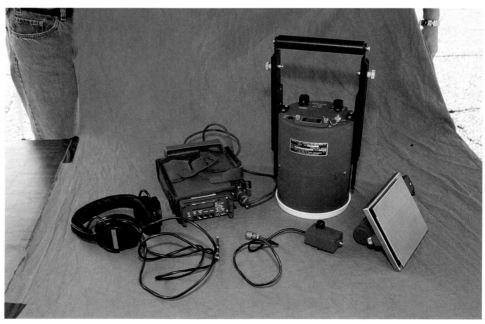

radiation received. These devices range from simple pencil-type dosimeters to more sophisticated and accurate thermoluminescent dosimeters. Pencil dosimeters have an ion chamber and give a rough estimate of the exposure to gamma rays (Figure 5.12). Thermoluminescent dosimeters use a crystal to accurately determine exposure (Figure 5.13). There are also electronic devices using newer technology that will sound an alarm when a high radiation dose rate or a particular dose is reached (Figure 5.14). Emergency personnel should wear whatever dosimetry is available when responding to any call involving explosions or unknown substances. Health physics technicians (responders who have special training in management of radiation hazards) can use the dosimetry data to estimate the whole-body exposure based upon the type of isotope involved. From this information they can determine the safe length of time for responders to work in the contaminated area. If the dose is high, then groups of responders should work in short shifts to minimize exposure. "Practical Skills: 6" discusses the use of specific radiation detection equipment.

Figure 5.12
Pencil dosimeters and calibrating device.

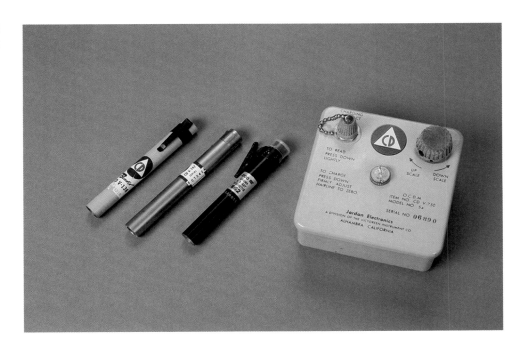

Figure 5.13
Thermoluminescent dosimeter.

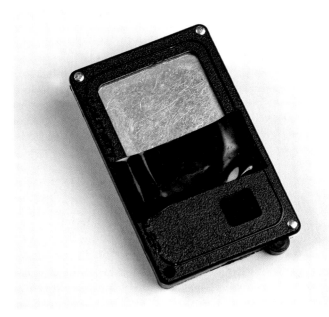

Figure 5.14
Modern alarming radiation
detection instrument
(radiation pager).

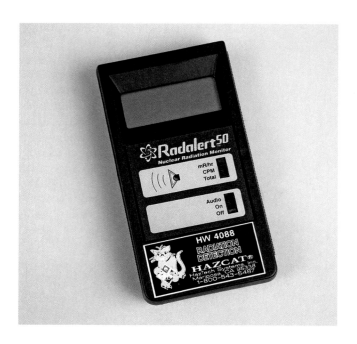

Emergency Response Issues

When responding to any explosion or report of an unusual substance, or when treating patients with an exposure to an unknown substance, you should conduct a survey for radiation contamination. This cannot be overemphasized!

RDDs using explosives present the same dangers as any other explosion (see Chapter 6), plus the dispersal of radioactive material. Depending upon the amount of explosive, the type and physical state of the radioactive materials, winds, and prevailing weather, a RDD might contaminate a large area, especially downwind from the site. Whenever possible, you should approach explosion sites from upwind. Contamination can be a long-lived event, and it can require both extensive and expensive decontamination efforts.

A crucial factor is realizing that a radiation hazard exists. Bomb squads, emergency management agencies, and hazardous materials units should have radiation detection instruments to allow trained emergency responders to test for a radiation hazard. Emergency responders must wear respiratory and protective clothing and use the four protective principles when dealing with radiation:

- *Quantity.* Remove contaminated clothes and wash contaminated material from the victim's body.

- *Time.* Work quickly to minimize time in contact with the contaminated area. Ask the walking wounded to leave the contaminated area. A health physics technician should determine how long it is safe for emergency responders to remain in the contaminated area. This may require multiple shifts working for short periods.

- *Distance.* Stay as far away from the contaminated area as possible. Radiation follows the inverse square law. If you double the distance, you have one-fourth the exposure.

- *Shielding.* Wear Level B PPE (Level C may be used if the APR is rated for radioactive material) so as not to inhale any radioactive dust. Try to maintain something dense, preferably large metal or concrete objects, between you and the source of contamination.

Once the hazards are known, you should enter the contaminated area only to save lives. You must minimize the dose of radiation you receive and prevent the spread of contamination. Female public safety personnel who are pregnant or who might want to have children should not enter the contaminated area or go near contaminated radiation victims or the decontamination area (hot and warm zones). The emergency limits of radiation exposure established by the Incident Commander should not be exceeded. The rule of thumb is that once the responder has been exposed to 50% of the allowable limit, the responder terminates his role and departs the hazard area. Emergency limits are set at 5 REM annually for occupational exposure and 25 REM for emergencies representing substantial risk to life and property (some say a limit of 10 REM) with up to 100 REM to save a life (some say a limit of 25 REM). In dangerous situations rotating personnel should help minimize radiation exposure. Older responders should be used when possible, as they are not as susceptible to radiation injury as younger responders. Any detection of neutron radiation is likely to be associated with a nuclear weapon or radiological dispersion device and requires immediate departure of all personnel from the hazard area. Notify the FBI immediately if neutron radiation is detected.

The North American Emergency Response Guide (NAERG) recommends a minimal isolation area of 25 to 50 meters (80 to 160 feet) in all directions from a radiation source (Figure 5.15). It is critical to remain upwind from radioactive material incidents and maintain an isolation distance of 1,000 to 1,500 feet if any explosives are involved. The only certain method to confirm or deny employment of radioactive materials is an appropriate radiation detection instrument used by a trained operator.

When surveying the scene, indications that radioactive materials may be involved are lead shielding or radiation placards with the yellow background and magenta propeller shape (Figure 5.16). However, it is unlikely terrorists would be so kind as to leave such clues at the scene.

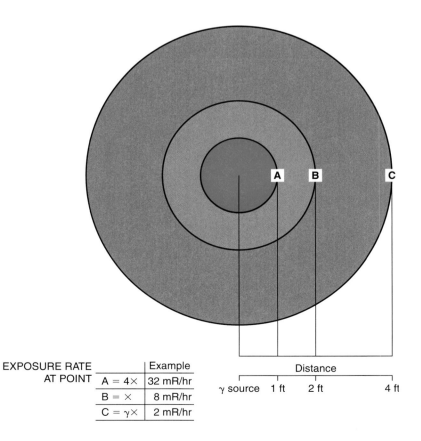

Figure 5.15
Increasing one's distance from a radioactive source is a very effective way to reduce one's radiation exposure. Moving 1 to 2 feet away decreases the dose to one-fourth. Moving to 4 feet away decreases the dose to one-sixteenth.

EXPOSURE RATE AT POINT		Example
A = 4×		32 mR/hr
B = ×		8 mR/hr
C = γ×		2 mR/hr

Figure 5.16
Examples of radiation
placards.

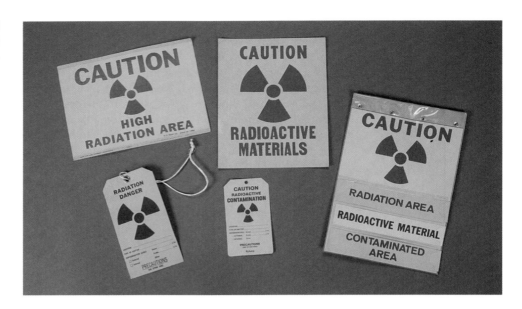

Decontamination

Trained health physics technicians, usually available from the hospital nuclear medicine unit, local HazMat response unit, or bomb squad, may be needed to direct any decontamination efforts. Uninjured, potentially contaminated persons should be segregated and detained. The removal of clothing plus a soap and water shower will remove most surface contamination. Radiation monitoring, using a "pancake probe," will be required of *all* persons and equipment to confirm that no contamination exists. Be sure to check the soles of shoes. To avoid possible ingestion of radioactive material, emergency responders and those potentially contaminated should not drink or eat until decontamination and monitoring confirms they are not themselves contaminated. Decontamination of the injured should have a high priority, not only to limit their own exposure but also to prevent further spread of contamination and cross-contamination to emergency responders. However, this should *not* prevent lifesaving medical treatment of traumatic injuries before decontamination. Early in the event, the nature of the hazard should be broadcast to all responders. The minimum protection that should be worn by responders is rated chemical protective apparel, dosimeters, and self-contained breathing apparatus (Level A or B). Level C may be used if the APR is rated for radioactive material.

Critical Actions at the Scene

If there is any indication that radioactive material is involved, you should immediately presume that all persons, vehicles, and materials within the site are contaminated. The use, by trained personnel, of instruments designed specifically to detect radioactive contamination is essential. All persons, vehicles, and materials to be removed from the incident must be tested to be determined that they are not contaminated. Scanning with a "pancake probe" can only progress at about 1 inch per second, and the entire surface area of a person, vehicle, or item must be scanned to rule out contamination. This slows the process of clearing persons from a scene.

Substantial amounts (90%) of contamination can be removed by simply removing clothing and shoes. All potentially contaminated persons should be instructed to remove their clothes immediately (blankets, paper gowns, or Doff-it kits should be provided—see "Practical Skills: 2"). Further decontamination is accomplished by washing with soap and water. Runoff water should be contained when possible but decontamination of patients should not be delayed if runoff containment is not available. Health physics personnel will need to perform tests to determine exactly what radioactive isotope is present and what is the maximum safe time allowed on scene. Individual body scans with sophisticated whole-body scanners may be required to determine the amount of radioactive material ingested.

Wound treatment can begin in the field setting. In many instances it is not possible to decontaminate wounds prior to transport. If the patient has a contaminated wound that cannot be decontaminated with gross decontamination techniques (clothing removal and flushing with water), you should dress and bandage the wound, clothe the patient in disposable paper coveralls, and wrap him in a sheet. When possible, cover open wounds prior to gross decontamination to prevent wound contamination. The process is to first cover the wound, then remove clothing and wash the body with soap and water, then remove the dressing and flush the wound (Figure 5.17).

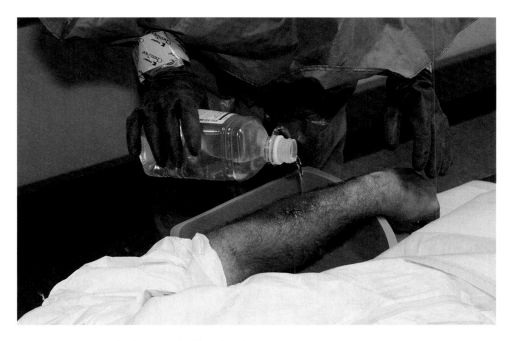

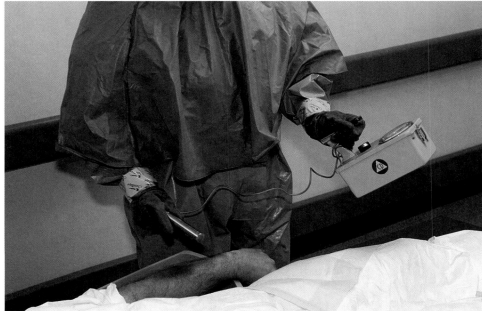

Figure 5.17
After cleaning a radiation-contaminated wound, you should recheck it with a radiation detection device to be sure the radioactive material has been removed.

Just because people are near a radioactive source for a short time or get a small amount of radioactive dust on their bodies does not mean they will get cancer. However, to limit contamination, patients should not be taken into the emergency department until they have been decontaminated. Contaminated patients should be taken to a special area for decontamination. *Life-threatening injuries or illness may require immediate treatment*; however, when possible, wound decontamination should take place first, followed by detailed or technical decontamination of other areas. Nuclear medicine personnel or health physics technicians are an invaluable resource in performing technical decontamination, which may involve debriding wounds, cutting hair, and/or mild scrubbing with detergents. Aggressive scrubbing of the skin can result in skin abrasions and internal contamination. Chemical agents and strong detergents should not be used unless recommended by a health physics technician. Hospital treatment of radiation injuries is beyond the scope of this course, but an excellent review of this is cited in the bibliography.

Box 5-1 discusses how to protect yourself in the case of a nuclear attack.

Box 5-1   Nuclear Attack—Advice to Citizens (and Off-Duty Public Safety Personnel) from the Department of Homeland Security

A nuclear blast is an explosion with intense light and heat, a damaging pressure wave, and widespread radioactive material that can contaminate the air, water, and ground surfaces for miles around. During a nuclear incident, it is important to avoid radioactive material, if possible. Although experts may predict at this time that a nuclear attack is less likely than other types of attack, terrorism by its nature is unpredictable.

If There Is a Nuclear Blast
If There Is Advanced Warning of an Attack

Take cover immediately, as far below ground as possible, though any shield or shelter will help protect you from the immediate effects of the blast and the pressure wave.

If There Is No Warning

1. Quickly assess the situation.

2. Decide whether you can get out of the area or if it would be better to go inside a building to limit the amount of radioactive material you are exposed to.

3. If you take shelter, go as far below ground as possible, close windows and doors, and turn off air conditioners, heaters, and other ventilation systems. Stay where you are, watch TV, listen to the radio, or check the Internet for official news as it becomes available.

4. To limit the amount of radiation you are exposed to, think about shielding, distance, and time.

   - **Shielding:** If you have a thick shield between yourself and the radioactive materials, more of the radiation will be absorbed by the shield and you will be exposed to less.

   - **Distance:** The farther away you are away from the blast and the fallout, the lower your exposure.

   - **Time:** Minimizing time spent exposed will also reduce your risk.

Use available information to assess the situation. If there is a significant radiation threat, health care authorities may or may not advise you to take potassium iodide. Potassium iodide is the substance added to your table salt to make it iodized. It may or may not protect your thyroid gland, which is particularly vulnerable, from

Box 5-1 *(continued)*

radioactive iodine exposure. Plan to speak with your health care provider in advance about what makes sense for your family.

Radiation Threats

A radiation threat, commonly referred to as a "dirty bomb" or "radiological dispersion device" (RDD), is the use of common explosives to spread radioactive materials over a targeted area. It is not a nuclear blast. The force of the explosion and radioactive contamination will be more localized. While the blast will be immediately obvious, the presence of radiation will not be clearly defined until trained personnel with specialized equipment are on the scene. As with any radiation, try to limit your exposure. It is important to avoid breathing radiological dust that may be released in the air.

If There Is a Radiation Threat or "Dirty Bomb"

1. If you are outside and there is an explosion or authorities warn of a radiation release nearby, cover your nose and mouth and quickly go inside a building that has not been damaged. If you are already inside, check to see if your building has been damaged. If your building is stable, stay where you are.

   Close windows and doors; turn off air conditioners, heaters, and other ventilation systems.

2. If you are inside and there is an explosion near where you are or you are warned of a radiation release inside, cover your nose and mouth and go outside immediately. Look for a building or other shelter that has not been damaged and quickly get inside.

   Once you are inside, close windows and doors; turn off air conditioners, heaters, and other ventilation systems.

3. If you think you have been exposed to radiation, take off your clothes and wash as soon as possible.

4. Stay where you are, watch TV, listen to the radio, or check the Internet for official news as it becomes available.

5. Remember: To limit the amount of radiation you are exposed to, think about shielding, distance, and time.

   - **Shielding:** If you have a thick shield between yourself and the radioactive materials, more of the radiation will be absorbed by the shield and you will be exposed to less.

   - **Distance:** The farther away you are away from the blast and the fallout, the lower your exposure.

   - **Time:** Minimizing time spent exposed will also reduce your risk.

As with any emergency, local authorities may not be able to immediately provide information on what is happening and what you should do. However, you should watch TV, listen to the radio, or check the Internet often for official news and information as it becomes available.

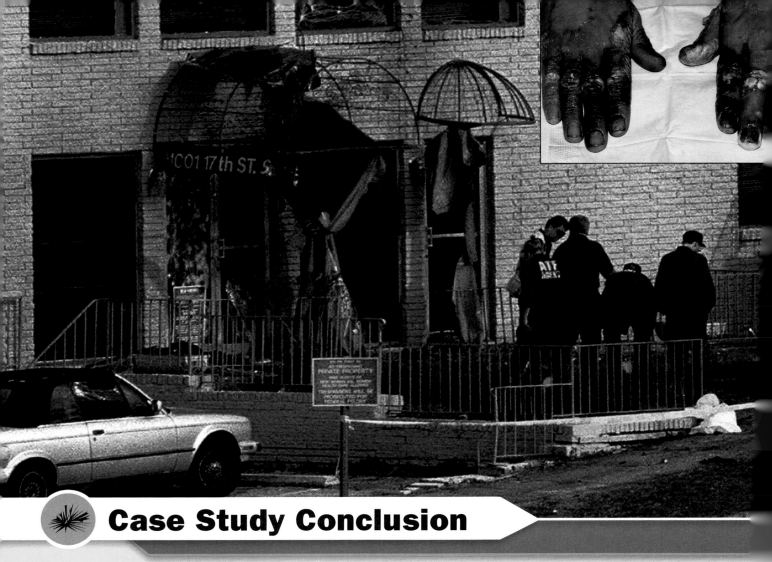

Case Study Conclusion

Abortion Clinic

Following the isolation of the passing motorist and withdrawal of emergency responders to a command post 1,500 feet away, bomb technicians enter the vicinity to check for additional explosives and to survey for toxic materials and radioactive materials. Police tactical members accompany them to search for and protect against armed assailants. The tactical officers are wearing Class III body armor over chemical suits with APRs, while bomb technicians are wearing search bomb suits over chemical suits with SCBAs. One bomb technician's radiation pager activates, and the bomb technicians and police immediately withdraw. The bomb technicians reenter the area carrying a radiation scintillation detector, which reacts and indicates gamma radiation in the area. The bomb technicians conduct a tactical retreat and notify the law enforcement incident commander.

With no persons to rescue, no fires to fight, and two indications for gamma radiation, the decision is made to extend the exclusion area, particularly downwind, and order an evacuation of those locations within it. The bomb technicians and police tactical members are surveyed with a pancake probe and no radioactive material is found. Fire service HazMat personnel then survey the motorist and his vehicle and detect gamma radiation, indicating that his vehicle and clothing are contaminated. The motorist removes and discards his clothing and is decontaminated by fire service HazMat technicians. He is resurveyed, paying

close attention to his hair and other body parts not covered with clothing during the exposure. There is now no indication of contamination. The runoff water is contained. The motorist is placed in disposable paper coveralls and taken to a local hospital equipped to handle radiation casualties, where he is held for observation and testing. His car is left in place.

A large-scale evacuation is undertaken, and the command post is moved to another location in a more distant structure with several landline telephones. The local public health department, emergency management agency, FBI, BATFE, and state radiological health department are all notified by landline telephone (to prevent the unauthorized release of information). Radio traffic is limited to encrypted traffic. The area radiation emergency response plan is activated. The scene rapidly escalates as local FBI agents arrive and assume incident command. At this point local responders move to a support role as state and federal assets flood the scene and unified command is established (NIMS—see Chapter 1). Media relations are handled in concert with federal authorities through a joint information center. The incident becomes the top news story nationwide for several days.

The radioactive contaminant is Cs-137 from a radiography source stolen from an area firm several weeks ago. It was dispersed by a pipe bomb using a hobby fuse and smokeless powder. The bomb also dispersed a gallon of butyric acid. Butyric acid has an overpowering nauseating odor that induces vomiting in most people. Although not particularly toxic, it is extremely irritating and long acting, and the nauseating odor is difficult to remove. It is prized by terrorists for its ability to render a facility unusable. It is speculated that the stolen sealed radioactive source was opened using brute force or sawed open with a metal-cutting saw. This suggests there is another location that is probably heavily contaminated, and that the persons who handled the source are probably contaminated also. There would have been significant external radiation exposure to the persons handling the source, and because it is a powder, it may have been inhaled with resultant substantial internal exposure of radiation. The use of the butyric acid was thought to be an effort to distract responders from the radioactive material and thus contaminate and injure them.

The site is isolated for 6 weeks, and the structure is decontaminated, razed, and buried in a radioactive waste landfill. The entire operation costs several million dollars, and the economic loss to the community is estimated to be even higher. The contaminated motorist received only a small external dose of radiation and has essentially normal internal body burdens of Cs-137 that should present no health hazard. His vehicle, however, is contaminated and must be disposed of in a radioactive waste landfill. The motorist is upset to find that his insurance policy does not cover such events. Investigation of the radiation exposures to bomb technicians reveals they received no appreciable radiation, as confirmed by the pencil dosimeters and thermoluminescent dosimeters they wear as a matter of routine on all calls. The local government expenditures are largely reimbursed by the Federal Emergency Management Agency (FEMA). The abortion clinic files bankruptcy because their insurance policy does not cover such events. No suspect is identified, and an intensive investigation continues, utilizing federal resources.

Emergency Department

The emergency department (ED) physician's interest is aroused by the injuries that are not explained by the patient's story. He consults the local burn center and discovers that the clinical picture suggests radiation exposure. The ED physician is concerned the patient might present a contamination hazard to the staff and has nuclear medicine personnel check him with a pancake probe. The wounds are positive for gamma radiation. The

physician institutes contamination protocols and isolates the patient. Local law enforcement is notified. The patient refuses to talk with police, who then notify the FBI. The patient's wounds are cleaned and decontaminated. Swabs of the wounds are examined by members of the nuclear medicine staff using a scintillation spectrometer that reveals the presence of Cs-137. The patient is transported, via medical helicopter and fixed-wing aircraft, to a specialized radiation treatment center. Several weeks later he succumbs to infection due to his neutropenia (low white blood cell count) and bone marrow depression induced by radiation exposure. His body is buried in a radioactive waste landfill due to its high body burden of Cs-137.

Because of his radiation contamination and refusal to talk with police, FBI agents investigating the RDD bombing at the abortion clinic obtain a search warrant for his house and barn. Members of the FBI Hazardous Materials Response Unit, local bomb technicians, Department of Energy Nuclear Emergency Search Team, and state radiological health department find the barn highly contaminated with Cs-137. The farmer's residence is lightly contaminated. The remains of the sealed radiography source and the hacksaw used to cut open the sealed source are found in the barn, along with bluish-colored Cs-137 powder scattered around a vise that was used to hold the sealed source. Cash register receipts reveal the suspect bought hobby fuse and smokeless gunpowder at a hobby shop under a false name and galvanized pipe from a local hardware store. A search of his computer reveals he has visited websites that demonstrate how to build a pipe bomb and RDD. Anti-abortion literature is found in his residence, and neighbors state he was greatly disturbed by the local abortion clinic. Cleanup of the barn and residence costs several million dollars. Most of the structures have to be razed and buried in a nuclear waste landfill.

Case Study Discussion

An explosion may be used to spread a chemical, biological, or radiological agent. All explosion scenes should be checked for chemical and radiological agents. The fact that you find one does not rule out the other. In this case the explosion dispersed both a chemical and a radiological agent. Radiation burns appear no different than flame burns and can't be diagnosed by examination. In this case the history was suspicious.

Pearls

- You cannot protect from radiation unless you detect it. Use a radiation detector to scan all suspicious substances, all explosion scenes, and suspicious scenes with mass casualties.

- Think "quantity, time, distance, and shielding" to protect from contamination and radiation. Get clothes off contaminated persons; minimize time spent in the contaminated area; stay upwind and as far away from the contaminated area as possible; try to keep dense objects (metal, concrete, terrain features) between you and the contaminated area, and wear proper personal protective equipment.

- Removal of a victim's clothing will usually greatly reduce the victim's radioactive contamination.

- Soap and water will remove most skin contamination.

- Decontaminate stable patients prior to treatment.

- Do not let your patient die of injuries while awaiting decontamination. Critical patients may require treatment before and during decontamination.

Want to Know More?

Bibliography

DeLorenzo, R.A. & R.S. Porter. *Weapons of Mass Destruction: Emergency Care,* Prentice-Hall Health, 2000.

Handling of Radiation Accidents by Emergency Personnel Course, Radiation Emergency Assistance Center/Training Site, Oak Ridge, Tennessee, 1987.

Koenig, K., et al. Medical Treatment of Radiological Casualties: Current Concepts. *Annals of Emergency Medicine* 45, no. 6 (June 2005): 643-652.

Oldfield, K.W. *Emergency Responder Training Manual for the Hazardous Materials Technician,* 2nd ed. Wiley Inter-Science, 2005.

TG 244 Med NBC Battle Book, U.S. Army, 2002.

U.S. Army, *Chemical and Biological Countermeasures Course,* 1997.

Internet Sources

Fact Sheet on Dirty Bombs
www.nrc.gov/reading-rm/doc-collections/fact-sheets/dirty-bombs.html

Military nuclear accidents
http://en.wikipedia.org/wiki/List_of_military_nuclear_accidents

Civilian nuclear accidents
http://en.wikipedia.org/wiki/List_of_civilizn_accidents

Advice to citizens from the Department of Homeland Security
www.ready.gov/america/nuclear.html
www.ready.gov/america/radiation.html

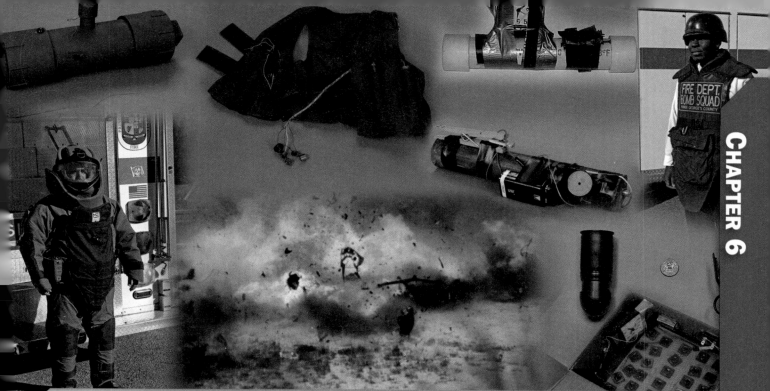

Incendiaries and Explosives

Chapter Objectives

Upon completion of this chapter you should be able to:

1. Discuss the characteristics of incendiaries and explosives and how they can be used by terrorists.
2. Discuss suicide bombers and how they operate.
3. Discuss the response to an explosion scene.
4. Discuss the dangers found at an explosion scene.
5. Generally discuss blast injuries.

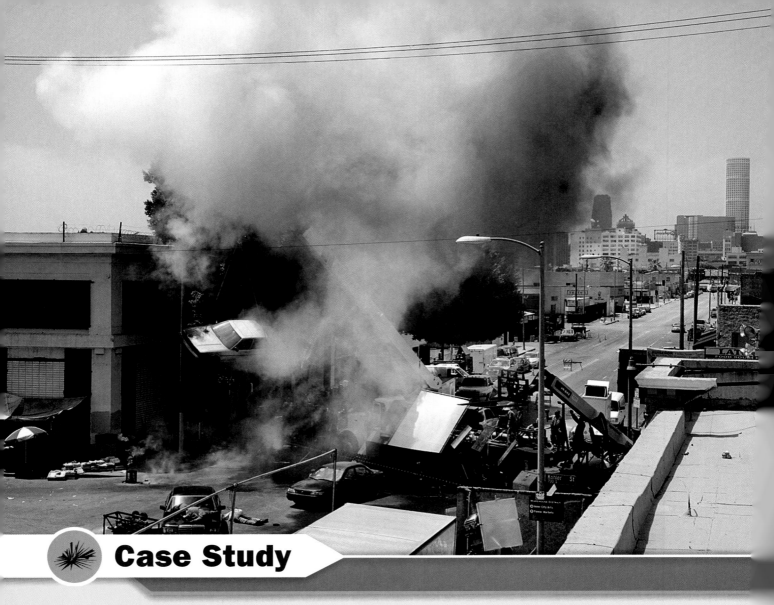

Case Study

You are returning from a call and are going by a construction site near a small but popular tavern on a busy side street. An explosion rips through the structure and rocks your vehicle. You are stunned and stop your vehicle. While engulfed in the enveloping dust cloud, you hear glass and other debris falling. As the dust begins to clear, you note several persons staggering away from the structure into the street and several persons down in front of the structure. The front wall of the structure has collapsed, and you also note a small fire inside. Nearby commercial structures have lost their front plate glass windows, and cars in front of the tavern have lost their windows.

Over your ambulance radio you hear an "Explosion" toned out for your location. You immediately confirm that an explosion has occurred; there are 10 to 15 persons down on the street in front of the tavern, and you have partial structural collapse with fire.

- What has happened? Is this a criminal act?
- Is a chemical agent or other toxic material involved?
- Are you in danger?
- What protective clothing is required?
- Where is the best location for triage and a command post?
- What resources are needed?

The Case Study will continue at the end of the chapter.

An incendiary is any device that can be used to start a fire. An explosive is any substance or device that, under the right circumstances, will explode. A bomb is an explosive device used as a weapon and fused to detonate under specified conditions. As far as terrorism is concerned, explosives almost always are bombs.

A bomb may be designed to injure and kill people, or to destroy property by explosive power alone; or it may be used as an incendiary to cause damage both by explosion and by fire. It also may be used to disperse some other toxic product, such as a radioactive material, toxic chemical, or biological agent. Incendiaries can be as simple as a kitchen match or as complicated as a remotely detonated incendiary bomb. Bombs have always been the weapon of choice of terrorists because they are cheap, easy to make, and easy to conceal. Used in crowded places, bombs cause significant loss of life and gruesome disfiguring injuries. Explosions often tear bodies apart so badly that only DNA testing can identify them. Some explosions are so powerful that many bodies are disintegrated and no parts are found to identify. During wartime this accounts for most of the soldiers listed as "missing in action." Bomb attacks get intense news coverage and are very successful in causing widespread terror.

Incendiaries

Molotov Cocktails

For terrorists, the "Molotov cocktail" is the most common incendiary. It comes in a variety of configurations, the most common being a flammable liquid in a glass bottle with a wick of cloth or paper (Figure 6.1). When the bottle is inverted, the wick becomes saturated with the flammable liquid, usually gasoline. The wick is then lit and the device hand-thrown. Upon impact the bottle shatters, spraying the area with flammable liquid and vapor, which ignites from the burning wick. Some variations include adding motor oil, wax, glycerin, soap powders, or other thickeners to the gasoline. This can make the ensuing fire hotter and of greater duration, as well as enable the burning liquid to adhere to surfaces.

A self-igniting Molotov cocktail can be assembled by mixing gasoline with sulfuric acid in a glass container. This mixture is a very unstable and very hazardous to make. The container is wrapped in paper, typically newspaper, that has been soaked in a mixture of sugar and potassium. Upon impact the container shatters, allowing the mixture of sugar and sulfuric acid to ignite and, with the potassium chlorate as an oxidizer, burn at a high temperature.

Molotov cocktails can be easily set as booby traps. When found, they should not be disturbed except by trained personnel.

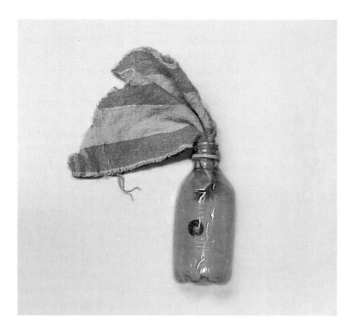

Figure 6.1
Example of a simple Molotov cocktail.

Injuries from Incendiaries

Most injuries from incendiaries are thermal burns. In rare circumstances there can be chemical burns from exposure to solvents, acids, or other chemicals used in the devices. Vigorous irrigation to remove caustic chemical agents may be needed, particularly in the case of bottle bombs (see page 125). Otherwise, standard burn treatment is indicated. Remember: incendiary devices may produce toxic fumes and gases, such as acid halogen gases, phosgene, and carbon monoxide (see Chapter 2). The emergency responder should use protective gear and an SCBA or APR (Level B or C) until it is known there are no toxic gases present.

Explosives (Bombs)

Bombs are the weapon of choice for terrorists because explosive materials are easy to acquire (purchase or steal), and bombs are simple to assemble, transport, and conceal. Bombs are reliable and anonymous and can be delivered through the mail or a package service. Bombs can be detonated remotely using sophisticated electronics or detonated personally by suicide bombers. Improvised explosive devices (IEDs) are homemade bombs, ranging from simple pipe bombs to vehicles loaded with explosives. Also, just because they are not made by the military does not mean they are simple or ineffective. Vehicle-borne IEDs (VBIEDs), commonly called car bombs or truck bombs, are most commonly used to attack structures and have been employed successfully worldwide. A bomb may serve to disperse other agents, such as radioactive material, biological agents, or chemical agents. According to the FBI Bomb Data Center, there are more than 2,000 bombings in the United States annually. These bombings result in an average of 70 fatalities per year. An alarming trend is that the lethality of bombings is increasing even though the overall number of bombings has decreased. Terrorists are becoming more brutal, more cunning, and more focused on casualties than on property damage. When responding to an explosion, you must consider the possibility of multiple bombs coupled with secondary devices and/or armed assailants targeting responders.

Basic Characteristics of Explosives

Explosives are materials that combust at an extremely fast rate to form a pressure-shock wave. Explosives can be classified into two groups: low explosives, with pressure waves traveling at less than 3,300 feet per second (fps), and high explosives, with transonic shock waves (>3,300 fps).

The faster the detonation shock wave, the more powerful the explosion. Low explosives, such as gunpowder, have to be confined so that the gases can build up enough pressure to shatter the container, thus producing the explosion. The damage from low explosives is from the thermal event (fireball and hot gases) and from fragments (shrapnel) produced by the explosion. High explosives need no container and produce a powerful transonic shock wave that can cause injury along with the thermal event and shrapnel.

The blast pressure wave, or shock wave, is a two-phase phenomenon in which the short (a few milliseconds), but intense, transonic blast from the high explosive washes over the surrounding environment with a positive-pressure wave, followed by a relatively negative-pressure wave of longer duration (Figure 6.2). The blast wave pushes air ahead of it, causing blast winds far more powerful than any hurricane. A blast wave of 100 pounds per square inch (psi) would produce a wind of over 1,500 miles per hour (and kill every human exposed to it). Solid objects may reflect blast waves, causing unusual damage and injury patterns.

Fragmentation or shrapnel comes in the form of primary fragments from the container and secondary fragments from nearby objects that are disrupted. Glass is deadly in the explosive environment, as it easily shatters into daggerlike fragments that travel some distance and can deeply penetrate the human body. Glass may also be shattered some distance away from the explosion site and fall from

Figure 6.2
The blast pressure wave reaches fatal levels in a few millionths of a second.

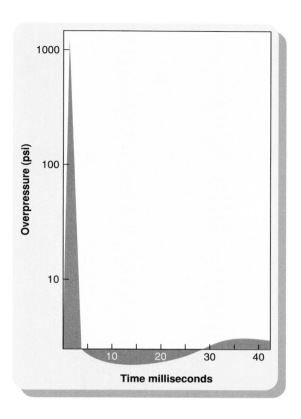

Figure 6.3
Injuries from explosions come not just from the pressure wave and collapsing structures, but also from both the primary fragments of the bomb itself and the secondary fragments (broken glass and other debris) that are propelled at extremely high velocities by the pressure wave.

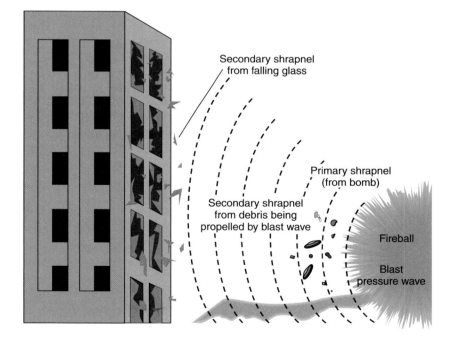

windows onto persons standing underneath (Figure 6.3). People hearing an explosion may run to a window to look out, just in time to be blinded by shattering glass from the blast wave. Fragment speeds may exceed 14,000 feet per second in the detonation of high explosives; the typical high-velocity rifle bullet has a velocity of less than 3,500 feet per second.

Another phenomenon that accompanies explosion is the thermal event, which may be observed as a fireball (Figure 6.4). Depending upon the type of explosive, the heat liberated may cause radiant heat intense enough to burn nearby persons

Figure 6.4
The heat of the explosion
fireball can cause thermal
burns and start fires.

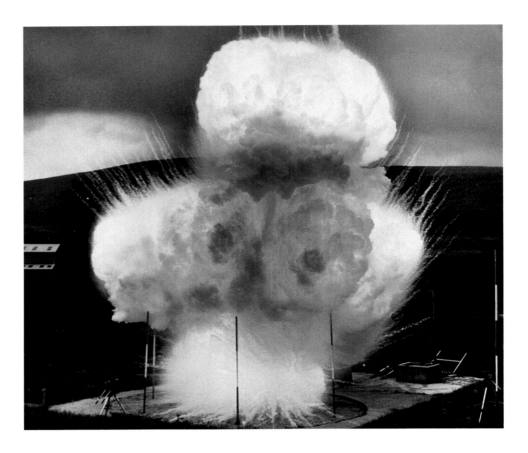

Figure 6.4
The heat of the explosion fireball can cause thermal burns and start fires.

or start fires. Ground shocks come from the shock wave interacting with the ground and nearby structures, and may cause failure of walls and damage the structural integrity of buildings.

Explosions are the ultrarapid oxidation of a fuel, and many toxic gases are produced as by-products. Explosions in confined spaces leave toxic carbon monoxide, carbon dioxide, and nitrogen oxides, along with a large quantity of soot and some acidic gases. Many explosives are toxic themselves. Persons covered in dust, soot, and debris following an explosion should be decontaminated by disrobing and showering with soap and water.

These factors should be remembered when effecting entry into any confined space following an explosion. Confined spaces present the dangers of lack of oxygen, presence of toxic gases, and danger of structure collapse. Chemical protective clothing and respiratory protection in the form of an SCBA (Level A or B) is required, along with the other precepts for entry into a confined space (see Chapter 7).

Types of Explosives

Explosives may also be classified as primary, secondary, and blasting agents, depending on their ease of detonation. Primary explosives are very sensitive to fire or impact and shock, while secondary explosives are less sensitive to such a stimulus. Examples of primary explosives are nitroglycerin or lead styphnate, both of which explode easily from impact, friction, or flame. More stable explosives, such as desensitized nitroglycerin in dynamite (Figure 6.5), trinitrotoluene or TNT, and cyclotrimethylenetrinitramine (RDX), require a primary explosive to detonate, usually in the form of a blasting cap (Figure 6.6). Blasting agents, such as ammonium nitrate–fuel oil (ANFO) mixtures are very insensitive; exploding them usually requires a primary explosive in the form of a blasting cap that detonates a secondary explosive in the form of a booster, such as pentaerythritetetranitrate (PETN). Just because blasting agents are difficult to detonate does not mean they aren't high explosives, capable of causing severe damage. The World Trade Center bomb

Figure 6.5
Sticks of dynamite.

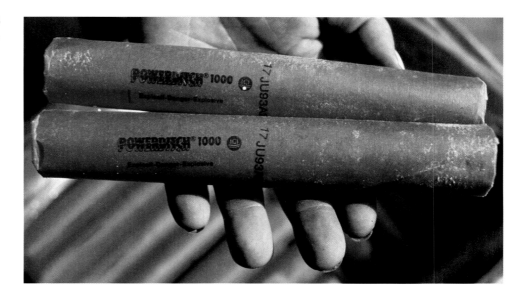

Figure 6.6
(a) Examples of blasting caps.

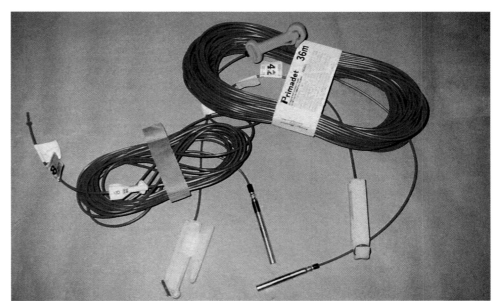

(b) A hand injury from holding a blasting cap that exploded.

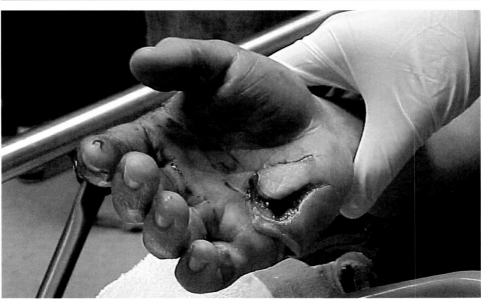

Figure 6.7
An example of the power of a vehicle-borne improvised explosive device (VBIED) made from ammonium nitrate and fuel oil.

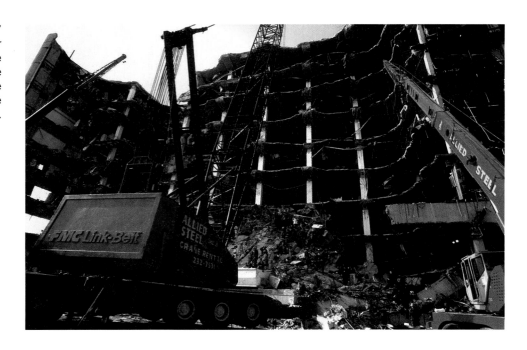

Figure 6.8
Vehicles can carry enough explosives to destroy large structures. Notice the distances the ATF recommends for evacuation.

ATF	VEHICLE DESCRIPTION	MAXIMUM EXPLOSIVES CAPACITY	LETHAL AIR BLAST RANGE	MINIMUM EVACUATION DISTANCE	FALLING GLASS HAZARD
	COMPACT SEDAN	500 Pounds 227 Kilos (*In Trunk*)	100 Feet 30 Meters	1,500 Feet 457 Meters	1,250 Feet 381 Meters
	FULL SIZE SEDAN	1,000 Pounds 455 Kilos (*In Trunk*)	125 Feet 38 Meters	1,750 Feet 534 Meters	1,750 Feet 534 Meters
	PASSENGER VAN OR CARGO VAN	4,000 Pounds 1,818 Kilos	200 Feet 61 Meters	2,750 Feet 838 Meters	2,750 Feet 838 Meters
	SMALL BOX VAN (*14 FT BOX*)	10,000 Pounds 4,545 Kilos	300 Feet 91 Meters	3,750 Feet 1,143 Meters	3,750 Feet 1,143 Meters
	BOX VAN OR WATER/FUEL TRUCK	30,000 Pounds 13,636 Kilos	450 Feet 137 Meters	6,500 Feet 1,982 Meters	6,500 Feet 1,982 Meters
	SEMI-TRAILER	60,000 Pounds 27,273 Kilos	600 Feet 183 Meters	7,000 Feet 2,134 Meters	7,000 Feet 2,134 Meters

in 1993 (1,200 pounds of urea nitrate) and the Oklahoma City bomb in 1995 (4,800 pounds of ammonium nitrate fertilizer) were nitrate-based blasting agents sensitized with other agents. Both did extensive property damage and created great loss of life (Figure 6.7). These bombs are examples of vehicle bombs, which can involve a large quantity of explosives (Figure 6.8). Remember, even though some explosives are fairly stable, *all* explosives can be detonated when exposed to fire.

Types of Bombs
Bottle Bombs
Bottle bombs do not appear at first glance to be hazardous devices. Usually they are bottles, plastic or glass, filled with a caustic liquid and aluminum foil (Figure 6.9). Bottle bombs self-detonate after the components are added, but the detonation occurs at unpredictable times. Bottle bombs may explode seconds, minutes, or

Figure 6.9
An example of an
exploded bottle bomb.

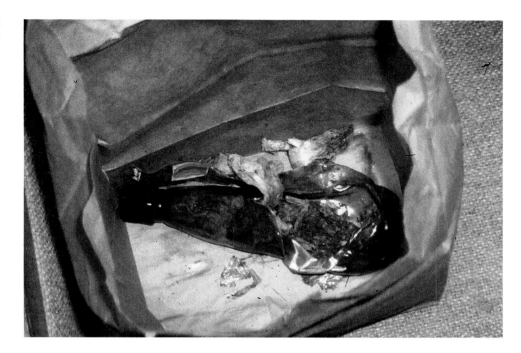

Figure 6.9
An example of an
exploded bottle bomb.

hours after they are made, depending upon the concentration of the corrosive material, the container strength, and the amount of reactants. The explosion of a bottle bomb made using an 8-ounce glass soft drink bottle can blow glass fragments more than 100 feet. Bottle bombs are not used just by terrorists; some inquisitive young people (almost always males) experiment with bottle bombs and may use them for destructive purposes.

Items commonly used to produce bottle bombs include liquids such as drain cleaner, hydrochloric acid, and lye mixed with aluminum foil as the metal reactant. Some more inventive experimenters have used isopropyl alcohol and HTH (high-test hypochlorite). The chemical reaction between these items generates heat and hydrogen gas, which is explosive. When the pressure reaches a certain point, the container will explode, spraying hot corrosive liquid, fragments, and hot aluminum foil fragments onto anything close by. A very few devices may reach the ignition temperature of hydrogen and generate a fireball, thus becoming an incendiary. High school chemistry textbooks and many Internet sites demonstrate how to make the chemical reaction that powers these devices. Be wary of any container that has a "muddy" looking liquid or aluminum foil within it. Any residue and fragments from such an explosion are usually covered in corrosive liquid.

Pipe Bombs

Pipe bombs are usually constructed of metal or plastic pipe and are filled with gunpowder (Figure 6.10). These are the most common homemade bombs, as they

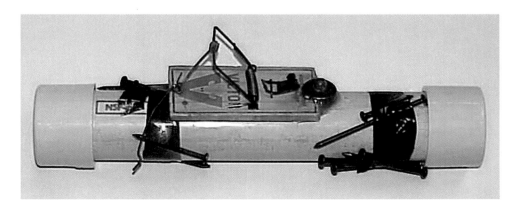

Figure 6-10
An example of a simple
pipe bomb.

Figure 6.11
An example of a letter
bomb.

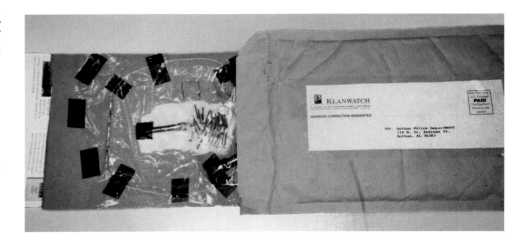

are easily made and simple to put in place and conceal. Metal pipe bombs using gunpowder produce a substantial amount of fragments and may contain additional shrapnel in the form of nails, screws, or wire. Simple burning fuses are used to detonate most pipe bombs. Pipe bombs are usually designed to attack people, because their ability to damage structures is limited unless a high explosive is substituted for gunpowder.

Letter, Package, and Briefcase Bombs

A letter bomb usually weighs less than a pound and can be mailed in a manila envelope (Figure 6.11). A package or briefcase bomb is a bomb built into a container with a size limitation of about 50 pounds total weight (Figure 6.12). These devices can be placed and set with a timer or antidisturbance booby trap, or simply sent through the mail or a package delivery service (Figure 6.13).

Vehicle-Borne Improvised Explosive Devices (VBIEDs)

Vehicle bombs have been used in the Middle East for many years and are very common there now, but they were not observed in the United States until the World Trade Center bombing in 1993.

Figure 6.12
(a) An example of a
package bomb.

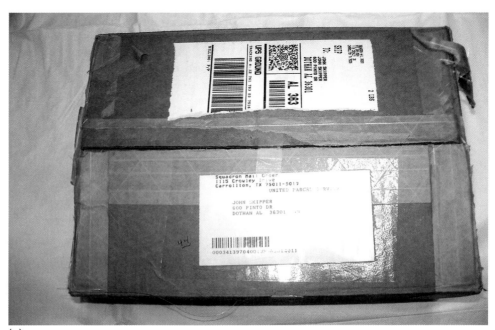

(a)

Figure 6.12 (*Continued*) (b) The inside of a package bomb.

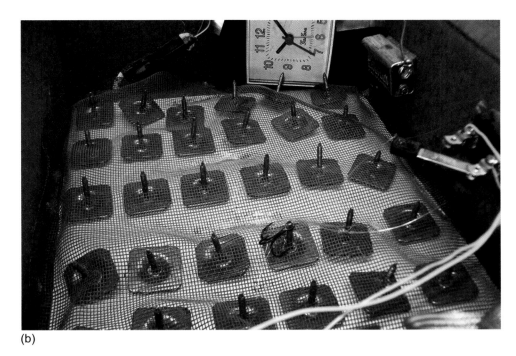

(b)

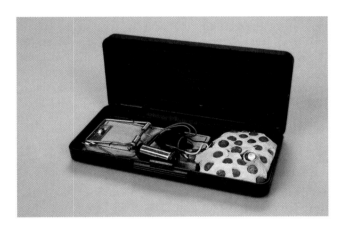

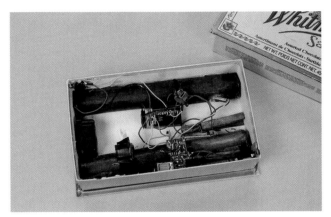

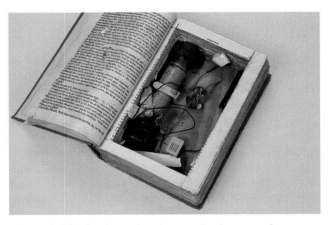

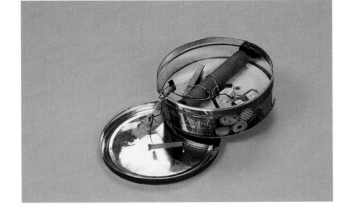

Figure 6.13 Package bombs can be in many forms.

In 1983, U.S. Marines were acting as peacekeepers in Beirut, Lebanon. At 6:17 a.m. a Mercedes truck identical to those used to deliver cargo from the Beirut airport drove up to the door of the Marine barracks and exploded. The truck was a specially constructed suicide VBIED containing a "shaped charge" of 300 kilograms (660 pounds) of hexogene with a booster of PETN. The bomb had a shape and composition that were designed to have greater effect on the building, and it was very successful. The building was demolished, killing 241 Marines and wounding another 146. The bomb used against the World Trade Center in February of 1993 was an exact copy of the Beirut bomb.

In the current climate of terrorism, the utilization of vehicles to deliver improvised bombs or other weapons of mass destruction is an issue. Vehicle bombs were used to attack the Murrah Federal Building in Oklahoma City, the World Trade Center, the U.S. Marine barracks in Beirut, and several U.S. embassies. As of this writing, car bombs are a daily occurrence in Iraq. The U.S. Department of Transportation Federal Motor Carrier Safety Administration states there are more than 230 million vehicles on U.S. highways, nearly 8 million of which are large trucks. The typical passenger car can be loaded with more than 500 pounds of explosives, and a large truck can hold up to 60,000 pounds of explosives. Vehicles may also be used by terrorists in other ways than for bombing attacks. A vehicle may be used to release flammable or toxic materials. Sometimes explosives are also used to enhance the dispersion of these toxic materials.

Potential targets include high-occupancy sites such as hospitals, shopping malls, government buildings, stadiums, theaters, schools, arenas, and transportation facilities. Some other potential targets might include hazardous materials storage sites or infrastructure such as pipelines, bulk petroleum storage facilities, water storage and purification sites, bridges, and communications facilities.

Some red flags for a possible vehicle bomb (VBIED) terrorist attack:

- Vehicles with explosives or anhydrous ammonia placards out of truck routes or in densely occupied areas.
- Vehicles with hazardous materials placards at a densely occupied location.
- Vehicles with cylinders of poison gas, such as hydrogen sulfide, chlorine, or other toxic gases, in nonindustrial settings.
- Rental vehicles with hazardous materials placards.
- Any unattended vehicle marked with explosives placards.

Suicide Bombers

A suicide bombing is a suicidal attack a using a bomb carried, worn, or, in the case of VBIED, driven by a person who is willing to kill himself or herself in order to kill others. Usually this is to further a cause. Some people call these "homicide bombers," but *all* bombers who intend to take human life are homicide bombers, so *suicide bomber* is a better term. The suicide bomber supposedly is making a political, ideological, or religious statement in killing members of what is considered the enemy. The fact that the bomber is killed negates the need for an escape plan and simplifies the operation. The resolve of the suicide bomber comes from indoctrination and reinforcement of the martyr complex. The suicide bomber can be used for a specific target or in a random attack. There is little consideration for bystanders, and in fact, the more carnage, the broader the media coverage and the more terror produced in the target population. Fanatical groups that do not have the resources to perform conventional attacks are more likely to use this brutal method of attack.

The suicide bomber is usually given the device and briefly trained in its use shortly before employment. The device will use a battery with a push button or

Figure 6.14
An example of a suicide bomb vest.

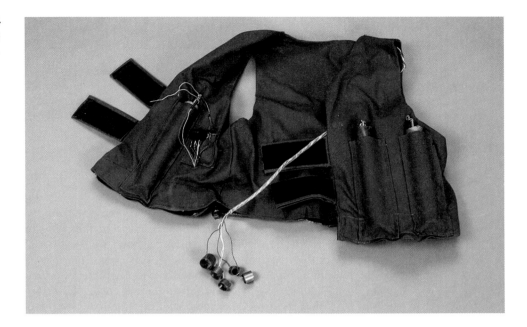

toggle switch to detonate blasting caps that are attached to the explosives. Members of the delivery team will survey the location and may use photographs or drawings to familiarize the bomber with the location. Some groups even do practice runs. In some cases a "minder" may be deployed to watch and confirm that the bomber completes his or her mission. Occasionally the minder will carry a simple radio remote control device to remotely detonate the explosive.

Suicide bombs are limited in size and complexity because most are worn or carried (Figure 6.14). However, more and more suicide bombers are using car bombs. These are much more powerful and can be more complex, although most remain simple devices. Normally the suicide bomber will be dressed to fit the setting, and *no single profile fits suicide bombers.* This eliminates the use of profiles as a reliable detection method. Good camouflage, such as wearing a uniform or being disguised as a pregnant female, is often used. Some suicide bombers use a vest worn over clothing to conceal or contain the explosives. The bomber may also wear loose or baggy clothing over the device to conceal it. The worn device may be detectable under the clothing as bulges, or the outer layer of clothing may be inappropriate, such as a coat or vest worn in warm weather. The worn device is normally limited to 10 to 30 pounds of explosive. The explosives in worn IEDs range from sophisticated high explosives using augmented shrapnel such as nails or screws, to homemade unstable explosives contained in pipe bombs. Backpacks and hand-carried devices such as laptop computers and radios or similar items can be used to hide bombs and would escape cursory inspection. For this reason, when you respond to any terrorist attack, you should not allow victims to carry out of the scene any personal items large enough to conceal a bomb or other dispersal device.

One problem facing responders to a suicide bombing is that the bomber or accomplices may have hidden other devices at the scene or there may be a follow-up bomber. The only effective method to protect a location from vehicle bombs is to exclude vehicles from within at least 300 feet of the target area.

Anytime you suspect a person of having a bomb on his or her person, you should immediately leave the area and notify law enforcement. Taking such a person into custody is very dangerous, because if the person is conscious and able, he or she will try to detonate the device. For this reason some law enforcement personnel have been instructed to shoot the suspected bomber in the head. This is a desperate measure and can lead to the shooting of an innocent person. The killing of a person mistakenly suspected of being a suicide bomber after the London subway attacks in 2005 is an example of the danger of this policy.

The 2002 bombing on the Indonesian island of Bali is an example of a suicide bombing followed by an ambush of rescuers. The initial bomb was in a backpack carried by a suicide bomber who detonated it in a crowded hotel bar. Later, as victims, hotel occupants, and would-be rescuers gathered outside the hotel, a much larger secondary device (in a van parked outside the hotel) was detonated, killing a majority of the 202 victims (another 209 were injured).

Responding to Explosions

Responder safety is paramount. Use extreme caution in approaching the site of any explosion. Unless immediate rescue and lifesaving patient care is required, do not enter the explosion area. Retreat outside the blast damage area. A good indicator of the blast damage area is broken glass. Survey the scene and look for things that might pose a danger. Look for people, vehicles, packages, or other suspicious activity. Make sure your operations area is secure. *Also make sure your ambulances are secure.* There have been instances of ambulances being stolen and used to make vehicle bombs. When doing your scene size-up, be alert for unusual factors, such as:

- Any prior threats to the location
- Any unusual item, containers, or vehicles that look abandoned or out of place
- Unusual odors
- Unusual tanks, attachments to utility poles, or items near sensitive areas such as ventilation systems or hazardous materials storage areas
- Packages with wires attached or protruding from the package
- Obvious bombs

The commitment of responders to scenes involving explosions should be based on a risk–benefit ratio. If there is no fire and no persons to be rescued, then do not enter the scene before the bomb squad clears the scene of secondary devices and partially consumed explosives. Know how to contact your local bomb squad and what their response time will be.

Explosion scenes are not secure until bomb squad members have thoroughly assessed them for additional bombs, unconsumed explosives, chemical devices, biological agents, and radioactive materials. Remember, secondary devices may be present or there may be assailants waiting in ambush.

The use of bomb threats is a common ploy to divert public safety resources while another location is attacked. A bank can be robbed while public safety personnel are dealing with a bomb threat at a school. Bombs can also be used as a diversion for the same reason.

The size of the bomb will affect the size of the evacuation area and subsequent damage should detonation occur. The minimum evacuation area for a small bomb is 300 feet, but 1,000 to 1,500 feet is preferred (Figure 6.15).

Structures with a dense occupancy, such as a shopping mall or stadium, structures that have hazardous materials present, or those with a fixed population such as a hospital or nursing home, present a special hazard. It may not be feasible to evacuate a hospital or nursing home following a bomb threat. Facilities that use or store hazardous materials may contain toxic agents that could be released by an explosion. Structures with large expanses of glass are also very dangerous, as the glass is likely to fragment and fall during an explosion.

Just as with radiation, three techniques are used to minimize potential injury from explosives. These are Time, Distance, and Shielding. If you are called to a bombing site, you should spend a minimum amount of time in the danger area (hot zone), which is the area usually within 1,000 feet of the device or blast site.

Figure 6.15
Trash can and
decontamination tent
viewed from 10, 100, 300,
and 1,000 feet.

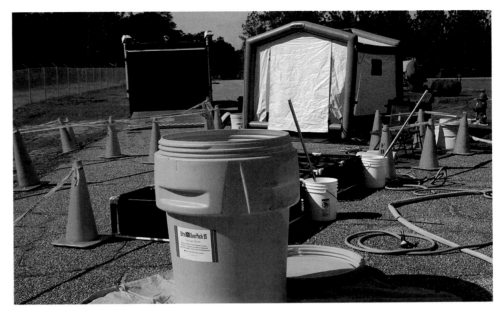

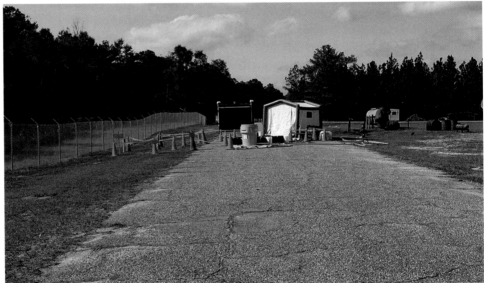

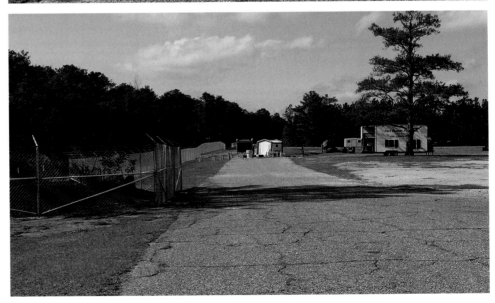

Figure 6-15 (*Continued*)

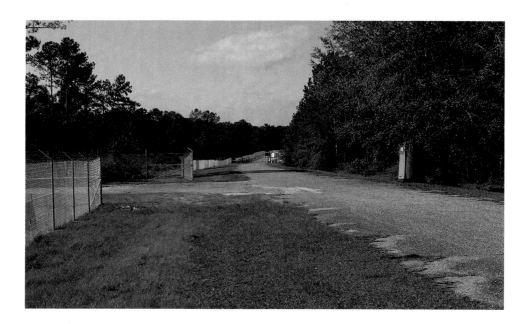

Try to stay outside this area. Use shielding, which includes keeping terrain features or structures between you and the danger area, while staying upwind and uphill and away from any glass that could fall on you if broken. Shielding also includes protective clothing and respiratory protection.

The rule of Time, Distance, and Shielding applies with this admonition: If you can see the device, you are too close; if you can see the bomb technician, you are too close; if you can see the structure, you are too close. You should stage vehicles and personnel out of sight of the scene and away from any glass, particularly overhead glass, that might fall onto personnel and vehicles.

Firefighting should be accomplished with remote appliances such as the water cannon (also called deck gun) of the fire truck. If there are no fires to fight, the fire service should remain out of the blast zone. Treat all explosions as a criminal act until proven otherwise. All bomb scenes are crime scenes and should be treated as such (see Chapter 1).

Scene Survey and Patient Rescue

The first emergency responders on-scene should do a scene survey and ascertain the scope of the incident. If help is needed, it should be requested before engaging in rescue activities. During your survey of the scene, if you discover a bomb or something you believe to be a bomb, immediately leave the area and notify Incident Command. The bomb should not be moved or tampered with in any manner, and nothing should be placed upon it.

The number of casualties may overwhelm initial responders, and help should be requested before you begin treating the patients. Many of the ambulatory injured will immediately approach any emergency responder, so having a safe triage area already set up is critical. A triage area should be established outside the blast zone. The blast zone is considered the area in which windows are broken. If possible, place the triage area out of direct line of sight of the incident. Identify the best area for a triage area and/or a command post, but do not use it. It is safer to pick an area that is not the obvious choice for triage or command. The terrorists may have planned a secondary attack on the most obvious place for triage. They may plant secondary explosive devices there or make an armed attack on that area. Security is critical; make certain you have a secure scene and a secure triage area.

Immediately perform "bullhorn triage." Take a bullhorn (loudspeaker) and announce that all patients who can walk are to follow a designated emergency responder to a safe place (the triage area). Identify those who are still alive prior to entry if possible. Again use the bullhorn to ask those who can't walk to raise their hands. This helps identify those persons who are still conscious but unable to stand. The best practice is to confirm that no chemical, biological or radiological hazards exist before entering the hot zone. However, if multiple people are injured and HazMat is not immediately available, you will be compelled to rescue the injured patients. If it is necessary to enter the blast zone to save lives, do so in Level B or C PPE. Minimize the number of personnel entering the blast area even if it appears safe to enter. Rapidly rescue patients who are too injured to walk using "load and go" tactics with expedient spinal motion–restriction techniques. The Israelis, from their vast experience with bombings, have found that the danger of a second bomb or an ambush is far more likely than a chemical or radiological attack and so they do no treatment or decontamination on-scene but instead immediately remove all living patients. They do not perform evaluation or treatment until the patient is in the ambulance. You and your medical director should decide ahead of time how your service will respond to a bombing scene with multiple injuries.

Blast Injuries

Blast injuries to victims are classified as primary, secondary, or tertiary (Figure 6.16).

Primary Blast Injuries

Primary injuries are from both the pressure wave and the fireball from the explosion. The fireball from the explosion usually causes flash burns of exposed skin but may also ignite clothing causing deeper more extensive burns. The pressure wave almost exclusively affects air-containing (hollow) organs. This is due to the

Figure 6.16
Explosions can cause injury by the primary blast wave and heat (primary injury), by the shrapnel thrown by the blast (secondary injury), or by the blast victim being thrown against a fixed object (tertiary injury).

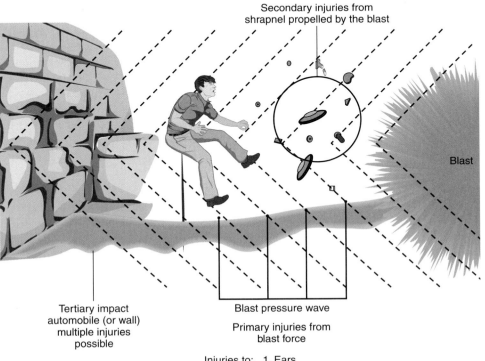

Secondary injuries from shrapnel propelled by the blast

Blast

Tertiary impact automobile (or wall) multiple injuries possible

Blast pressure wave

Primary injuries from blast force

Injuries to: 1. Ears
2. Lungs
3. G. I. Tract

Table 6.1	Effects of Blast Pressure Wave
Blast Pressure Wave in psi	**Effects**
0.5 to 1.0 psi	Glass breaks.
Greater than 1.0 psi	People are blown to the ground.
1.0 to 2.0 psi	Wood siding is damaged.
Greater than 2.0 to 3.0 psi	Nonreinforced cinder block walls collapse.
Greater than 5.0 psi	Eardrums are ruptured.
Greater than 15 psi	Lung injuries begin.
Greater than 35 psi	Fatal injuries begin.
Greater than 50 psi	50% fatality rate of those exposed.
Greater than 65 psi	99% fatality rate of those exposed.

interface effect: when the pressure wave passes from one type of medium to a different type of medium, the interface point receives significant damage. In the human body, these areas include eardrums, lungs, and intestines. The longer the duration and intensity of the pressure wave, the greater the injury. When the pressure wave exceeds 50 pounds per square inch (psi) about 50% of the victims will die (LD50) (Table 6.1).

Explosions within structures generate complex pulse waves with multiple peaks. Repetitive pulses cause significantly more damage and injury. Body orientation also plays a significant role in the seriousness of the injury. Obviously the transonic pressure wave from high explosives is more likely to cause damage to internal organs than a small pipe bomb made from gunpowder. Always suspect lung injuries in a blast victim. Primary blast injuries are often immediately fatal.

Secondary Blast Injuries

Secondary injuries are caused by shrapnel thrown by the blast. Shrapnel is common in both high and low explosives, but the higher the velocity of the shrapnel the more likely it is to cause serious injury. The shrapnel itself is classified as primary and secondary. Primary shrapnel is from the explosion itself and tends to impact at high velocity (up to 14,000 fps). Secondary shrapnel is from broken glass or falling debris from the blast pressure wave. While such shrapnel (especially glass) may be just as deadly, it tends to travel at a lower velocity. The injuries produced from missile impacts may appear superficial, small pieces of shrapnel, particularly projected or falling glass can penetrate deeply into internal organs. Law enforcement tactical teams routinely undertake explosive breaching. This process uses an explosive charge to cut through or deform doors, windows, walls or other barriers to allow entry into structures. There is some risk for overpressure injuries if a person is very close to the explosion site, but the more common risk is injury from debris projected from the explosion itself in the form of shrapnel.

Tertiary Blast Injuries

Tertiary injuries are caused when the victim's body is thrown against a solid surface such as a wall or a tree. Essentially the victim becomes secondary shrapnel. These injuries are much the same as those seen after a person is ejected from an automobile during a high-speed collision. Commonly seen are broken bones, traumatic amputations, and head/brain injuries. Because of their transonic pressure wave, high explosives frequently cause tertiary injuries (Figure 6.17).

Other Injuries

If the explosion is confined in a structure or other confined space then significant amounts of toxic combustion products may also be present. Patients trapped in these areas may have poisoning from inhalation of these toxic gases. When there is structural collapse you may have patients with crush injuries. Persons with crush

Figure 6-17
A tertiary injury from being
blown against a wall by an
explosion.
Photo: Roy Alson, MD.

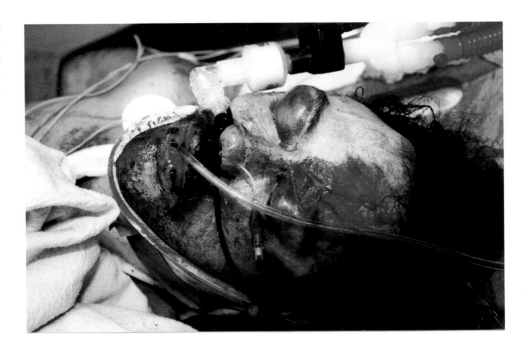

Figure 6-17
A tertiary injury from being blown against a wall by an explosion.
Photo: Roy Alson, MD.

injuries may require large amounts of IV fluids. If possible, give IV fluid and sodium bicarbonate before extricating the patient. Contact Medical Direction early for these patients.

Any patient injured in an explosion should have a rapid trauma survey as taught in the International Trauma Life Support Course. This is a rapid head-to-toes survey for life-threatening injuries.

Significant findings that indicate the potential for severe injury include:

- A decreased level of consciousness (LOC) and/or hearing loss.
- Bleeding or penetrating injuries to the head, face, neck, chest, pelvis, or abdomen.
- Burns or crush injuries.

Box 6-1 discusses what to do if you are caught in an explosion.

Box 6-1   Advice for the Individual (or Off-Duty Public Service Personnel) from the Department of Homeland Security

If You Are Caught in an Explosion
- Take shelter against your desk or a study table.
- Exit the building as soon as possible.
- Do not use elevators.
- Check for fire and other hazards.
- Take your emergency supply kit if time allows.

If There Is a Fire
- Exit the building as soon as possible.
- Crawl low if there is smoke.
- Use a wet cloth, if possible, to cover your nose and mouth.
- Use the back of your hand to feel the upper, lower, and middle parts of closed doors.
- If the door is not hot, brace yourself against it and open slowly.
- If the door is hot, do not open it. Look for another way out.
- Do not use elevators.

Box 6-1   (*Continued*)

- If you catch fire, do not run. Stop, drop, and roll to put out the fire.
- If you are at home, go to a previously designated meeting place.
- Account for your family members and carefully supervise small children.
- Never go back into a burning building.

If You Are Trapped in Debris

- If possible, use a flashlight to signal your location to rescuers.
- Avoid unnecessary movement so that you don't kick up dust.
- Cover your nose and mouth with anything you have on hand. (Dense-weave cotton material can act as a good filter. Try to breath through the material.)
- Tap on a pipe or wall so that rescuers can hear where you are.
- If possible, use a whistle to signal rescuers.
- Shout only as a last resort. Shouting can cause you to inhale dangerous amounts of dust.

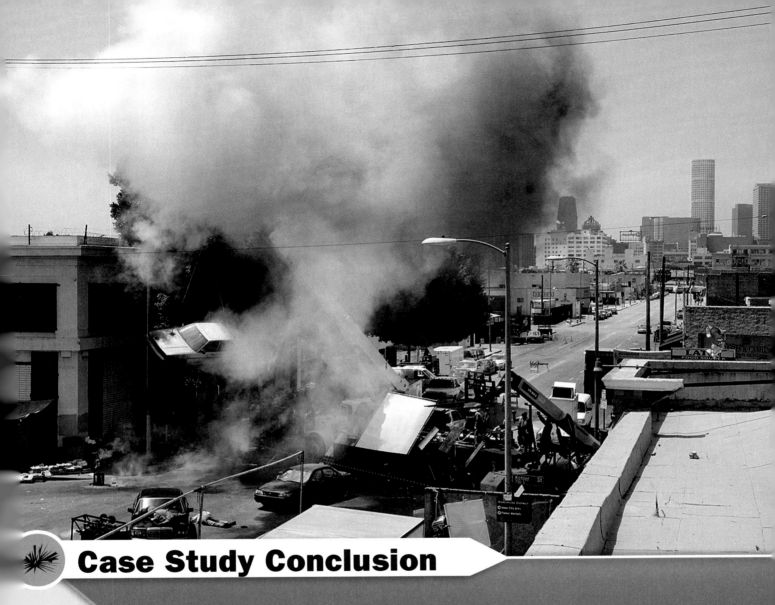

Case Study Conclusion

You immediately call over the loudspeaker for those who can walk to come to the vehicle while your partner confirms that additional EMS support, law enforcement, bomb squad, and fire department personnel are en route. Several of the nearby construction workers ask if they can help. You quickly have the walking wounded, some eight persons, loaded into the vehicle with the assistance of the construction workers and carefully back away from the scene. You pull into the parking lot of a commercial structure out of sight of the tavern while your partner begins assessment of the injured. You establish the triage area there, some 800 feet from the scene. You advise your on-line medical direction physician that you have multiple injured patients and to expect up to 50 patients may be transported. You find that your eight walking wounded mainly have lacerations, but one is suffering serious bleeding from the scalp. You control the bleeding with pressure. This patient is also complaining of hearing loss. The first arriving EMS supervisor assumes Incident Command, and your patient with hearing loss is transported to a nearby hospital by another EMS unit. The fire department arrives and uses its water cannon to extinguish the fire in the tavern. Against your better judgment, you and your partner, along with several

firefighters and the construction workers, remove five of the persons that are down in front of the structure. You note additional persons partially covered with debris both inside and outside the structure but can hear no calls for help. Of those five persons recovered, two are dead and three are critically injured and unresponsive. You note that patient 1 has no visible injuries but does have decreased breath sounds over one side of the chest and is breathing rapidly, is hypotensive, and has distended neck veins. You suspect a tension pneumothorax from blast overpressure and successfully relieve it. You also suspect that this patient may have additional internal injuries such as shock lung and gastrointestinal injury from blast overpressure. The patient improves when you decompress the tension pneumothorax. Patient 2 has multiple puncture wounds (no bleeding) along her anterior torso. She has no palpable blood pressure and subsequently suffers cardiac arrest. You suspect these are primary shrapnel wounds and turn to treat patient 3, who is now conscious and is complaining he cannot hear. You find no obvious external injuries and suspect that blast over-pressure has ruptured his eardrums and that he has a concussion or other closed head injuries. When additional EMS resources arrive, you transport your surviving patients to the hospital. The emergency physician confirms that patient 1 has a tension pneumothorax and shock lung. He replaces your decompressing needle with a chest tube. The patient also is discovered to have a ruptured liver and is taken to surgery, where he dies from internal hemorrhage. Patient 3 survives with substantial permanent hearing loss in both ears.

In the meantime the fire department engine backs away from the scene, leaving their supply line after shutting down their water cannon. Law enforcement begins to secure a much larger perimeter some 1,500 feet away, and the bomb squad arrives some 15 minutes later. The triage area and command post are moved farther back to a more distant location. The local emergency department reports that they have twelve walk-in patients with minor to moderate injuries. The injuries are mainly lacerations to pedestrians who were near the blast site. Bomb technicians wearing bomb suits, chemical protective clothing, and SCBAs enter the blast area and report that the fire is out, there are multiple victims present, but no signs of life are obvious. The bomb technicians also note no chemical agents, radioactive material, or toxic industrial chemicals. The bomb technicians continue to search the area and find no additional explosives. They declare the scene to be clear.

Firefighters who have requested mutual aid descend upon the scene and begin to clear debris from the street. The city engineering department uses a front-end loader to clear a path to the structure while wreckers remove vehicles near the scene that are impeding heavy equipment. The city's engineer examines the structure from the exterior and pronounces it safe to conduct rescue. Firefighters gingerly remove several persons from the debris in front of the structure, but all are dead from crush injuries. Heavy equipment is needed to remove some debris, and the rescue effort continues over the next 12 hours. Bomb technicians and law enforcement investigators work alongside firefighters recovering evidence. No survivors are found by firefighters, but some twelve additional bodies are recovered.

The Bureau of Alcohol, Tobacco, Firearms, and Explosives sends its National Response Team to investigate and along with the local bomb squad concludes that the cause of the blast was in a bomb. This is confirmed by metal fragments recovered from bodies and from the scene. Chemical tests reveal that commercial dynamite was used in the device. The device is reconstructed and determined to be a briefcase with three galvanized metal pipe bombs filled with commercial dynamite using conventional electric blasting caps, 9-volt batteries and a mechanical egg timer. The investigation centers on the motive for the bombing. Investigators interview scores of persons and learn that a recently terminated employee who was caught skimming money from the owner vowed vengeance. The employee has fled town. Investigators obtain a search warrant for his home and find receipts for galvanized pipe from a local hardware store. In the interim a local construction company notes that one of its explosives magazines has been burglarized and that dynamite and blasting caps were stolen. Tool marks found on wires of the device are matched with wire cutters and wire found in the suspect's home. A warrant for the suspect is issued, and he is arrested without incident at a relative's home in a nearby state. He is convicted of capital murder and executed some 5 years later. The owner who fired the suspect was not present at the time of the bombing and is uninjured. Feeling responsible, he becomes very depressed about the incident and later commits suicide. The insurance company for the tavern pays its maximum liability benefit of one million dollars.

Case Study Discussion

This is an example of a revenge bombing with a briefcase bomb. Luckily for the EMS squad there were no chemical, biological, or radiological agents employed and there was no second bomb. The ambulance unit showed poor judgment in entering the scene without at least Level C protection and would have been contaminated if any other CBRNE agent had been used. They compounded their poor judgment by treating the patients on-scene rather than transporting immediately. An explosion scene is always complex and requires EMS, fire, HazMat, bomb technicians, and law enforcement. Triage and the command post should be placed at least 1,000 feet away and out of sight of the scene. Explosions in enclosed spaces (building, tunnels, etc.) tend to cause higher casualty rates than those outside.

Pearls

- If you detect or confirm an explosion, have dispatch notify other responders, law enforcement, the bomb squad, the fire service, the on-line medical direction physician, receiving hospitals, and the HazMat team.

- Stop outside the area where broken windows begin and observe the scene. As a general rule, if you can see the device, the bomb technician, or the structure, you are too close.

- Identify the best location for the command post, staging, and triage, and select another one (to avoid preplaced secondary devices or ambush). Stage at least 1,000 feet away from the scene, if possible. Stay alert and look around you for suspicious persons, vehicles, or objects.

- Stay upwind and uphill, away from liquids, mists, smoke, and fog. Bombs may be used to disperse chemical, biological, or radioactive materials.

- Wear Level B or Level C PPE. Think about toxic agents.

- *Remember Time, Distance, and Shielding!*

- Proceed cautiously while staying alert for physical hazards such as falling glass, leaking natural gas, or structural collapse. The blast area may contain unconsumed explosives, secondary devices, toxic materials, collapse hazards, and other substantial hazards.

- If you find an unexploded bomb, immediately retreat at least 1,000 feet and call for help.

- Coordinate your actions with other responders.

- Instruct the ambulatory to walk out of the danger area to a triage area.

- *Enter the blast area only to save lives.* If possible wait until the scene has been cleared by bomb technicians and the HazMat team. Use "load and go" tactics with expedient spinal precautions. Leave the dead behind.

- All penetrating injuries, even minor surface injuries, need hospital evaluation.

- Injured persons' clothing may contain evidence of interest to law enforcement. Do not discard.

- Treat all explosions as crime scenes.

- Keep entry and exit points open for emergency traffic.

- Always have an escape plan in case you are attacked.

Want to Know More?

Bibliography

Akhavan, J. *Chemistry of Explosives.* Royal Society of Chemistry, 1998.

Campbell, J. *Basic Trauma Life Support,* 5th Edition, Prentice-Hall Health, 2003.

De Lorenzo, R.A. *Tactical Emergency Care.* Prentice-Hall, 1991.

DeLorenzo, R.A. & R.S. Porter, *Weapons of Mass Destruction: Emergency Care.* Prentice Hall Health, 2000.

Meidl, J.H. *Explosive and Toxic Materials.* Glencoe Press, 1970.

Yinon, J. Toxicity and Metabolism of Explosives. CRC Press, 1990.

Internet Sites

Blast Injuries

   www.emedicine.com/emerg/tompic63.htm

Dirty bombs

   www.nrc.gov/reading-rm/doc-collections/fact-sheets/dirty-bombs.html

Advice to citizens from the Department of Homeland Security

   www.ready.gov/america/explosions.html

Notes

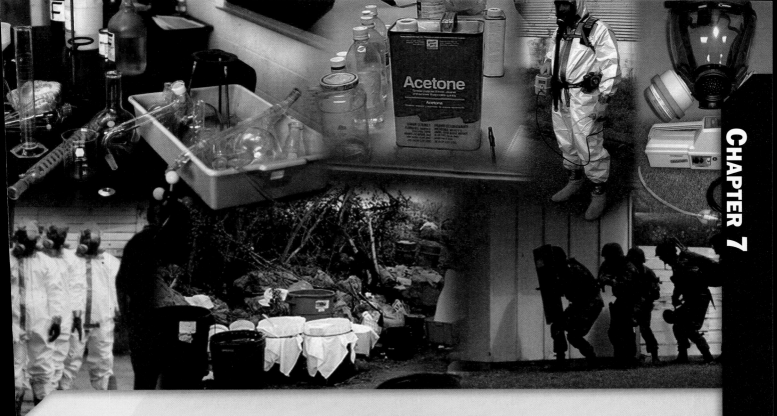

CHAPTER 7

Clandestine Drug Laboratories

Chapter Objectives

Upon completion of this chapter you should be able to:

1. Recognize the signs of a clandestine drug laboratory (CDL).

2. Discuss the dangers associated with a CDL.

3. Discuss the special hazards of underground and single-entry labs.

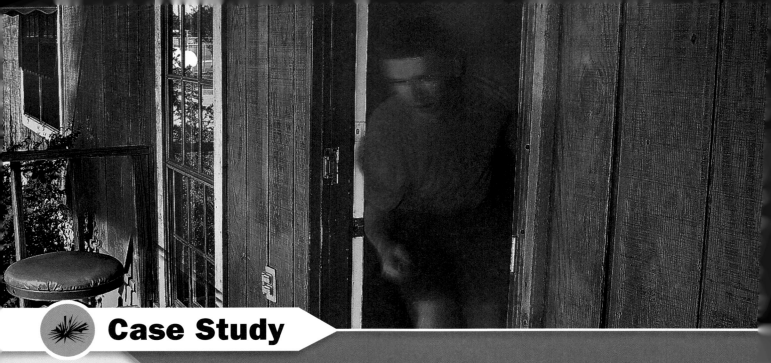

Case Study

Your fire engine company responds to a reported fire in a rural area. Upon your arrival, neighbors point to a residence that has dark smoke streaming from an open front door. They state they heard an explosion and then saw the resident come staggering out, get into a truck, and leave. As you approach the structure, you note an odor similar to fingernail polish remover.

- What has happened?
- Is a chemical agent or other toxic material involved?

- Are the responders on-scene in danger?
- What protective clothing is required?
- What is the next step for responders?
- What resources are needed?

The Case Study will continue at the end of the chapter.

Clandestine drug laboratories (CDLs) are not commonly associated with terrorism, but they present the same hazards for public safety personnel. When responding to the scene of a CDL, you will follow the principles for response to a chemical weapon attack. Because CDLs are so common, you are likely to be called to the scene of a fire or explosion at a CDL, and you may be asked to team with law enforcement and fire personnel in a raid on a CDL.

Overview of Clandestine Drug Laboratories

Clandestine drug laboratories (Figure 7.1) are usually used to manufacture methamphetamine or other illegal drugs. Rarely, a clandestine laboratory may be used to manufacture explosives such as TATP (a white to yellow colored powder and a very unstable explosive), biological agents such as ricin, or chemical agents such as sarin. What is originally thought to be a CDL could in fact have another use, or multiple uses. These laboratories can present multiple hazards, and it is very dangerous to approach them unless you are properly trained and equipped. The hazards include explosion and toxic chemicals plus armed criminals who are likely to be under the influence of the drug being produced. Remember that methamphetamine produces paranoid behavior. Many laboratories and marijuana-growing operations will be booby-trapped and may contain bombs or chemical devices. A substantial number of laboratories are discovered following explosions or fires (Figure 7.2). In some rural areas methamphetamine labs are so common that any report of a mobile home on fire is assumed to be a CDL until proven otherwise.

Figure 7.1
Clandestine drug
laboratory in a house.

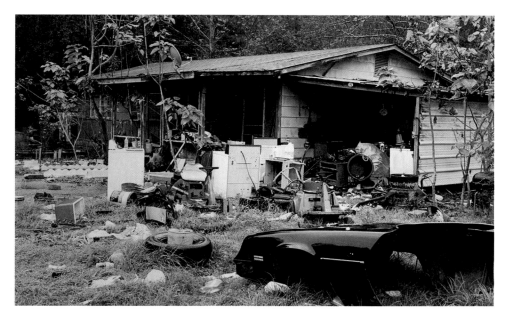

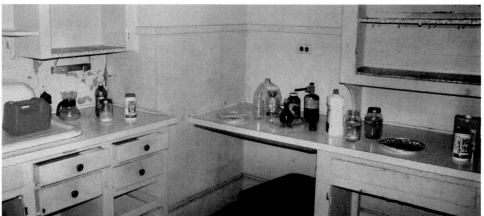

Figure 7.2
Remains of a CDL
explosion and fire.

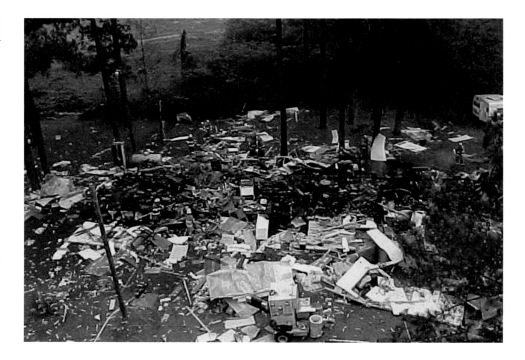

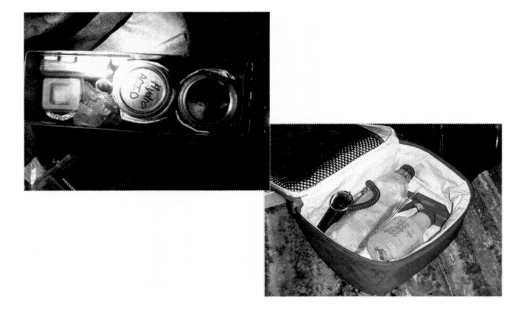

Laboratories may be found occupying rental property, motel rooms, and mobile homes. Portable labs may be found in vehicles such as RVs, and boxed labs may be transported in a passenger vehicle (Figure 7.3). All public safety personnel who respond to a suspected CDL should be trained and certified in clandestine drug laboratory safety. Such responders should be equipped with the appropriate chemical protective clothing, chemical detection equipment, respiratory protection equipment, and needed backup personnel. If you respond to a CDL, you may face a range of problems that include:

- Toxic, potentially carcinogenic, and explosive chemicals
- Booby traps
- Leaking pressurized gas cylinders
- Confined spaces
- Armed, paranoid laboratory operators

All the chemicals used to produce methamphetamine and other related drugs are flammable, toxic, corrosive, explosive, and potentially carcinogenic. These dangers make personal protective equipment essential (see Chapter 1).

During planned raids, a Site Safety Officer from the clandestine laboratory entry team should be designated to determine what level of protection is needed during the raid and subsequent laboratory assessment. This individual must be well trained and certified in the CDL hazards and should have the authority to decide whether it is safe to enter the area. The Site Safety Officer should also make decisions regarding the decontamination of suspects and responders and should supervise air sampling and the assessment for chemical and physical hazards.

Law enforcement officers raiding a CDL may elect to wear an APR (Level C PPE), flame resistant clothing, and body armor in lieu of chemical protective clothing if they expect to encounter armed suspects (Figure 7.4). This will facilitate mobility and their ability to perform tactical tasks.

Some laboratories are found during unrelated events, such as calls to a chemical odor, medical emergency, fire, or explosion. In these circumstances a tactical retreat by public safety responders is in order until appropriate resources can arrive. Any citizen who stumbles onto a possible CDL should immediately retreat and call 911. Do not seek to investigate the situation yourself.

Figure 7.4
(a) Police officer in Level C PPE. (b) Officer in Level C PPE and holding a PID to test the atmosphere in the CDL.

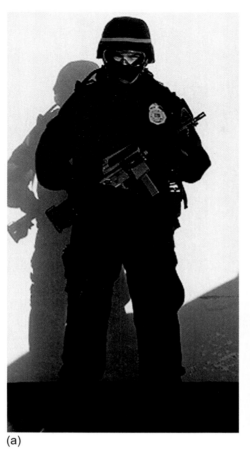

(a)

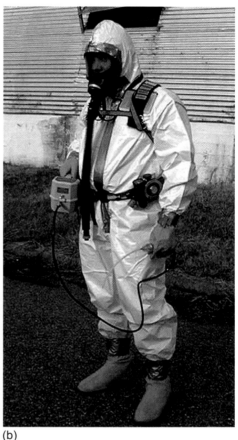

(b)

Planned raids are deliberate operations with all the required assets (fire, EMS, and police teams) in place. A Medical Threat Assessment (MTA) should be performed before law enforcement begins their operation. The MTA should assess all aspects related to medical support, including threats, planned response, treatment and transportation of potential victims, and other important issues related to the mission. In many instances fire and EMS may be staged some distance away and called when suspects are secured. Close-up medical support may be provided by personnel specially trained in tactical EMS, who may remain with the law enforcement unit before, during, and after the search warrant is served.

Suspects would usually have clothing removed and replaced with disposable paper coveralls (dry decontamination) and then be transported to a detention facility where they are showered. Most CDLs do not require wet decontamination (showering) on-scene. The Site Safety Officer should determine what type of decontamination method is required.

Physical Hazards

Numerous physical hazards may be present in a CDL, one of which is armed suspects who may be under the influence of methamphetamine with its induced paranoia. Explosive vapors from the solvents used in the manufacturing process as well as incompatible chemicals (when mixed, these cause fire, toxic fumes, or explosion) are common in CDLs, as most operators are not trained chemists and have little regard for safety.

Booby traps, chemical devices, trip-wired firearms, and bombs may be present on the site (Figure 7.5). This is particularly true if the operators have military

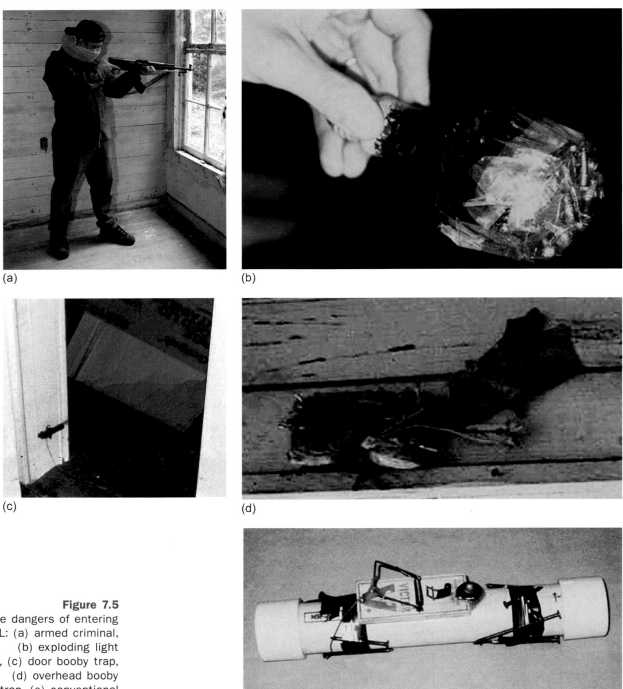

(a)

(b)

(c)

(d)

Figure 7.5
Some dangers of entering
a CDL: (a) armed criminal,
(b) exploding light
bulb, (c) door booby trap,
(d) overhead booby
trap, (e) conventional
booby trap.

(e)

training, a history of violence, or gang affiliation. CDL operators commonly use infrared sensors, video surveillance, trip wires, guard dogs, and electronic devices to detect intrusion. Dangerous booby traps such as fishhooks on monofilament lines, chemical booby traps for generating cyanide gas, explosives, and pipe bombs are possible. Responders should always be alert for trip wires and booby traps. When entering a building containing a possible CDL, there are several things you should NOT do:

- Do not turn power or switches on or off.
- Do not turn off cooling water to laboratory apparatus.

- Do not touch anything in the lab.
- Do not sniff containers.
- Do not open or move containers of chemicals or suspected chemicals.
- Do not eat, drink, smoke, or chew anywhere around a CDL.
- Do not open refrigerators or other electrical appliances.

Confined Spaces

If the CDL is below ground level, is well sealed, or has only one entry/exit point, it should be considered a confined space. Confined spaces often trap toxic gases, and the gases often displace the oxygen in the air. Well-sealed and below-ground laboratories (Figure 7.6) are often oxygen deficient. It is prudent to ventilate such an area with fresh air prior to entry if possible. Prior to entering such areas the atmosphere must be tested for oxygen level, toxic chemicals, and explosive vapors. The use of an SCBA (Level A or B PPE) is required even if oxygen levels are adequate, because any release of chemicals will be concentrated in the confined space. Underground labs are often damp, and toxic molds may grow there.

An emerging trend among CDL operators is to use an underground laboratory for concealment purposes. Most are makeshift laboratories that may collapse easily, have noncode wiring, and grow toxic molds, all in addition to standard CDL hazards. The access to the lab is usually through a single opening by way of a home-made ladder. There is usually no forced ventilation system. This results in high carbon dioxide levels if occupied, or carbon monoxide levels if open flames are used for heating chemicals. The laboratory might not be drained. Operators might wade in water and dump used chemicals onto the floor. If you suspect an underground CDL, use caution driving a vehicle over the site because doing so might precipitate a collapse.

Inadequate ventilation can result in a buildup of explosive solvent vapors. If the red phosphorus method is being used, phosphine gas can result, leading to a toxic and oxygen-deficient atmosphere. The Nazi or Birch method uses anhydrous ammonia, which, if released, can result in a toxic and explosive atmosphere. Hydrochloric acid is used in most processes and corrosive vapors may be present.

Because of the danger of entering a confined space (Figure 7.7a,b), OSHA has developed strict requirements for responding public safety personnel. There must be careful planning with immediate rescue resources and backup personnel available. Sometimes it is better not to enter underground laboratories by

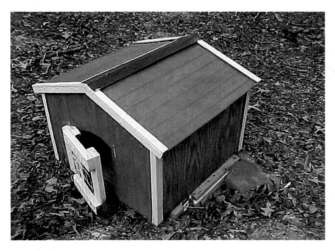
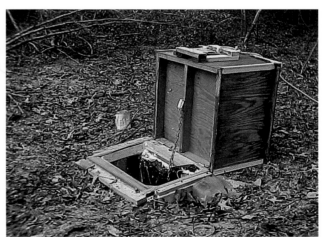

Figure 7.6
Underground CDL hidden under hinged dog house.

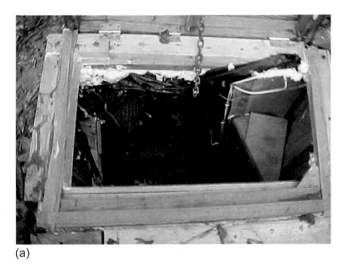

(a)

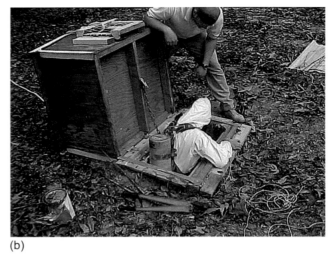

(b)

Figure 7.7
(a) Underground CDL with difficult egress. (b) Officers carefully enter underground CDL.

way of the regular entrance. In these cases you would use heavy equipment to literally remove the laboratory roof and slope the earth to the sides of the underground room to prevent collapse of the earthen walls. If available, a structural engineer should be consulted to evaluate the underground CDL as a collapse hazard. If you choose to enter an underground or tightly sealed lab through the regular entrance, entry personnel not only must be certified for CDL entry, but they must also be certified for confined-space entry. Planning must address contingencies, and a rescue team must be immediately available and suited to make entry. The responder who enters must wear a lifting apparatus and harness. If the responder collapses in the room, he is dragged out by his harness rather than by another responder going into the room. Remember, an underground CDL presents all the common hazards plus entry/exit issues, rescue hazards, higher levels of toxic chemicals, and an oxygen-deficient atmosphere.

Other CDL Hazards

Other CDL hazards include the following:

- Noncode wiring and switches present an explosion hazard (electrical spark) and a shock hazard (especially if there is water on the floor).
- Explosive, heavier-than-air solvent vapors make ventilation of the CDL important. If possible, air sampling should be undertaken to determine what hazards are present.
- Slip and fall hazards are present, and there may be standing water.
- Compressed gas cylinders present a hazard if unsecured.
- Compressed gas cylinders containing anhydrous ammonia may present a cryogenic (cold injury) hazard. The liquid anhydrous ammonia is very volatile and, like liquid nitrogen, will immediately freeze the skin.
- Wearing chemical protective clothing and respiratory protection increases heat stress, limiting work time. Normal stay time is less than 30 minutes. EMS personnel should assess entry personnel for vital signs prior to entry and following exit. Anyone experiencing signs or symptoms of heat-related illness, including nausea, vomiting, high pulse rate, weakness, dehydration, light-headedness, or abnormal vital signs, should be removed from service and medically assessed.

Chemical Hazards

Chemicals found in the CDL include flammable, explosive, corrosive, water reactive, carcinogenic, and caustic chemicals (Figure 7.8). Also present may be high-pressure gases in cylinders. These present both an explosion and an inhalation hazard (Figure 7.9). The manufacturing method being used will determine what chemicals are present.

- Chemicals used in a CDL are toxic and include cyanide, red phosphorus, mercuric chloride, chloroform, and methanol.
- All the solvents are flammable/explosive, making testing for an explosive atmosphere critical. Some CDLs use anhydrous ammonia and hydrogen, both of which are flammable.
- Acids and caustic materials are present. These can cause burns or react with other chemicals to cause an explosion. Common corrosives include hydrochloric acid, sulfuric acid, and sodium hydroxide (lye).
- Metallic sodium or metallic lithium will explode if exposed to water.
- Many of the chemicals will produce toxic gases when heated. An example is phosphine gas from red phosphorus.

Anhydrous Ammonia

Anhydrous ammonia is a caustic chemical that is used in large commercial refrigeration systems and in the manufacture of fertilizer. It may be stored in containers ranging in size from large pressurized tanks carried by trucks or rail cars down to small, towable agricultural tanks.

Because it is used as a precursor chemical for the manufacture of methamphetamine, anhydrous ammonia is commonly stolen from industrial or agricultural sites. It presents a significant hazard through illegal transport and theft.

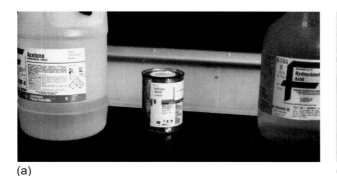
(a)

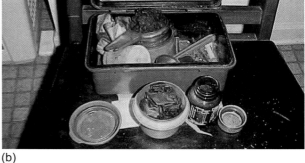
(b)

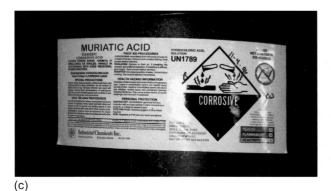
(c)

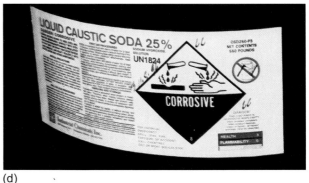
(d)

Figure 7.8
Some chemical hazards of CDLs: (a) acetone, sodium metal, and hydrochloric acid; (b) red phosphorous; (c) muriatic acid; (d) sodium hydroxide.

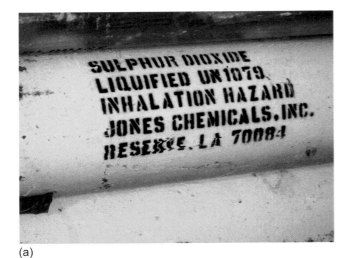

(a)

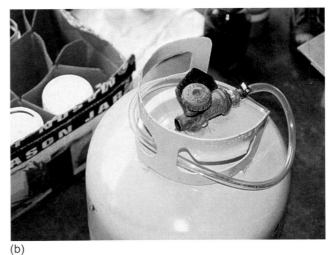

(b)

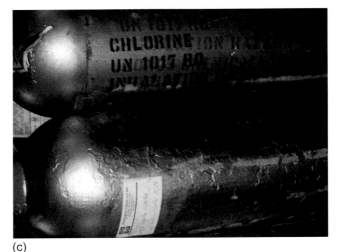

(c)

Figure 7.9
Some inhalation hazards of
CDLs: (a) sulfur dioxide,
(b) anhydrous ammonia,
(c) chlorine.

Valves may be left open or broken off, and large amounts of the product may be released. Individuals involved in the theft can be injured or killed. Persons with cryogenic injuries (cold injuries to the skin—these look like regular thermal burns) or lung injuries involving ammonia may be involved in the manufacture of methamphetamine.

The U.S. Department of Transportation classifies anhydrous ammonia as a non-flammable gas in Class 2.2. When transported, the tank should display a green background placard with the drawing of a compressed gas cylinder and the four digit code "1005." Some tanks are labeled "Anhydrous Ammonia." Though rated as nonflammable, anhydrous ammonia is flammable and explosive when confined and exposed to a very high-temperature ignition source. It is also corrosive and toxic to breathe. If anhydrous ammonia is released from a pressurized tank, its temperature can be −28 degrees Fahrenheit. It is very volatile (expands 850 times from a liquid to vapor state), so it will rapidly freeze whatever it touches. The product is devoid of water and will concentrate in locations where water is available. When mixed with water it produces ammonium hydroxide, which is corrosive. Roughly 1,300 gallons of ammonia vapor will dissolve in one gallon of water. Ammonia has a strong odor that is easily detected. Inhaled ammonia vapors react with the water in the moist lungs and upper airway to produce ammonium hydroxide, causing tissue burns and pulmonary edema. Ammonia vapor will also burn the delicate tissues of the eyes.

A variety of containers are used to steal anhydrous ammonia, the most common being a portable liquid propane gas (LPG) cylinder. This tank has a nonsparking brass valve that reacts chemically with the ammonia, leaving a bluish

Figure 7.10
Anhydrous ammonia stored in an LPG cylinder. Note the blue discoloration on the valve.

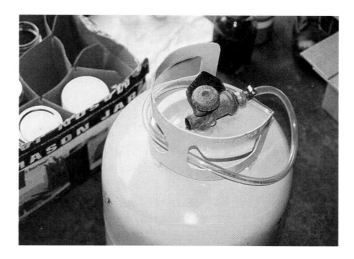

corrosion product (Figure 7.10). Any LPG cylinder with bluish discoloration of the valve should be assumed to contain anhydrous ammonia. Corrosion will eventually cause valve failure, suddenly releasing all of the stored anhydrous ammonia. Fatalities have been associated with the transport of anhydrous ammonia in LPG cylinders.

Patients who have been exposed to anhydrous ammonia and who complain of stinging or burning of the eyes should be decontaminated by flushing the eyes with saline or water for at least 20 minutes. Their clothing should be removed, and they should be given total-body decontamination by showering. If exposure to liquid anhydrous ammonia has occurred, then the person has probably also suffered cryogenic injury and their clothes might be frozen to their skin. The affected area should be flushed with water and the clothing removed to prevent off-gassing ammonia vapors. The injured site should be left uncovered to allow off-gassing. Persons exposed to the vapor should be given high-flow oxygen and evaluated for pulmonary burns and edema. Mucous membranes exposed to the vapor or liquid should be flushed for 20 minutes with water.

Types of Clandestine Drug Laboratories

Methamphetamine Laboratory

Methamphetamine is a potent stimulant that until the late 1980s was relatively unknown except along the West Coast. Its use began to spread across the United States during the 1990s. By 2004, forty-one states reported a significant number of seizures of local methamphetamine laboratories. About two-thirds of methamphetamine sold in the United States is produced in large labs in Mexico and California. Local methamphetamine labs are usually not a part of the organized trafficking by the large labs, but instead are operated by poorly educated criminals who both use and sell their product locally. Methamphetamine has become a popular recreational drug because it gives the same euphoric state as cocaine but lasts longer and is cheaper. Methamphetamine overdose or chronic abuse can cause paranoia, toxic psychosis, hallucinations, seizures, and coma. There are several methods of producing methamphetamine, including the red phosphorous method, the Nazi or Birch method, the thionyl chloride method, the phenyl-2-propanone (P2P) method, and the phenylacetic acid method.

Red Phosphorous Methamphetamine Laboratory

Expect to find the following in a red phosphorous methamphetamine laboratory:

- *Flammable solvents, acetone, toluene, etc.* These would usually be in labeled solvent cans.

- *Red phosphorus.* You may see many matchboxes or matchbooks with the striker strip removed. The phosphorus may cause red stains on floors, cabinets, or microwave ovens. When overheated, red phosphorus produces phosphine gas. Phosphine gas smells like rotten fish and is extraordinarily toxic. It can cause death in minutes at concentration of 2,000 ppm. Phosphine is also flammable.

- *Iodine and hydriodic acid.* These are both corrosive and toxic. Iodine may cause purple stains on floors, cabinets, or microwave ovens.

- *Sodium hydroxide or lye.* Lye is very caustic and will dissolve flesh. It is the active ingredient in drain cleaners, and you may find containers of drain cleaners in the lab.

- *Sulfuric acid, hydrochloric acid, or muriatic acid.* All of these are corrosive. Acids may explode if mixed with sodium hydroxide or metals.

- *Hypophosphorus acid.* This is rarely used, but presents an extreme explosion hazard.

- *Pseudoephedrine.* Sudafed, or cold or allergy remedies containing ephedrine or Sudafed.

- *Laboratory-type glassware.*

Ammonia Methamphetamine Laboratory using Nazi or Birch Method

Expect to find the following in an ammonia methamphetamine laboratory using the Nazi or Birch Method:

- *Flammable solvents, such as toluene, lighter fluid, or acetone.* These will usually be in labeled containers.

- *Lithium.* This is usually obtained from lithium batteries but may be present as a gray colored metal. Metallic lithium will explode on contact with water.

- *Anhydrous ammonia.* This may be stored in an LPG gas cylinder with blue discoloration of the valve. Anhydrous ammonia presents a toxic and explosive gas with an extreme respiratory hazard.

- *Hydrochloric acid (or hydrogen chloride gas from gas generators).* You may find pressurized cylinders of hydrogen chloride. It is more common to find hydrogen chloride gas generators using rock salt and sulfuric acid. These are usually made from plastic gasoline containers or sprayer bottles hooked together with plastic tubing (Figure 7.11). Either of these presents a respiratory hazard.

Figure 7.11
An example of a hydrogen chloride gas generator.

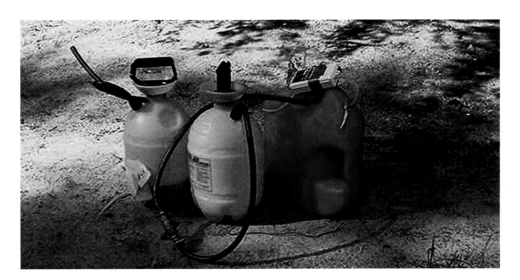

- *Pseudoephedrine.* Sudafed, or cold or allergy remedies containing ephedrine or Sudafed.
- *Laboratory-type glassware.*

Thionyl Chloride Methamphetamine Laboratory (Uncommon)

Expect to find the following in a thionyl chloride methamphetamine laboratory:

- *Flammable solvents.* These will include chloroform, methanol, or ethanol. Chloroform may be carcinogenic.
- *Palladium black.*
- *Thionyl chloride.* This will explode on contact with water.
- *Hydrogen gas.* This is normally contained in a red cylinder. This is a very explosive gas.
- *Paint shakers.* These labs are called "shaker labs."
- *Pseudoephedrine.* Sudafed, or cold or allergy remedies containing ephedrine or Sudafed.
- *Laboratory-type glassware.*

Phenyl-2-Propanone (P2P) Methamphetamine Laboratory (Rare)

The phenyl-2-propanone (P2P) process results in a toxic atmosphere. Expect to find the following in this lab:

- *Mercuric chloride and methylamine.* Both are toxic and corrosive.
- *Alcohol.*
- *Aluminum foil.*
- *Hydrogen chloride gas or hydrogen chloride gas generator.*
- *Pseudoephedrine.* Sudafed, or cold or allergy remedies containing ephedrine or Sudafed.
- *Laboratory-type glassware.*

Phenylacetic Acid Methamphetamine Laboratory (Unusual)

Expect to find in the lab:

- *Phenylacetic acid and acetic anhydride.* Acetic anhydride reacts violently with water.
- *Sodium hydroxide or lye.*
- *Pseudoephedrine.* Sudafed, or cold or allergy remedies containing ephedrine or Sudafed.
- *Laboratory-type glassware.*

Methylenedioxymethamphetamine (MDMA) or Ecstasy

MDMA and its demethylated metabolite 3,4-methylenedioxyamphetamine (MDA) are known on the street as "Ecstasy." MDMA and MDA are amphetamine derivatives similar to methamphetamine and the hallucinogen mescaline. MDMA was first synthesized in 1914 but found no use until the 1970s when it began to be used in psychotherapy. During this time it began to be used as a recreational drug by young professionals who mistakenly thought it was safe and nontoxic. Because of the potential for huge profits, it was soon being sold on the street. In 1985 it was found to cause long-term brain damage in laboratory animals. The Drug Enforcement Administration declared MDMA illegal in 1986. However, by this time the drug had already developed into a popular recreational drug.

The effects of MDMA and MDA are both stimulating and hallucinogenic. The drugs have become very popular at "raves," where young adults gather to dance and do drugs for hours. Users report that MDMA not only produces stimulation and euphoria but also increased tactile sensation as well as loss of inhibitions.

Box 7-1   Evidence Suggesting an Ecstasy Laboratory

- The precursor, isosafrole
- Formic acid
- Hydrogen peroxide
- Sulfuric acid
- Methanol
- Benzene (benzene is thought to be a carcinogen)
- Ammonium formate

High doses cause paranoia and anxiety. Abuse of MDMA and MDA has become a worldwide problem. For a list of substances to expect to find in an Ecstasy lab, see Box 7-1.

Phencyclidine (PCP) or Angel Dust

Phencyclidine was originally developed as an anesthetic agent. It produces a dissociative anesthesia, meaning that a person's mind is separated from his or her body (out-of-body experience) and thus does not notice pain. It appeared to be a useful anesthetic agent because in therapeutic doses it did not depress respiration. However, there were so many reports of patients having hallucinations, agitation, and disoriented behavior that its use on humans was discontinued in 1965. It was quickly re-released as a veterinary anesthetic agent. It began to be abused as a recreational drug and by 1978 it had developed such a bad reputation that it was completely withdrawn from the market. Since then all PCP has been made by CDLs.

In low to moderate doses, PCP causes hyperactivity and mood elevation. At higher doses PCP causes hallucinations, paranoia, and bizarre, often violent, behavior. Because of its anesthetic effects, people who abuse PCP feel no pain and are very difficult to subdue when they become violent. The adverse psychological effects can last for days.

Abuse of PCP began in the 1960s in California, but even in that drug culture it was soon recognized as being too dangerous to use. Since then its use has waxed and waned, but the drug has never gained great popularity. For a list of substances you would expect to find in a PCP lab, see Box 7-2.

Gamma-hydroxybutyrate (GHB)

In the 1960s GHB was developed as an anesthetic agent. Like PCP, it had serious side effects (seizure-like activity) and its use was discontinued. In the 1980s GHB was sold in the health food industry as a "growth hormone stimulator" and was supposed to help body builders gain muscle mass. It was also sold as a sleep aid. It became a popular recreational drug because in low doses it can have an aphrodisiac effect as well as cause relaxation and euphoria. However, at higher doses it causes coma and amnesia. These effects made it effective as a "date rape"

Box 7-2   Evidence Suggesting a PCP Laboratory

- The precursor, piperidine
- Potassium or sodium cyanide (if mixed with an acid, forms lethal cyanide gas)
- Sodium bisulfate
- Sodium hydroxide
- Petroleum ether
- Magnesium metal (magnesium fires are very difficult to extinguish)

Box 7-3   Evidence Suggesting a GHB Laboratory

- Gamma-butyrolactone
- Lye or sodium hydroxide

drug. The coma produced by GHB can be deep enough to cause death from respiratory depression.

GHB was banned by the FDA in 1991 but has continued to be a popular recreational drug, especially among college students. For a list of substances common in GHB labs, see Box 7-3.

Personal Protective Equipment

The Site Safety Officer should determine what level of personal protective equipment is used. Each service may use a different level. Law enforcement may elect to use APRs (Level C), ballistic helmets, body armor, flame-resistant gloves and flame-resistant clothing for the entry team, whereas the chemist will wear chemical protective clothing and an SCBA (Level B) for the initial assessment but may downgrade to Level C after the assessment. Fire service personnel should not depend upon structural firefighting turnout gear to give them chemical protection. The hands and feet are the areas most likely to be contaminated in a CDL, making chemical boots and substantial chemical gloves a necessity. Safe CDL habits include:

- No eating or drinking in contaminated areas.
- Frequent hydration and rest breaks.
- Use of proper respiratory and protective clothing.
- A shower with soap and water after leaving the site.

Decontamination

Dry decontamination is defined as the removal of contaminated items and the washing of the hands and face. A full shower should follow when possible. In most circumstances this technique is adequate for CDL exposures.

The decontamination sequence for responders with no significant contamination known, other than to the chemical boots and gloves, is listed below:

- Place any equipment in the proper location.
- Remove outer gloves.
- Remove outer chemical suit.
- Remove chemical boots.
- Remove respiratory protection.
- Remove inner gloves.
- Wash face and hands.
- Shower completely when possible.

The only items decontaminated by washing, not disposed of on-site by the cleanup contractor, are the respirator and chemical boots. Any badly contaminated items should be left on-site. If an APR is used, leave the filters on-site. Electronic instruments should be placed in clean bags and tested to confirm that they are not contaminated.

Wet decontamination should occur when ordered by the Site Safety Officer. Wet decontamination requires showering on-site with control of runoff water. A HazMat team will be needed to assist.

A chemist trained for CDL should be available and may be part of a forensic team or part of a law enforcement agency. The chemist should conduct an on-site assessment of the chemicals, including identification and segregation. The chemist reports to the Site Safety Officer.

Role of the Fire Service and EMS

Fires or explosions occasionally occur in CDLs, and sometimes this is how a CDL is discovered. Always be suspicious of explosions and fires in unusual settings or without an obvious explanation.

Fires in CDLs can spread rapidly. If significant quantities of chemicals are present, efforts should be limited to protecting responders from exposure. Consider evacuation of personnel from downwind of the area. It is best to be upwind and on higher ground. Fire service personnel should consider a defensive mode in a known CDL. This means that they do not enter the structure but fight the fire from outside (surround and drown). Runoff water can be contaminated and needs to be controlled. Notify the EMA and environmental protection agencies early into the incident. Law enforcement should make certain that EMS and firefighters know that a suspected or known CDL is involved. If EMS or fire personnel (or private citizens) accidentally discover a CDL, they should retreat and call law enforcement.

Medical emergencies involving the CDL entry team will normally be heat related. Heat-related medical events require removal from the laboratory, emergency removal of protective equipment or dry decontamination, cooling, hydration, and transport to a medical facility. Any chemical contamination on skin, eyes, or mucous membranes should be irrigated for no less than 20 minutes. Identification of the contaminant is important.

Any exposure to toxic gases or vapors requires EMS assessment after removal from the laboratory and emergency decontamination. High-flow oxygen and transport to a medical facility are indicated. Remember that exposure to some agents such as phosphine may produce delayed problems such as pulmonary edema. Medical evaluation is required for everyone exposed to toxic gases.

CDL Operator Appearance and Clinical Presentation

Those persons operating a CDL frequently have some form of skin lesions, such as allergic dermatitis, rashes, open sores, and/or burns from exposure to the acids or caustics. Paranoid behavior with hallucinations is common following periods of intense methamphetamine use. Sleep deprivation and altered sleep patterns are common among methamphetamine users. If using methamphetamine regularly, they may be underweight, even to the point of emaciation. Dental problems are normally present. The chronic inhalation of toxic fumes may present as bronchitis or pneumonia. Pulmonary edema and respiratory burns result from exposure to phosphine and hydrochloric acid. Bone marrow depression, thrombocytopenia, and other blood disorders may be present. Children living in a building housing a CDL may have many of the symptoms of methamphetamine use and usually screen positive for methamphetamine.

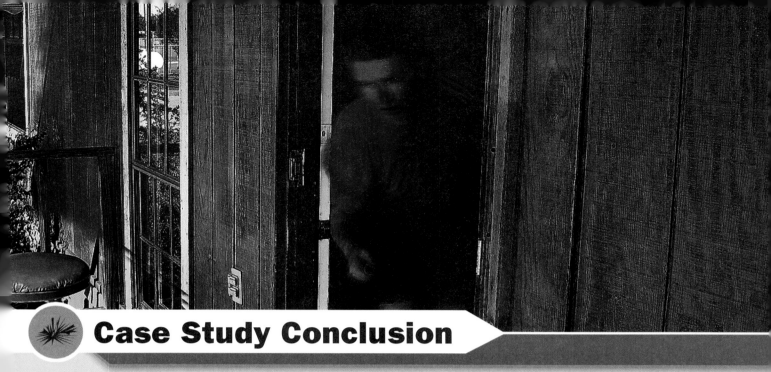

Case Study Conclusion

You know that the smell of fingernail polish remover is likely from methyl ethyl ketone, a solvent commonly used in CDLs. You notify other responders that a CDL is probably involved. The fire department conducts a defensive exterior operation, and within minutes the fire is contained and then extinguished. The small amount of water runoff is contained by the fire department. You telephone the local emergency center to advise them that a patient may be reporting with burn and explosion injuries and that a CDL is probably involved. They report that a male with burn injuries is presently being treated and the emergency physician requests that you and law enforcement respond to the hospital. By the time you arrive, the emergency physician has removed gray metallic particles from several locations on the victim's arm and face. The patient complained bitterly to the emergency physician that the areas were burning him. The physician asks you to observe, and he places a small part of one of the objects in water. You notice vigorous bubbling. You realize the explosion has propelled metallic lithium strips from a battery into the victim's skin. This means the Nazi or Birch method was being used in the CDL and anhydrous ammonia is likely to have been present. The emergency physician also informs you the victim has some respiratory injury. The law enforcement clandestine laboratory entry team, along with arson and fire investigators, soon confirms that a CDL was involved, and they recover several LPG cylinders that probably contain anhydrous ammonia. The anhydrous ammonia is vented into water to create ammonia, which is then disposed of by a HazMat cleanup vendor. The victim recovers after a 3-day stay in the hospital and is prosecuted for manufacturing methamphetamine, possession of anhydrous ammonia, and operating a clandestine drug laboratory. He receives a 35-year sentence. The clean up cost is $45,000.

Case Study Discussion

This is an example of an explosion and fire in a CDL. There is always the possibility of toxic, flammable, or explosive chemicals in a CDL. This laboratory contained anhydrous ammonia and the flammable solvent methyl ethyl ketone. Responders on-scene were in danger from fire and explosion as well as from the toxic chemicals in the lab. Until the lab had been evaluated for chemicals and oxygen level, it was best for anyone who entered to wear Level B PPE. The correct response upon recognizing a possible CDL was to retreat to a safe distance while awaiting HazMat, law enforcement, and the CDL entry team. In this case, the fire department was able to extinguish the fire without entering the residence.

Pearls

- Consider a clandestine laboratory when called to unexplained explosions or fires in residential homes, motels, or vehicles.

- Unexplained chemical odors or the smell of ammonia may indicate a CDL.

- Toxic and explosive chemicals are present in a CDL.

- Booby traps and bombs can be in a CDL.

- Armed paranoid persons are often present at a CDL.

- Unexplained and bizarre behavior may be due to methamphetamine use.

- When a CDL is discovered, leave the area until the police declare that the situation is stable.

- Stay upwind and uphill of a potential CDL.

- Use an SCBA and chemical protective clothing for initial entry into a CDL, especially an underground CDL.

- Remember "Time, Distance, and Shielding." Remain in the danger area only for the minimum time, stay upwind and as far away as feasible, and wear respiratory protection along with PPE.

- Use defensive firefighting techniques in fires involving a suspected CDL.

- Removal of clothing will remove most contamination.

- Soap and water will remove contamination from chemicals found in CDLs.

- Runoff water from a CDL is contaminated.

Want to Know More?

Bibliography

Oldfield, K. W. *Emergency Responder Training Manual for the Hazardous Materials Technician,* 2nd ed. Wiley Inter-Science, 2005.

Clandestine Drug Laboratory Training, Network Environmental Services, 2005.

Internet Sites

GHB
www.aafp.org/afp/20001201/2478.html

Methamphetamine
www.usdoj.gov/dea/pubs/cngrtest/ct062705.html
http://nida.nih.gov/infofacts/methamphetamine.html
www.emedicine.com/emerg/topic859.htm

PCP
www.emedicine.com/med/topic3118.htm

Ecstasy
www.emedicine.com/emerg/topic927.htm

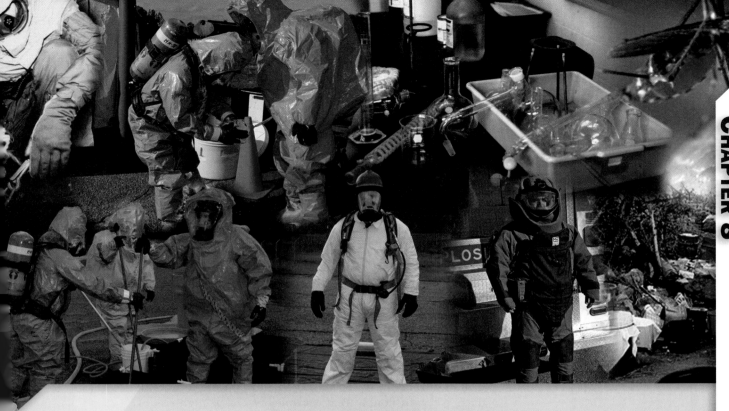

CHAPTER 8

Putting It All Together

Chapter Objectives

At the end of this chapter you should be able to:

1. Discuss the general assessment and management of an emergency scene.
2. Discuss the recognition and response to a chemical weapon attack.
3. Discuss the recognition and response to a biological weapon attack.
4. Discuss the recognition and response to a radiological-nuclear weapon attack.
5. Discuss the recognition and response to an explosives attack.
6. Discuss the recognition and response to a potential clandestine drug laboratory.

General Scene Assessment and Management

Before You Arrive at the Scene

Gather information about the call via radio, computer-aided dispatch, and personal knowledge. When other responders are on-scene, communicate with them to obtain more information. If the Incident Command System has already been established, report to the command post or staging area.

Based on the information you have obtained en route to the scene, you should be able to differentiate between a high-risk call, a suspicious call, and a routine call.

- *High-risk call.* High-risk calls include situations of known violence, a location flagged for prior violence, problems reported by on-scene personnel, hazardous materials, or large numbers of persons sick or down with an unexplained illness. You should also be very suspicious if the call is from a high-risk area, such as a government facility, strategic industry, controversial facility, or densely populated location such as a stadium or auditorium.

- *Suspicious call.* Suspicious calls include those where the information about the call is unknown, incomplete, or contradictory and there is insufficient data to fully determine what hazards exist. Also be suspicious if the information is not logical based upon the location and known data. When in doubt, treat a suspicious call as high risk.

- *Routine.* Routine calls include those with a known medical or other problem in a low-risk location with no unusual factors. This does not mean that you let your guard down when approaching the scene.

When responding to any call, shut down emergency equipment (turn off lights and siren, turn radio down) before the scene comes into view. Slowly approach the scene using your observational skills (binoculars are recommended), looking for any indicators of hazards, such as:

- Persons fleeing
- Persons concealing themselves
- Armed persons
- Disorderly crowds
- The demeanor of persons present (angry, scowling)
- Absence of people

Listen for shouts, altercations, gunshots, or other audible information as you observe the scene. If there is any doubt as to scene safety, stop and wait for law enforcement to clear the scene. If the scene needs assessment by specialized personnel (bomb technicians, HazMat technicians, technical rescue personnel, law enforcement, or CDL entry team), withdraw until they have finished their mission and give you the OK to enter.

While you continue your observation of the scene, communicate with dispatch and with other responders to obtain any additional information.

When You Arrive at the Scene

If it appears safe to approach the scene, do so from upwind and uphill, when possible. Look for any mists, fogs, vapors, smoke, or persons down, fleeing, or injured. If you note any of these things you should stop, continue the assessment, and if you decide the scene is not safe, retreat upwind while notifying dispatch, the command post, and other responders.

If you are the first unit responding and you identify the scene as a potential terrorist attack, immediately call dispatch and have them notify all of the appropriate agencies. It is essential that a HazMat team immediately test the area for CBRNE.

Continually assess what resources are needed and what resources are available. Before leaving your vehicle, call for additional resources as required to control hazards and to perform patient rescue and treatment.

Identify physical hazards, including terrain features such as ravines, bodies of water, streams, large structures, unstable vehicles, downed power lines, fires, hazardous materials, and collapsed buildings.

Identify potentially dangerous people from the presence and demeanor of persons on scene, or the lack of persons on scene. Scan anyone present, including the injured, for weapons. Disorderly persons or a crowd may require law enforcement to secure the scene before you approach. Armed persons mandate an immediate retreat out of sight of the scene. If they can see you, they can shoot you. Do not allow yourself to develop tunnel vision but rather continue to survey the whole scene for hazards and threats. Keep an escape route in mind.

You should be able to identify a potential cause of the attack (nerve agent exposure, cyanide poisoning, multiple gunshot wounds, explosion syndrome, etc.) by the number and types of injuries or by the signs/symptoms of patients.

From your survey you should decide what level of personal protective equipment to use. Put on your PPE prior to scene entry or patient contact. When the threat is unknown, the correct PPE is Level A for those trained to use it. This will usually require calling in the HazMat team. When the need for vapor protection is not high, those responders equipped and trained for it should use Level B. When the threat is known and minimal you may use Level C. You must have the correct filters for the known threat to use Level C PPE.

After your survey of the scene you should plan an escape route and communicate this plan to other responders. Stay in contact with, and make regular reports to, the command post and/or dispatch.

When You Enter the Scene

When you enter the scene, coordinate your mission with other responders on-scene. Following the Incident Command System, you should conduct rescue, triage, patient decontamination, assessment and care, and patient transport as needed. Avoid contaminated areas if possible.

Practice scene safety by minimizing the time spent in the hazard area, by staying as far away from the hazard area as possible, and by using the appropriate PPE (time, distance, and shielding).

Preserve the crime scene using the following guidelines:

- Establish and secure scene boundaries.
- Leave the dead where they are found.
- Be aware of potential physical evidence and avoid touching or moving it.
- Document who and what was removed from the scene.
- Document the name, unit, and phone number of all responders who entered the scene.
- Document the names of all victims and the destinations they were transported to.
- Be aware of any statements or comments made by victims, suspects, or witnesses of the scene. Document these statements when this does not interfere with your mission.
- Do not "clean up" the scene.
- Do not allow unauthorized persons to enter the scene.

When You Leave the Scene

When you leave the scene, proceed to decontamination and perform wet decontamination if possible. Always report to your supervisor and to Incident Command.

Responding to the Chemical Attack Scene

Before You Arrive at the Scene

Because public safety responders are likely to be first on the scene of a chemical attack, your recognition of the incident as a chemical attack can prevent contamination of responders, including yourself. In a chemical attack there are usually reports of a number of persons reported to be "sick" or down. If dispatch states that you are responding to a scene of multiple people down, you know you are responding to a high-risk call. Keep in mind that in addition to the chemical attack, there may be other hazards:

- Additional explosive or chemical devices, designed to attack responders
- Terrorists lying in ambush to shoot responders
- Scene contamination by radiation or biological agents

When responding the call, shut down emergency equipment (turn off lights and siren, turn radio down) before the scene comes into view. Slowly approach the scene using your observational skills (binoculars are recommended), looking for any indicators of hazards, such as:

- Persons fleeing
- Persons concealing themselves
- Armed persons
- Disorderly crowds
- The demeanor of persons present (angry, scowling)
- Absence of people

Listen for shouts, altercations, gunshots, or other audible information as you observe the scene. If there is any doubt as to scene safety, you should stop and wait for law enforcement to clear the scene. This scene needs assessment by HazMat technicians. You should stage in a safe place uphill and upwind until they have finished their mission and give you the OK to enter. While you continue your observation of the scene, communicate with dispatch and with other responders to obtain any additional information.

When You Arrive at the Scene

When you survey the scene, look for other evidence that you are dealing with a chemical attack, such as the presence of mists, smoke, fogs, or liquids at the scene.

Following are the common signs and symptoms of various chemical agents:

- Nerve agents cause eye pain, dimness of vision, and shortness of breath. Patients will exhibit the DUMBELS or SLUDGEM signs.
- Blister (vesicant) agents cause burning of eyes, cough, and burning and then blistering of skin. The symptoms can be delayed for several hours.
- Cyanide causes gasping for air; red eyes, skin, and lips; seizures; unconsciousness; and death.
- Pulmonary agents (phosgene, phosphine, chlorine, anhydrous ammonia, etc.) cause irritation of eyes and throat and then coughing, tightness in chest, and difficulty breathing.
- Riot control agents generally cause *immediate* burning of eyes and skin but no blistering.

As soon as you suspect you are dealing with a terrorist attack, you should immediately notify dispatch and have them notify all appropriate agencies and local hospitals.

Resist the urge to rush into the scene and rescue the victims. Immediately withdraw to a safe place and wait for the HazMat team to enter and size up the scene. They will test for chemical and radiological hazards as well as search for bombs and booby traps. If people are dying on-scene and HazMat is not available within minutes, you may have to don your PPE and rescue those patients who cannot walk from the scene (see the next section).

While HazMat is performing the scene size-up, you should establish the Incident Command System and find a safe place for the command post and for decontamination, evaluation, and treatment of patients. Remember to choose a **good** place upwind, upstream, and uphill but not the **best** place. Terrorists are clever and they may have already scouted the best place and targeted it.

Depending on wind conditions, consider evacuation of nearby areas using the North American Emergency Response Guide (NAERG) section on evacuations. Remember that slow steady winds cause higher concentrations for a greater distance. No wind will cause a high concentration locally, but a smaller hot zone. High or gusty winds will rapidly clear the area of the gas or aerosol but will increase the size of the hot zone in the short term.

Ambulatory victims may see you and approach you. They are likely contaminated with the chemical agent, so you should direct them to a safe place for decontamination, but do not approach them or let them approach you until you are in at least Level C PPE. A bullhorn (loudspeaker) can be used to direct these patients to the decontamination area.

When You Enter the Scene

Once the HazMat team has identified the chemical agent, don the appropriate PPE (see Chapter 1). If you are using Level C attire, you must also use a full-face shield to protect you from liquid splashes. Keeping the number of responders to a minimum, enter the scene from upwind, uphill, and upstream. Continually observe for hazards while on-scene. Have a planned escape route.

Ambulatory patients should be directed to the decontamination area. They should have a thorough wet decontamination as soon as possible. Alive but nonambulatory patients should be removed rapidly from the scene using "load and go" principles. They should have a thorough wet decontamination as soon as possible. If the weapon is a nerve agent, some critical patients may need the Nerve Agent Antidote Kit before they are moved. Do not put these patients in your ambulance until they have been decontaminated. Leave the dead in place until law enforcement personnel have investigated the crime scene.

While on-scene, avoid contact with any contaminated areas and avoid liquids or powdered materials. Persons fleeing from the event may be contaminated and should be isolated until they can be examined and cleared. This may be very difficult because terrified victims may refuse to obey orders. Law enforcement is responsible for scene security.

Preserve the crime scene by doing the following:

- Establish and secure scene boundaries.
- If the delivery device for the chemical attack is unknown, do not allow the ambulatory patients to take anything with them (handbags, briefcases, backpacks, shopping bags, baby carriages, etc.) that could conceal a delivery device.
- Leave the dead where they are found.
- Be aware of potential physical evidence and avoid touching or moving it.
- Document who and what was removed from the scene.
- Document the name, unit, and phone number of all responders who entered the scene.
- Document the names of all victims and the destinations they were transported to.
- Be aware of any statements or comments made by victims, suspects, or witnesses of the scene. Document these statements when this does not interfere with your mission.

- Do not "clean up" the scene.
- Do not allow unauthorized persons to enter the scene.

When You Leave the Scene

Proceed to decontamination and perform wet decontamination if possible. Always report to your supervisor and to Incident Command.

Decontamination of Victims

Victims of chemical attack require very thorough decontamination. Use soap and lots of water for victims. Up to 10 to 15 minutes of irrigation with soap and water may be needed. The victims' clothes can be a source of cross-contamination. Using hazardous material bags, double-bag all clothes. Control water runoff if possible, but do not delay decontamination of patients. When performing decontamination you must wear protective clothing, respiratory protection of at least Level C, and a full-face hood or shield.

If you find casualties who have oily liquids on their clothing and skin, wipe the liquid from their skin and have the patient shower with soap and water. The clothing should be removed and double-bagged. Avoid becoming contaminated yourself. Soap and water is best in the initial decontamination efforts, but as a minimum a rinse with water is required.

Hypochlorite (bleach) can be used at full strength for clothing or environmental decontamination. Consider cross-ventilation to blow contaminated vapors away from personnel and equipment being decontaminated.

Responding to a Biological Attack

Biological agents generally don't cause immediate symptoms, so a bioweapon attack will *not* likely be called in as multiple patients sick at a single location. Most bioterrorism attacks will present as multiple people (usually not from the same location) who become sick at about the same time. They may present to their regular doctor or to an emergency department (perhaps at multiple hospitals). Unless it is an unusual disease (anthrax, smallpox, or viral hemorrhagic fever), the illnesses may not be recognized as an attack for days after patients begin to seek treatment. Usually victims of a biological attack will have something in common, such as attending the same church or school, working in the same building, having attended the same event, or riding the same public transportation.

Prehospital EMS providers may or may not see these patients, depending on how ill the victims feel when the disease presents itself. Many patients will likely use personal vehicles to seek medical care. Many health care providers may be exposed before anyone recognizes that a biological attack has occurred.

The biological agents with short incubation periods (minutes to hours) that might present as a call for multiple people sick at the same location are inhaled ricin, trichothecene mycotoxin T2, and staphylococcal enterotoxin B (SEB). It is understandable that these act like chemical poisons because all of them are toxins (poisons made by living organisms) and not infectious agents. If dispersed as aerosols, ricin and SEB would present much like a pulmonary agent chemical attack, whereas mycotoxin T2 would appear more like a vesicant agent attack. None of these would be detected by the chemical agent detectors. Ricin and staphylococcal enterotoxin B may also be placed in food and be ingested. In this case, they would present like staphylococcal food poisoning. Field personnel would likely not recognize this as an attack. Treating such patients would not put responders in danger, because they would have to ingest the contaminated food to be affected.

Use the following protocol when responding to a biological attack with aerosolized ricin, trichothecene mycotoxin T2, or staphylococcal enterotoxin B.

Before You Arrive at the Scene

Gather information about the call via radio, computer-aided dispatch, and personal knowledge. If the call comes in as multiple people with respiratory symptoms, you would likely think of a hazardous material spill or a chemical weapon attack and recognize it as a high-risk call. Keep in mind that in addition to the possible chemical attack, there may be other hazards, including:

- Additional explosive or chemical devices designed to attack responders
- Terrorists lying in ambush to shoot responders
- Scene contamination by radiation or biological agents

Just as when responding to any other call, shut down emergency equipment (turn off lights and siren, turn radio down) before the scene comes into view. Slowly approach the scene using your observational skills (binoculars are recommended), looking for any indicators of hazards, such as:

- Persons fleeing
- Persons concealing themselves
- Armed persons
- Disorderly crowds
- The demeanor of persons present (angry, scowling)
- Absence of people

Listen for shouts, altercations, gunshots, or other audible information as you observe the scene. If there is any doubt as to scene safety, stop and wait for law enforcement to clear the scene. If this call came in as multiple people with difficulty breathing, you would request a HazMat team to check the scene while you stage upwind and uphill. While HazMat is sizing up the scene, you should establish the Incident Command System and find a safe place for the command post and for decontamination, evaluation, and treatment of patients. Remember to choose a **good** place upwind, upstream, and uphill but not the **best** place. Terrorists are clever, and they may have already scouted the best place and targeted it.

While you continue your observation of the scene, communicate with dispatch and with other responders to obtain any additional information.

When You Arrive at the Scene

If the complaints were pulmonary, when you survey the scene you should look for other evidence that you are dealing with a chemical attack, such as mists, smoke, fogs, or liquids.

Because the victims complain of coughing and difficulty breathing, you may misinterpret the signs and symptoms as being from a chemical pulmonary agent (phosgene, phosphine, chlorine, anhydrous ammonia, etc.). In an attack by myco-toxin T2, the victims would be mainly complaining of burning of the skin and eyes and you would tend to think of the riot control or vesicant chemical agents. You would thus choose to wait for HazMat to evaluate the scene before considering entering. You may be forced to don PPE and perform patient rescue if HazMat is not available within a reasonable time.

When HazMat reports no chemical agents are detected, you would suspect either that the agent is a chemical the detection equipment will not recognize or that it is a biological agent (ricin, trichothecene mycotoxin T2, or staphylococcal enterotoxin B). Some agencies may be able to do field tests for ricin or staphylococcal enterotoxin B. Depending on wind conditions, consider evacuation of nearby areas using the North American Emergency Response Guide (NAERG) section on evacuations.

Ambulatory victims may see you and approach you. They are likely to be contaminated with the chemical or biological agent, so you should direct them to a safe place for decontamination, but do not approach them or let them approach you until you are in at least Level C PPE. A bullhorn (loudspeaker) can be used to direct these patients to the decontamination area.

When You Enter the Scene

With an unknown chemical or biological agent in mind, put on chemical-rated Level B PPE with a full-face hood so that no area of your skin is exposed. Keeping the number of responders to a minimum, enter the scene from upwind, uphill, and upstream. Continually observe for hazards while on-scene. Have a planned escape route.

Ambulatory patients should be directed to the decontamination area. They should have thorough wet decontamination if possible. Alive but nonambulatory patients should be removed rapidly from the scene by "load and go" principles. They should have thorough wet decontamination if possible. Patients should not be placed into your ambulance until they have been decontaminated. Leave the dead in place until law enforcement has made an investigation of the crime scene.

While on-scene, avoid contact with any contaminated areas and avoid liquids or powdered materials. Persons fleeing from the event may be contaminated and should be isolated until they can be examined and cleared. This may be very difficult, because terrified victims may refuse to obey orders. Law enforcement is responsible for scene security.

Preserve the crime scene using the following guidelines:

- Establish and secure scene boundaries.
- If the delivery device for the biological is unknown, do not allow any of the ambulatory patients to carry anything with them (handbags, briefcases, backpacks, shopping bags, baby carriages, etc.) that could conceal a delivery device.
- Leave the dead where they are found.
- Be aware of potential physical evidence and avoid touching or moving it.
- Document who and what was removed from the scene.
- Document the names, units, and phone numbers of all responders who entered the scene.
- Document the names of all victims and the destinations they were transported to.
- Be aware of any statements or comments made by victims, suspects, or witnesses of the scene. Document these statements when this does not interfere with your mission.
- Do not "clean up" the scene.
- Do not allow unauthorized persons to enter the scene.

When You Leave the Scene

Proceed to decontamination and perform wet decontamination if possible. Always report to your supervisor and to Incident Command.

Radiological Attacks

Because radiation does not cause immediate symptoms, a radiation attack will not present with the report of multiple people sick or down at a single location. You should recognize a scene with *potential* radioactive contamination. This will include all explosions of unknown origin, bombings, unknown substances, particularly those received by mail or package, or other suspicious circumstances with an unknown substance. In all of these cases, the HazMat team should test for radiation as well as for chemical and biological agents. If a scene is positive for radiation, all responders who enter the hot zone must wear radiation dosimeters and must limit time on-scene to the very minimum for lifesaving operations.

It is possible there could be a radiation attack that would not become known until the local medical community began to find multiple patients with signs of radiation sickness—nausea and vomiting, anemia and leukopenia (low white blood cells), hair loss, and possibly radiation burns. An attack with lower doses of radiation might show up only years later with an increase in cancer in the community.

When you are called to evaluate a suspicious powder, think of anthrax spores and radioactive material. You can use the anthrax test kit (see "Practical Skills: 4") and a radiation detection device ("Practical Skills: 6") for field testing.

When responding to any call involving an explosion or patients being sprayed with a liquid or powder, always think of a chemical, biological, or radiological attack.

Before You Arrive at the Scene

When responding to the call, shut down emergency equipment (turn off lights and siren, turn radio down) before the scene comes into view. Slowly approach the scene using your observational skills (binoculars are recommended), looking for any indicators of hazards, such as:

- Persons fleeing
- Persons concealing themselves
- Armed persons
- Disorderly crowds
- The demeanor of persons present (angry, scowling)
- Absence of people

You should listen for shouts, altercations, gunshots, or other audible information as you observe the scene. If there is any doubt as to scene safety, stop and wait for law enforcement to clear the scene. The scene will need assessment by HazMat technicians and law enforcement. Withdraw until they have finished their mission and give you the OK to enter. While you continue your observation of the scene, communicate with dispatch and with other responders to obtain any additional information.

When You Arrive at the Scene

While HazMat is sizing up the scene, establish the Incident Command System and find a safe place for the command post and for decontamination, evaluation, and treatment of patients. Remember to choose a **good** place upwind, upstream, and uphill but not the **best** place. Terrorists are clever, and they may have already scouted the best place and targeted it.

Depending on wind conditions, consider evacuation of nearby areas using the North American Emergency Response Guide (NAERG) section on evacuations. Ambulatory victims may see you and approach you. They are likely to be contaminated with a chemical, biological, or radiological agent, so you should direct them to a safe place for decontamination, but do not approach them or allow them to approach you until you are in at least Level C PPE. A bullhorn (loudspeaker) can be used to direct these patients to the decontamination area.

Once the HazMat team has identified the powder as radioactive, put on Level C attire with a radiation dosimeter. The main danger is inhaling any of the powder. Because nobody is injured, do not enter the scene but instead position yourself upwind and use a loudspeaker to direct all the victims to the decontamination area. The patients should be decontaminated by having them remove their clothes and personal effects and shower with soap and water.

If you respond to a bomb scene where there are multiple injured victims who must be rescued and it is determined that the bomb was also a dispersal device for radioactive material:

- You may enter the scene wearing Level C PPE with a radiation dosimeter.
- You should enter the scene only for lifesaving reasons.

- Minimize your time on-scene.
- All nonambulatory patients should be removed by load-and-go principles. If there is known radiation contamination, do not place any patients into your ambulance until they have been decontaminated.
- Prevent external contamination (which can be washed off) from becoming internal contamination (which cannot be removed):
  - Wipe off the patient's face before applying an oxygen mask or attempting intubation.
  - Carefully wash the skin before inserting an IV line.
  - Remove the patient's clothes, jewelry, and shoes as soon as possible (this will remove 80% of contamination).
  - Brush off any powder on the skin or blot with an absorbent material any liquid on skin.

Response to an Explosives Attack

Before You Arrive at the Explosion Scene

Gather information about the call via radio, computer-aided dispatch, and personal knowledge. When you are told that you are responding to an explosion scene, you immediately know it is a high-risk call. When you get close to the address, shut down emergency equipment (turn off lights and siren, turn radio down) before the scene comes into view. Slowly approach the scene using your observational skills (binoculars are recommended), looking for any indicators of hazards, such as:

- Persons fleeing
- Persons concealing themselves
- Armed persons
- Disorderly crowds
- The demeanor of persons present (angry, scowling)
- Absence of people

Listen for shouts, altercations, gunshots, or other audible information as you observe the scene. If there is any doubt as to scene safety, stop and wait for law enforcement to clear the scene. The scene will need assessment by bomb technicians, HazMat technicians, and law enforcement. You should stage nearby in a safe area until they have finished their mission and give you the OK to enter.

While you continue your observation of the scene, communicate with dispatch and with other responders to obtain any additional information. Be sure all appropriate agencies and local hospitals have been notified.

When You Arrive at an Explosion Scene

You should be familiar with the potential hazards at an explosion site, including:

- Secondary explosive devices
- Possible ambush
- Structural collapse
- Fire
- Unconsumed explosives
- Radioactive materials
- Toxic chemicals
- Biological agents
- Natural gas leaks
- Body fluids
- Debris and glass

You should be able to define the blast zone (a minimum of 300 feet, but 1,000 feet is preferred). If Incident Command has not been established, you should initiate the system. If no patient decontamination and evaluation area has been selected, you should do this before entering the scene.

Park your ambulance or rescue vehicle as near the scene as is safe and facing in the direction in which you can exit most easily. It is usually best to park near the area where patient decontamination and evaluation will be done.

You must decide whether to enter the blast zone. It is best to have a HazMat team test for CBRNE agents before entering the scene. If there are multiple injured victims, you may have to suit up and rescue them before HazMat has completed their evaluation of the scene. Communicate with your supervisor and other responders, especially law enforcement, before entering.

Select the appropriate PPE for the scenario:

- Use Level A if the danger is unknown (usually worn by HazMat team).

- Use Level B if vapor danger is not too great and you have this equipment.

- You may use Level C if the dangers have already been identified and you have the correct filters for your APR/PAPR. Because of the dust in the air after an explosion, you will usually have to use this level of PPE even if HazMat finds no toxic chemicals.

When You Enter the Scene

Enter the scene from upwind, uphill, and upstream. Continually observe for hazards in the blast zone. Have a planned escape route. Direct the ambulatory injured to the decontamination area outside of the blast zone. Keeping the number of responders to a minimum, enter the blast area to rescue those who are alive but unable to stand or walk. Use "load and go" principles to remove nonambulatory patients. Perform no treatment until you are in a safe place. Leave the dead in place until law enforcement personnel have investigated the crime scene.

When You Leave the Scene

When you leave the scene, proceed to decontamination and perform wet decontamination if possible. Always report to your supervisor and to Incident Command.

Evaluation and Treatment of Victims

To properly assess blast injury patients, you must be familiar with the method of injury and injury syndromes seen in persons in the post-explosion environment. The primary blast or pressure wave injures air-containing organs (eardrums, lungs, and less commonly intestines). The debris or shrapnel propelled by the blast travels at very high velocities and can cause deep penetrating wounds as well as blunt force injuries. If there is a fireball or thermal event, the patients may also receive thermal burns. The blast wave may throw the victim for some distance, causing impact with the ground or other solid objects. This causes blunt force injuries like those seen in a fall from a height or from being ejected from an auto in a high-speed motor vehicle collision.

As you assess the patients, be aware that early causes of death in these patients are due to lung injuries, neurological injuries, and hemorrhagic shock. You may have to support respiration, but do so very carefully because positive-pressure ventilation may cause a pneumothorax in the lung-injured patient.

Patients who are entrapped (structure collapse) will frequently have crush injuries and may require sodium bicarbonate and large amounts of IV fluids. If possible, fluids should be given before the patient with crush injuries is extricated.

Clandestine Drug Laboratory (CDL) Recognition

Signs of a clandestine drug laboratory include the following:

- A suspicious fire or explosion in a home, mobile home, or motel
- A call for suspicious activity in any of the above
- A call for someone with paranoid behavior
- A call for persons complaining of difficulty breathing, especially if they are young with no history of asthma
- A call for persons found unconscious in a building
- A call for strange chemical odors coming from a building

The dangers of a CDL scene include the following:

- Chemical hazards such as carcinogenic materials
- Flammable and explosive chemicals
- Toxic chemical and gases
- Oxygen-deficient atmosphere
- Armed criminals who may be paranoid
- Booby traps (explosive, chemical, other)
- Vicious guard dogs
- Collapse of underground structures

Materials and chemicals commonly used in a CDL include the following:

- Pseudoephedrine
- Lithium batteries
- Red phosphorus, often from matches
- Organic solvents
- Iodine
- Sodium hydroxide (lye)
- Various acids
- Rock salt

Be able to identify drug-making apparatus, such as:

- Pill grinders
- Compressed LPG cylinders (especially if there is blue discoloration on the valve)
- Acid generators
- Filters
- Laboratory equipment

If you are making an emergency call and determine that you may be at a CDL, you should immediately retreat and call law enforcement to investigate. If it is determined that a CDL is probably present, a trained CDL entry team should be called to enter and evaluate for dangers.

If you must enter a single-entry CDL, you should wear the appropriate PPE (Level A or B) and a rescue harness. Once the atmosphere in the CDL has been tested for toxic gases, you may be able to wear an APR/PAPR (Level C) with the appropriate filter.

The most common contamination will be of your hands and/or feet, so you should wear chemical boots and chemical-rated gloves. If you remove contaminated patients from a CDL, you should decontaminate them by removing their clothes and having them shower. If no shower is available on-scene, they should wash their hands and face and then shower as soon as possible. Patients complaining of eye pain or irritation should have their eyes irrigated with saline or water for 20 minutes. Patients complaining of difficulty breathing should get 100% oxygen and should be transported to an emergency department for further evaluation.

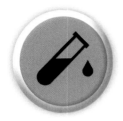 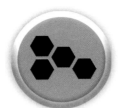 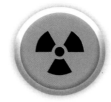 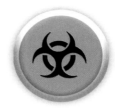 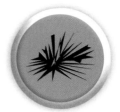

Selection and Use of Personal Protective Equipment

Chapter Objectives

At the end of this practical skill station you should be able to:

1. Determine when personal protective equipment (PPE) is needed.
2. Determine the level of PPE needed.
3. Properly put on Level C PPE.
4. Properly remove Level C PPE
   A. While performing wet decontamination
   B. While performing dry decontamination

Disaster scenes are always dangerous—bloodborne pathogens, sharp edges, moving vehicles, chaos, dust, electrocution hazards, environmental dangers such as hypothermia and disease—and that is without any terrorists! When you add terrorists, the list grows dramatically—bullets, secondary explosions, suicidal bombers who may be HIV-AIDS positive, CBRNE agents, and other things. You MUST wear protective clothing that matches or exceeds the threats. Public safety personnel are vitally important in the management of these situations, and most communities cannot afford to lose them. If responders are injured because they rashly entered a dangerous environment, they not only add to the number of victims but also there may be few, if any, trained individuals who can replace them. It is important that every public safety responder know what protective gear to use, as well as when and how to use it. It is also crucial that all public safety responders have their protective gear immediately available to them.

The most common contamination exposure is by the respiratory route. Most chemical and biological agents are dispersed by aerosol, and most explosion scenes are very dusty and may contain toxic airborne particles. Bombs can be used to aerosolize chemical and biological agents. Clandestine drug labs frequently have caustic or toxic fumes or vapors.

Some chemical and biological agents are caustic to the skin and others can be absorbed through the skin, so total body protection is needed until the dangers have been identified.

INDICATIONS FOR WEARING PPE

As discussed in Chapter 1, situations requiring HazMat evaluation and wearing of appropriate PPE include:

- Scenes in which there are multiple people "sick" or "down"
- All explosions of unknown origin
- Bombings
- Suspicious circumstances with an unknown substance, particularly one received by mail or package
- Suspicious scenes in which you encounter mists, smoke, fogs, or liquids

In these situations you should not enter the scene until the HazMat team (wearing Level A PPE) evaluates it and determines the correct level of PPE to wear. If you are first to arrive on-scene, and must enter to save lives, you *should* wear at least Level B PPE; however, Level C may be all that is available to you.

USE OF LEVEL A PROTECTIVE EQUIPMENT

When the threat is unknown but suspected to be very dangerous, it is prudent to wear the highest level of protection (Level A) until the threat is identified. Because it is difficult to work while wearing this material, its use is usually limited to HazMat specialists in the fire service. At a dangerous scene the HazMat team will don Level A PPE and then evaluate the scene to identify the dangers. Depending on the findings of the HazMat team, other responders may be able to wear lower levels of protection. Level A protection is a totally encapsulated chemical suit that requires use of a self contained breathing apparatus (SCBA) inside the suit. *Because of the specialized nature of this level of PPE, its use is not covered in this course.*

USE OF LEVEL B PROTECTIVE EQUIPMENT

Although is is not quite as good as Level A PPE this level provides protection against liquids and most vapors. Unless there is strong evidence of a severe risk, this level is usually adequate. EMS, hospital, and law enforcement personnel require a level of dexterity to perform their duties that precludes the use of Level A PPE. If HazMat evaluation determines that the scene is too dangerous for Level B PPE then victims will have to be removed from the scene before evaluation by EMS. Level B PPE is a

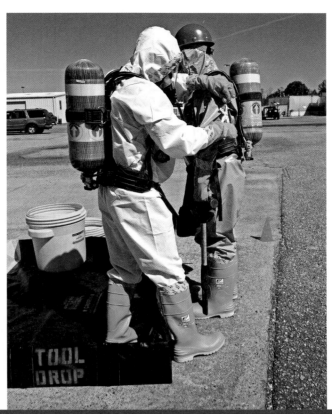

Figure S1.1 Two rescuers in Level B PPE.

chemical suit with the SCBA worn externally (Figure S1.1). Because this level of protective equipment is rarely used by EMS, hospital, and law enforcement personnel, it will only be taught if your service uses this level (see Appendix A: Optional Skills).

USE OF LEVEL C PROTECTIVE EQUIPMENT

Level C PPE is composed of a chemical suit worn with an air-purifying respirator (APR) or with a powered air-purifying respirator (PAPR) (Figure S1.2). It is usually easier for public safety personnel to perform their duties in this level of PPE. The APR (gas mask) requires a fit test, but the hood-type PAPRs do not and many services prefer them for this reason. These respirators do not provide oxygen and so cannot be used in an oxygen-deficient atmosphere. They should not be used in the presence of some gases, especially toxic but odorless gases. The filters lose their effectiveness quickly when exposed to cyanide gas.

APR/PAPRs must have the correct filters for the toxic atmosphere you will be entering. APR/PAPR canister filters are made up of a material that absorbs toxic chemicals and a particulate air filter that will filter particles of 0.3 microns and higher. There are many different kinds of filter canisters made for special situations. The military-type chemical warfare filters are effective against most chemical agents and will filter biological agents and radioactive particles. These NATO-specification filters can be used for most terrorist events. The filters that are made for use in entering clandestine drug laboratories are rated for volatile organic solvents and acids but will also work fairly well for chemical warfare agents, and they also filter small particles. Remember that all filters have an expiration date (usually 5 to 10 years) and a limit for how long they can be used once the seals are removed. Be sure that your filter canister is fresh when you use it. If in doubt, discard it and get a new one.

PAPRs do not increase the work of breathing, like APRs do; however, they are limited by their battery life. There are two types of PAPR batteries. The best is the lithium battery, which has a shelf life of 8 to 10 years and lasts from 8 to 10 hours

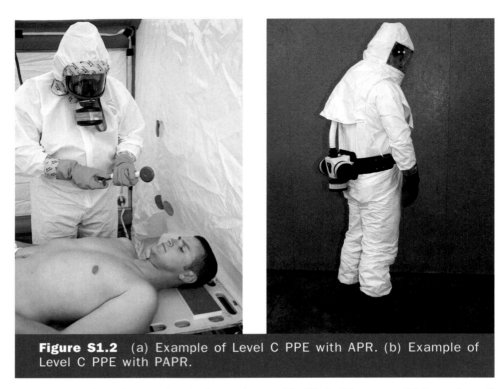

Figure S1.2 (a) Example of Level C PPE with APR. (b) Example of Level C PPE with PAPR.

when new. The other option is the rechargeable Ni-Cad battery, which works well for several hours if it is properly stored and kept adequately charged. However, this maintenance is often difficult to continue, and these batteries are better used for training, not actual disasters. A good plan would be to use Ni-Cads for routine training and drills and use lithium batteries for actual incidents.

Level C PPE does not require as much training to use and is preferred by EMS, hospitals, and law enforcement. The drawback is that Level C PPE should not be worn when the nature of the gas or vapor is not known.

LEVEL C PROTECTIVE EQUIPMENT

Procedure: Putting on Level C with PAPR

You should have a partner to assist you with this.

1 Remove and secure jewelry (including rings, earrings and any body piercings) and other personal items. When possible, remove and secure clothing and don hospital scrub attire or service clothing. Remember that your clothing should be appropriate to the ambient temperature.

2 If you wear eyeglasses, either secure them with a retaining band or tape them in place. Apply antifogging material to the lenses to prevent fogging or condensation when you sweat. Secure long hair. Check your hydration state. It is recommended that you consume 300–500 ml of water. *Remember that the time to visit the bathroom is prior to putting on PPE.* Also, before you don PPE, you should have your baseline vital signs (pulse rate, respiration rate, oral temperature, and blood pressure) taken and recorded. However, even though this is important, there may be emergency situations when you don't have the time to do this.

3 Select appropriate-size PPE. Be sure you know your size before the emergency. Confirm that all components are serviceable: inspect for defects, such as tears or holes, and make sure the PAPR/APR filters (the same filters are used for both) have not expired and are appropriate for the hazard (Figure S1.3). Be sure the batteries are charged or that you have new lithium batteries. Use chemically rated tape to make the seals on your PPE. Follow the manufacturer's recommendations for inspection and donning of the PAPR.

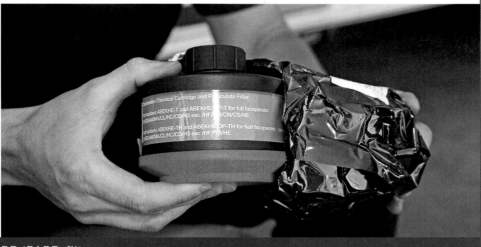

Figure S1.3 Checking APR/PAPR filters.

4 While sitting, remove your footwear if you are going to don chemical boots or if the PPE has integral boots. If you are going to wear shoes make certain they will not puncture the chemical suit.

5 Put on a pair of nitrile undergloves. Do not use latex gloves, as they offer no chemical protection (Figure S1.4).

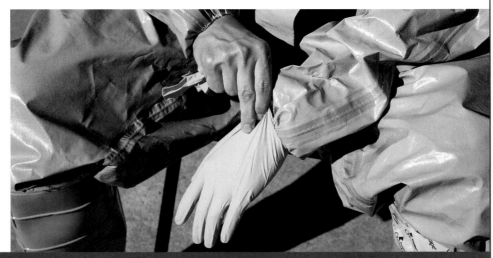

Figure S1.4 Nitrile undergloves.

6 Step into the legs of the suit, pull up the suit to your waist, and then pull on the integral boots or put on chemical boots and tape in place using chemically rated tape. Normally duct tape or paper tape is not used. Make certain to leave a tab so the tape can be easily removed.

7 Finish donning your chemical suit, including the hood. Zip up the suit and seal the seam of the suit with tape, leaving a removable tab. You do not have to tape around the hood (Figure S1.5).

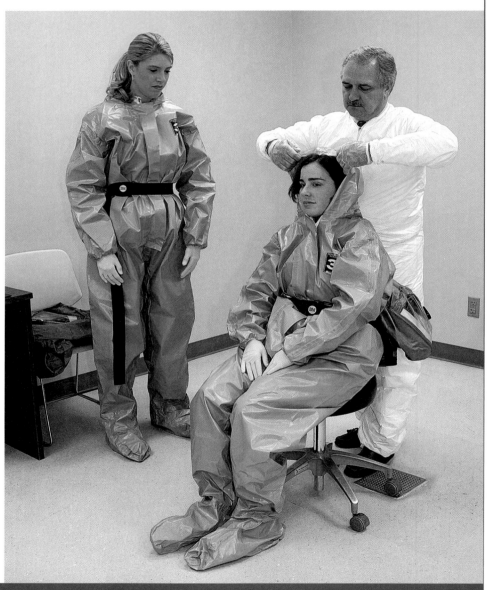

Figure S1.5 Don chemical suit.

8 Put on the PAPR hood (Figure S1.6). Place the PAPR battery and unit around your waist and secure them with the belt so that the unit rides above the buttocks (Figure S1.7). Place the battery in the unit and

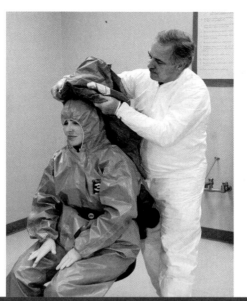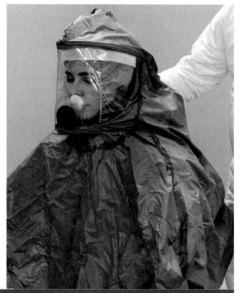

Figure S1.6 (a) Second person places PAPR hood over suit hood. (b) PAPR hood in place.

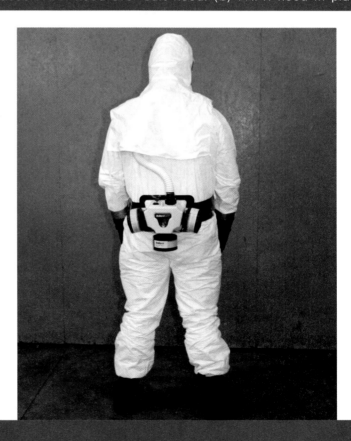

Figure S1.7 PAPR unit in place.

attach the air hose over your shoulder. Activate the unit and confirm airflow. *Make certain the filter seals (caps) are removed* (Figure S1.8). If you fail to remove the filter seals, no air can enter the filter and you will smother. **Deaths have occurred from failure to complete this step.** For this reason, unless absolutely necessary, you should never put on a gas mask while alone.

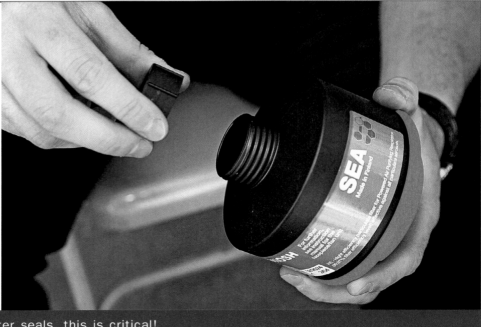

Figure S1.8   Remove filter seals, this is critical!

9   Don the appropriate second pair of gloves and tape in place, leaving a removal tab (Figure S1.9). For chemical incidents, the usual recommendation is one set of nitrile gloves followed by a set of butyl rubber gloves. Otherwise two pairs of nitrile gloves are recommended. Avoid ill-fitting vinyl gloves.

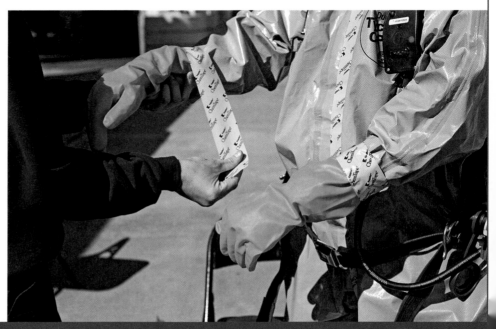

Figure S1.9   Taping butyl gloves.

10   It is wise to tape or attach a knife or shears to your boot (Figure S1.10) so that in an emergency you can get out of your suit without help (the zipper is often in the back).

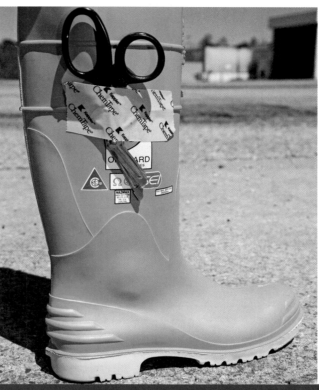

Figure S1.10   Scissors taped to boot.

11   Have someone attach a piece of tape with your name on the sleeve of your suit (Figure S1.11). If multiple agencies are involved, also note the name of your agency on the tape. Always work in pairs. If one partner becomes disabled, the other can bring help.

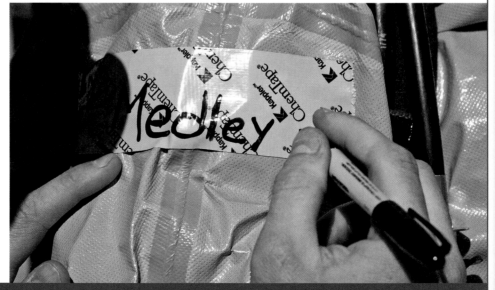

Figure S1.11   Marking identification information on tape.

Procedure: Putting on Level C with APR

You should have a partner to assist you with this.

1 Remove and secure jewelry (including rings, earrings and any body piercings) and other personal items. When possible, remove and secure clothing and don hospital scrub attire or service clothing. Remember that your clothing should be appropriate to the ambient temperature.

2 If you wear eyeglasses, either secure them with a retaining band or tape them in place. Apply antifogging material to the lenses to prevent fogging or condensation when you sweat. Secure long hair. Check your hydration state. It is recommended that you consume 300–500 ml of water. *Remember that the time to visit the bathroom is prior to putting on PPE.* Also, before you don PPE, you should have your baseline vital signs (pulse rate, respiration rate, oral temperature, and blood pressure) taken and recorded. However, even though this is important, there may be emergency situations when you don't have the time to do this.

3 Select appropriate-size PPE. Be sure you know your size before the emergency. Confirm that all components are serviceable: inspect for defects, such as tears or holes, and make sure the PAPR/APR filters (the same filters are used for both) have not expired and are appropriate for the hazard (Figure S1.3). Use chemically rated tape to make the seals on your PPE.

4 While sitting, remove your footwear if you are going to don chemical boots or if your PPE has integral boots. If you are going to wear shoes make certain they will not puncture the chemical suit.

5 Put on a pair of nitrile undergloves. Do not use latex gloves, as they offer no chemical protection (Figure S1.4).

6 Step into the legs of the suit, pull up the suit to your waist and then pull on the integral boots or put on chemical boots and tape them in place using chemically rated tape. Normally duct tape or paper tape is not used. Make certain to leave a tab so that the tape can be easily removed.

7 Finish donning your chemical suit. Zip up the suit and seal the seam of the suit with tape, leaving a removable tab. Do not pull up the hood until after you don the APR mask.

8 Put on the APR mask (Figure S1.12). Attach the filter(s) to the mask. *Make certain the filter seals (caps) are removed. If you fail to remove the filter seals, no air can enter the filter and you will smother.* **Deaths have occurred from failure to complete this step.** For this reason, unless absolutely necessary, you should never put on a gas mask while alone. Grasp the attaching straps and invert them over the outside of the mask. Place the mask on your face, pull the straps over your head, and then securely tighten them. Test to be sure that there is no air leak and that you can breathe with the mask in place. Then pull up the hood and tape it around the mask. Make certain to leave tabs for easy tape removal.

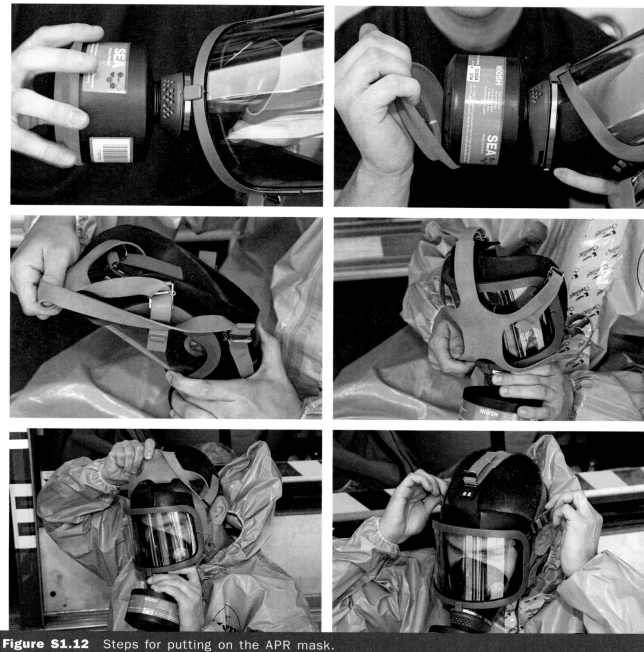

Figure S1.12 Steps for putting on the APR mask.

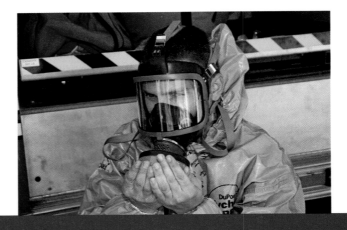

Figure S1.12   (Continued)

9   Don the appropriate second pair of gloves and tape in place leaving a removal tab (Figure S1.9). For chemical incidents, the usual recommendation is one set of nitrile gloves followed by a set of butyl rubber gloves. Otherwise two pairs of nitrile gloves are recommended. Avoid ill-fitting vinyl gloves.

10   It is wise to tape or attach a knife or shears to your boot (Figure S1.10) so that in an emergency you can get out of your suit without help (the zipper is often in the back).

11   Have someone attach a piece of tape with your name on the sleeve of your suit (Figure S1.11). If multiple agencies are involved, also note the name of your agency on the tape. Always work in pairs. If one partner becomes disabled, the other can bring help.

Procedure: Wet Decontamination and Removal of PPE

1   Report to the decontamination area and indicate that you wish to be decontaminated. Ensure that you have adequate breathing air in the SCBA or battery time on the PAPR. If you do not have adequate air or battery time, or if you are in medical distress, indicate this and then emergency procedures should be used to immediately remove the PPE using heavy-duty shears to cut away the PPE (Figure S1.13), followed by emergency decontamination.

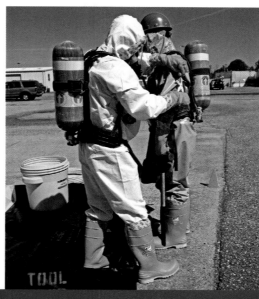

Figure S1.13 Emergency removal of suit.

2 Place any equipment in a plastic HazMat container or in a hazardous waste bag held open by one of the persons assigned to the area (Figure S1.14). Hazardous waste bags are available from HazMat vendors; they are 5 or 6 times as thick as ordinary garbage bags. Continue into the decontamination line as directed. The procedure may vary, depending upon the type of contamination and degree of contamination.

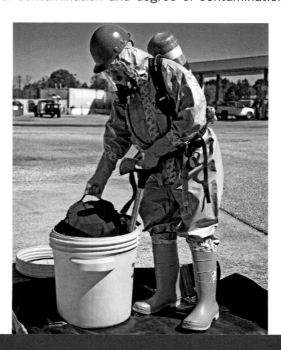

Figure S1.14 HazMat container.

3   Scrub your boots and rinse them (Figure S1.15).

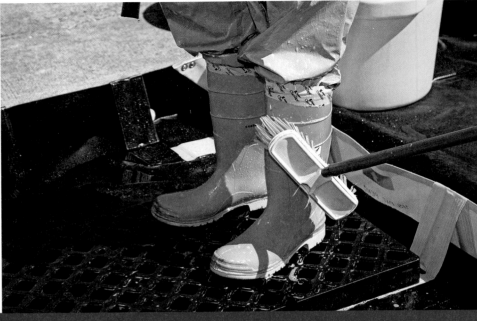

Figure S1.15 Cleaning boots.

4   Proceed to the first wash and rinse to clean and rinse your chemical suit. Scrubbing may be needed on some areas of contamination (Figure S1.16).

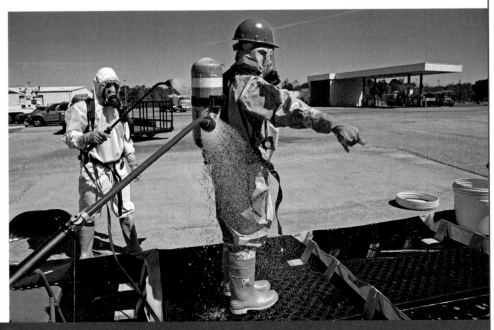

Figure S1.16 Cleaning chemical suit.

5   Proceed to the second and third wash and rinse, as directed.

6   Remove your outer gloves.

7   Assist with the removal of your chemical suit, leaving in place your SCBA or APR (the PAPR will come off with the suit). You may be required to sit for this part of the process (Figure S1.17).

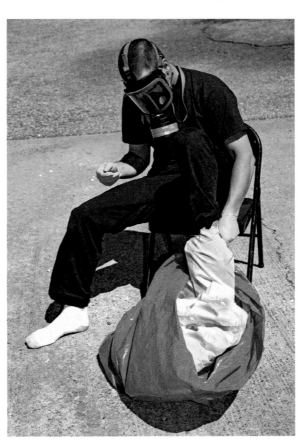

Figure S1.17   Removing chemical suit and placing it in a hazardous waste bag.

8   Remove your next set of gloves.

9   Step out of the chemical suit and boots.

10 Remove your SCBA or APR and place it in the HazMat bag or container (Figure S1.18).

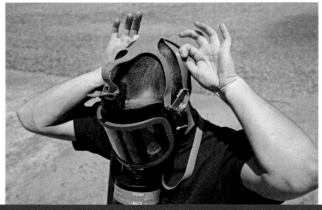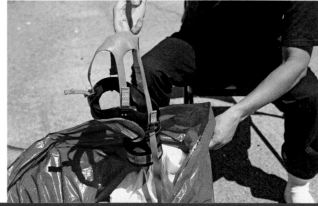

Figure S1.18 Proper removal and disposal of an APR.

11 Remove your inner gloves.

12 Your vital signs are taken and compared against your baseline vital signs. Any abnormalities should be evaluated by EMS personnel. Vital signs that are considered abnormal include a sustained pulse rate of more than 100 bpm after 5 minutes of rest, an oral temperature of 100° Fahrenheit or higher, signs of dehydration such at skin tenting, severe thirst, dizziness, visual difficulties, trembling, nausea, or pale skin (Figure S1.19).

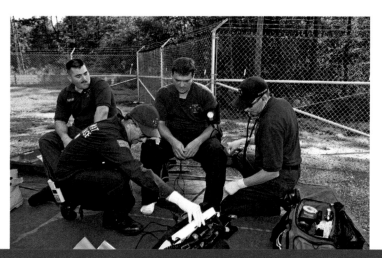

Figure S1.19 EMS personnel taking vital signs.

13 Shower with soap and water.

In some circumstances it may not be possible to perform wet decontamination, and dry decontamination may have to be performed.

Procedure: Dry Decontamination and Removal of PPE

1 Report to the decontamination area and indicate that you wish to be decontaminated.

2 Place any equipment in a plastic HazMat waste bag held open by one of the persons assigned to the area.

3 Continue into the decontamination line as directed.

4 Step into a HazMat waste bag and stand in front of ventilation fan for at least 2 minutes (Figure S1.20).

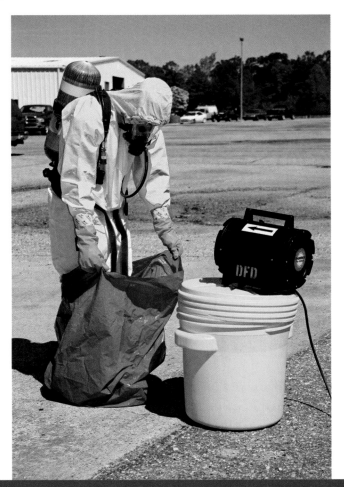

Figure S1.20 Stand in front of fan for at least two minutes.

5 Remove your chemical suit (and PAPR if wearing one) and boots and drop them into the HazMat waste bag.

6 Remove your outer gloves and drop them into the bag, which is then sealed and double-bagged.

7 Remove your APR or SCBA and drop it into a HazMat waste bag that is then sealed and double-bagged.

8 Remove your outer and inner gloves and dispose of them into the appropriate container.

9 Your vital signs are taken and compared against your baseline vital signs. Any abnormalities should be evaluated by EMS personnel. Vital signs that are considered abnormal include a sustained pulse rate of more than 100 bpm after 5 minutes of rest, an oral temperature of 100° Fahrenheit or higher, signs of dehydration such at skin tenting, severe thirst, dizziness, visual difficulties, trembling, nausea, or pale skin.

10 Shower with soap and water as soon as possible.

Want to Know More?

Bibliography

Hawley, C. *Special Operations for Terrorism and HazMat Crimes.* Red Hat Publishing, 2002.

Initial Response to Hazardous Materials Incidents. FEMA, 1992.

Meyer, E. *Chemistry of Hazardous Materials,* 3rd ed. Prentice-Hall, 1998.

Oldfield, K.W. *Emergency Responder Training Manual for the Hazardous Materials Technician,* 2nd ed. Wiley Inter-Science, 2005.

U.S. Army Chemical School. *Domestic Preparedness Training Manual.* 1997.

Varela, J. *Hazardous Materials Handbook.* John Wiley and Sons, 1991.

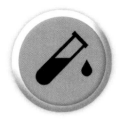 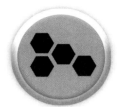 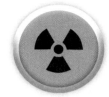 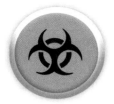 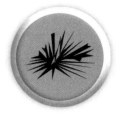

Decontamination of Patients

Chapter Objectives

At the end of this practical skill station you should be able to:

1. Perform wet decontamination of ambulatory patients in the field setting.
2. Perform emergency or expedient wet decontamination of ambulatory patients in the field setting.
3. Perform emergency or expedient dry decontamination of ambulatory patients in the field setting.
4. Perform wet decontamination of nonambulatory patients in the field setting.
5. Perform expedient dry decontamination of nonambulatory patients in the field setting.

Principles of Decontamination of Victims

Physical decontamination of victims is the removal of hazardous substances to prevent or reduce toxicity. Decontamination reduces the amount of toxic material to which the victim is exposed and also reduces the risk of secondary contamination (cross-contamination) of rescuers and others at the scene or the hospital. Time is critical for patients needing decontamination, so all the equipment necessary to perform mass decontamination is best carried in a special vehicle such as a decon trailer or decon truck (Figure S2.1).

There are four methods of decontamination:

1. **Dilution** is the application of large volumes of water to the contaminated patient. This is called wet decontamination. If possible it should be used with soap to make it more effective. If performed soon enough and well enough, this will reduce the concentration of the material on the skin by 99%. If water is not available, dry decontamination can be performed using a combination of absorption, isolation/disposal, and standing in front of a fan. Wet decontamination will then have to be done upon arrival at the emergency department at the hospital.

2. **Absorption** is the use of some substance (fuller's earth, flour, M291 kit, towels, etc.) to blot up the liquid material. This would usually be done when water is not available (dry decontamination) or if there is persistent oily liquid on the skin after showering. It is more commonly used for decontamination of equipment.

3. **Neutralization** is the eliminating of toxicity of a chemical by applying another chemical that reacts with it, such as neutralizing an acid with an alkali. These reactions can produce heat that is potentially as damaging as the original chemical. This method is almost never used on contaminated victims and is more applicable to decontaminating environmental surfaces.

4. **Isolation/disposal** is the separating of the patient from the hazardous substance. This means first removing the patient from the hot zone and then removing the patient's clothing and jewelry. All contaminated items should be properly stored in hazardous material bags.

Combinations of the above methods may be used in any particular situation.

Important Points About Decontamination

1. The most important thing is getting the agent off the skin as quickly as possible:
   a. For vapors, get the victims away from the vapor and then get their clothes off.
   b. If the victims still have liquid on their skin, more decontamination is needed quickly.

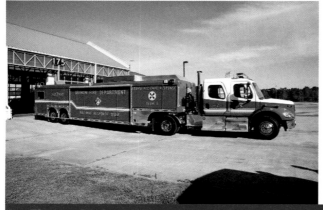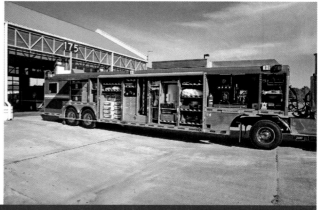

Figure S2.1   Example of a decontamination vehicle. Having all of the equipment together allows rapid response and setup.

2. If available, a soap-and-water shower or a shower with lots of water (high volume, low pressure) is best to get liquids off the skin.
3. Try to respect modesty by separating males and females. The Doff-it kits are helpful because the victims can wear the ponchos during wet decontamination.
4. Try to control run-off water, but victim's lives are the most important priority.
5. Everything that touches contaminated patients (clothes, tissues, towels, rescuers) is contaminated and must be decontaminated or placed in hazardous waste bags.
6. Vomitus may contain the chemical agent, so it should be collected in hazardous waste bags.
7. All contaminated equipment should be cleaned with 5% hypochlorite solution (except for those contaminated with vesicant agents—use soap and water)

Procedure

A. Wet Decontamination of Ambulatory Patients in the Field Setting

1 Identify those persons who are ambulatory and can assist with their decontamination. Have them report to the decontamination area (Figure S2.2).

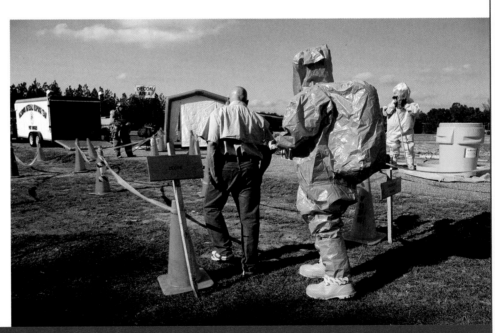

Figure S2.2 Contaminated ambulatory patient being led to decontamination tent.

2 If they have open wounds, cover the wounds with dry bandages to prevent further contamination of the wounds as the clothing is removed.

3 Have them remove their clothing, jewelry, and other items, including footwear and underwear, and place them in appropriate hazardous material bags that are labeled with the patient's name (Doff-it kits are good here). If at all possible, separate male and female patients during decontamination to respect modesty. You should be in Level B attire unless it has been determined that Level C is adequate (Figure S2.3).

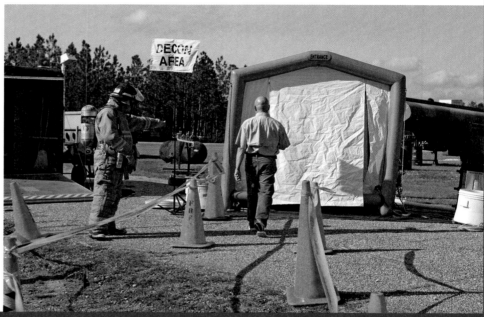

Figure S2.3   Patient entering a decontamination tent to remove clothes and shower.

4 Have the patients shower with soap and water, paying close attention to their hair, hands, face, and body creases and folds (Figure S2.4).

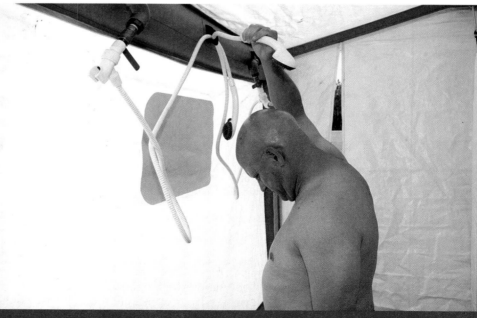

Figure S2.4   Patient showering after placing clothes in hazardous materials bag.

5 Have them put on disposable paper coveralls (or other temporary clothing) and move to a safe area (cold zone) (Figure S2.5).

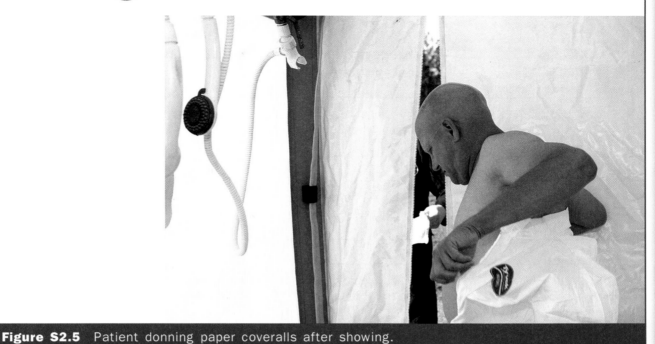

Figure S2.5 Patient donning paper coveralls after showing.

6 Perform patient assessment and emergency treatment at this time. You can usually do this while wearing your usual uniform (Level D), but some prefer to wear Level C attire if the agent was particularly toxic (Figure S2.6). Responders who have been in the hot or warm zones must go through decontamination and leave their contaminated equipment before entering the cold zone.

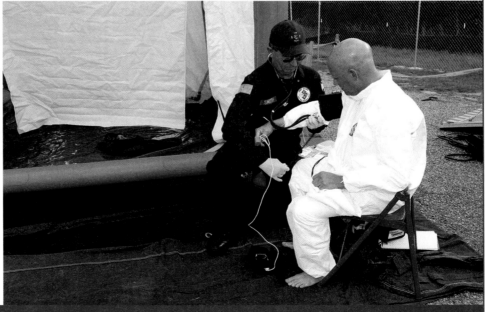

Figure S2.6 After the patient has showered, rescuers can perform assessment wearing Level D attire.

7   Transport patients to the hospital or other appropriate facility.

B. Emergency (Expedient) Wet Decontamination of Ambulatory Patients in the Field Setting

1   Identify those persons who are ambulatory and can assist with their decontamination.

2   If they have open wounds, cover the wounds with dry bandages to prevent further contamination of the wounds as the clothing is removed.

3   Have them remove their clothing, jewelry, and other items, including footwear and underwear, and place them in appropriate hazardous material bags that are labeled with the patient's name (use Doff-it kit if available). If at all possible, separate male and female patients during decontamination to respect modesty. You should be in Level B attire unless it has been determined that Level C is adequate.

4   Use any source of water available to wash (rinse, if no soap) the patients down. A full minute of water application is recommended. Have them wash their hands thoroughly in the water flow. You should be in Level B or C attire (Figure S2.7).

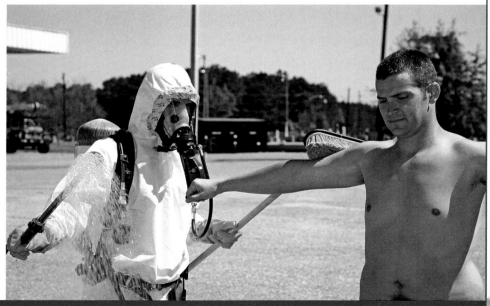

Figure S2.7   If no decontamination facility is available, any source of water can be used for wet decontamination.

5 Have them put on disposable paper coveralls or other temporary clothing and move to the cold zone.

6 Perform patient assessment and emergency treatment. Because this decontamination is not as effective as showering, you should perform the assessment while wearing Level C attire to prevent cross-contamination (Figure S2.8). Responders who have been in the hot or warm zones must not enter the cold zone until they have been decontaminated and left their contaminated equipment.

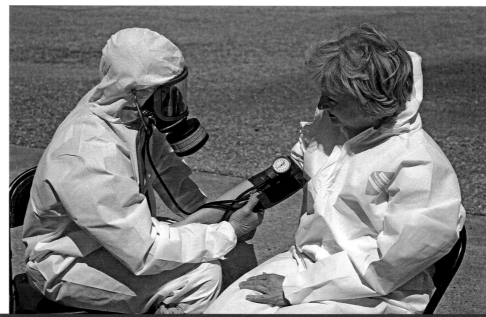

Figure S2.8 Because expedient wet decontamination is not as effective as a shower, rescuers should wear Level C attire while performing assessment.

7 Upon arrival at a hospital or other facility, have the patients shower with soap and water, paying close attention to their hair, hands, face, and body creases and folds.

C. Emergency Dry Decontamination of Ambulatory Patients in the Field Setting (When No Water Is Available)

1 While wearing Level B or C attire, identify those who are ambulatory and can assist with their decontamination.

2

If they have open wounds, cover the wounds with dry bandages to prevent further contamination of the wounds as the clothing is removed (Figure S2.9).

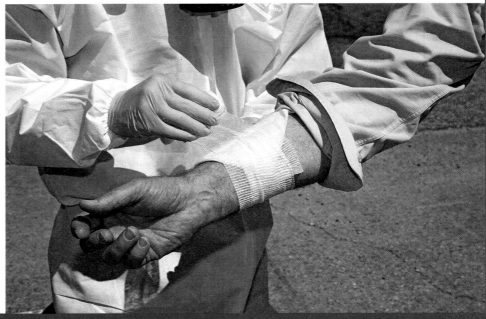

Figure S2.9 To prevent further contamination of the wound, a patient's open wound should be covered with a dry dressing before the patient's contaminated clothing is removed.

3

Have them remove their clothing, footwear, underwear, and personal items. Either leave these items in place or place them in a hazardous material bag labeled with the patient's name (use Doff-it kit if available).

4

Manually brush off any obvious contaminated material from the patient's body.

5

If there is liquid on the skin, it may be absorbed by fuller's earth or flour and then wiped off with a pad or towel. An M291 pad could also be used.

6 Move to the second station and, if available, use a ventilation fan for 2 minutes to remove any gaseous and particulate matter (Figure S2.10).

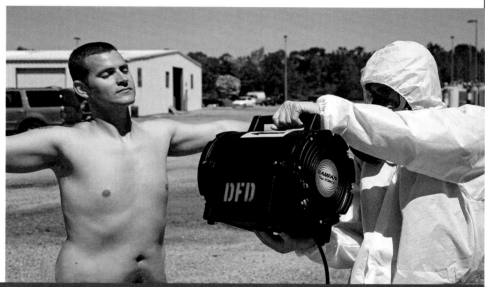

Figure S2.10 If water is not available, contaminated patients should stand in front of a fan for 2 minutes to remove gaseous and particulate matter.

7 Have the patients put on paper coveralls with a hood, surgical mask, and disposable gloves (if these supplies are available) (Figure S2.11) and move to the cold zone.

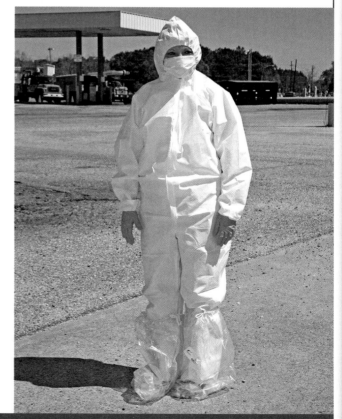

Figure S2.11 Until the patient can have wet decontamination it is best to have them wear paper coveralls with a hood, surgical mask, and disposable gloves. This helps prevent cross-contamination of rescuers.

8 While wearing Level C attire, EMS personnel in the cold zone perform patient assessment and emergency treatment.

9 Upon arrival at a hospital or other facility, have the patients shower with soap and water, paying close attention to their hair, hands, face, and body creases and folds.

D. Wet Decontamination of the Nonambulatory Patient in the Field Setting

1 Personnel in the appropriate protective clothing (usually Level A or B) should find those persons who are alive but not ambulatory. The rescuers should remove them from the scene using a long backboard or other improvised stretcher (Figure S2.12). Only lifesaving medical treatment (airway management, bleeding control, use of NAAK) is performed at this time. Victims who are unresponsive with no pulse should be left on-scene at this time.

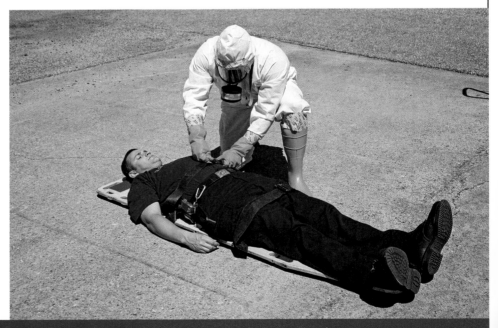

Figure S2.12 Use load-and-go techniques to move all nonambulatory patients.

2 Once you have removed the patient from the hot zone, you may immobilize obvious fractures and cover any wounds with dry bandages to prevent further contamination of the wounds as the clothing is removed.

3 At the first decontamination station, place the patient and backboard on the portable roller system and cut clothing away, log-rolling the patient as needed to accomplish this. Discard clothing into a hazardous material receptacle and personal items into labeled hazardous material bags to further limit cross-contamination. Persons working the decontamination line should wear Level B protective clothing. If tests have shown that it is appropriate, Level C protective clothing can be used (Figure S2.13).

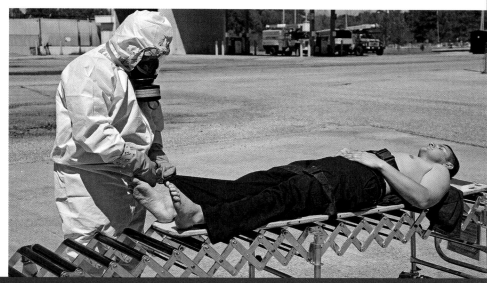

Figure S2.13 At the first station, remove the clothes and place them in HazMat bags. Rescuers should wear Level B or C attire.

4 Move the patient to the second station and use a water source to first rinse, then wash with soap, paying attention to hair, hands, and body creases and folds. Rinse again and also rinse the backboard (Figure S2.14). Contaminated wounds may be carefully cleaned and dressed at this time.

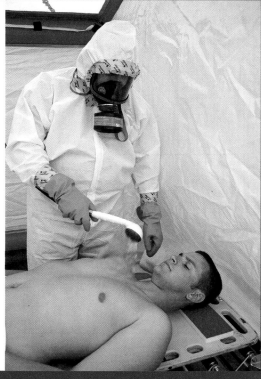

Figure S2.14 At the second station, carefully wash and rinse the patients. Wounds can be dressed at this time.

5   Move the patient to the end of the decontamination line, place the patient on a clean stretcher, cover with a sheet, and move the patient to the cold zone. EMS personnel in the cold zone may now perform assessment and emergency care of the patient. It should be safe to do this wearing Level D attire (Figure S2.15). Responders who have been in the hot or warm zone cannot enter the cold zone until they have been decontaminated and left their contaminated equipment.

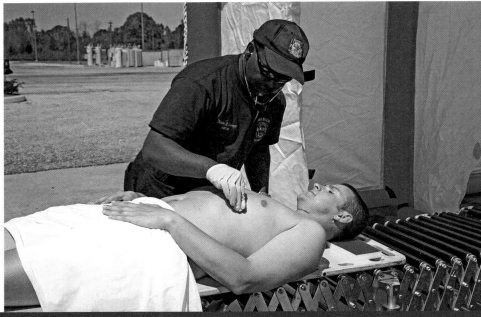

Figure S2.15   After the patients have been washed, you may move them to the cold zone, where they can be assessed by EMTs wearing Level D attire.

E. Dry Decontamination of the Nonambulatory Patient in the Field Setting

1   Personnel in the appropriate protective clothing (usually Level A or B) should find those persons who are alive but not ambulatory. The rescuers should remove them from the scene using a long backboard or other improvised stretcher. Only lifesaving medical treatment (airway management, bleeding control, and use of NAAK) is performed at this time. Victims who are unresponsive with no pulse should be left on-scene at this time.

2   Once out of the danger area, you may immobilize obvious fractures and control any visible serious bleeding. If the patient has open wounds, cover the wounds with dry bandages to prevent further contamination of the wounds as the clothing is removed.

3   At the first decontamination station, place the patient and backboard on the portable roller system (if available) and cut clothing away, log-rolling the patient as needed to accomplish this. Discard clothing into a hazardous material receptacle and personal items into labeled hazardous material bags to further limit the spread of contamination. Persons working the decontamination line should wear Level B protective clothing. If tests show that it is appropriate, Level C protective clothing can be used.

4   Move to the second station and (if available) use a ventilation fan for 2 minutes to remove any gaseous and particulate matter (Figure S2.16). Brush off any obvious contaminated material. Liquid material on the skin can be removed by using fuller's earth, flour, or the M291 kit and then wiping with a towel. Log-roll the patient as needed to remove contaminants.

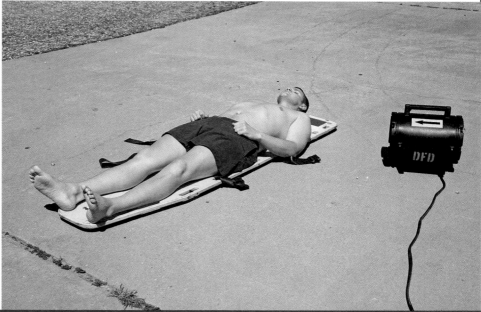

Figure S2.16   At the second station, keep the patient in front of a fan for 2 minutes. Remove any liquid contaminant with a towel or with fuller's earth, flour, or an M291 kit and then a towel.

5   Move the patient to the end of the decontamination line, place the patient on a clean stretcher, cover with a sheet, and move the patient to the cold zone. EMS personnel in the cold zone may now perform a thorough assessment and emergency care of the patient. They should do this while wearing Level C attire.

6   As soon as possible, use wet decontamination techniques to ensure contamination control.

PRACTICAL SKILLS: 2

Want to Know More?

Bibliography

Copenhaver, R.C. *Agent Characteristics and Toxicology First Aid and Special Treatment.* Oak Ridge National Laboratories, 1997.

Jensen, R.A. *Mass Fatality and Casualty Incidents: a Field Guide.* CRC Press, 1999.

MacArthur, S. *Preparing for Mass-Casualty Incidents: Hospital Readiness for Biological, Chemical, and Radiological Disorders.* Opus Communications, 2002.

Managing Hazardous Materials Incidents: Medical Management Guidelines for Acute Chemical Exposure, Health and Human Services, 2002.

Marrs, T.C. *Chemical Warfare Agents: Toxicology and Treatment.* John Wiley and Sons, 1996.

Roy, M.J. *Physician's Guide to Terrorist Attack.* Humana Press, 2004.

U.S. Army. Chemical and Biological Countermeasures Course, 1997.

Internet Sources

Decontamination of chemical casualties:

www.wnh.org/CHEMCASU/08Decontamination.html

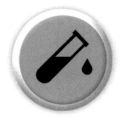 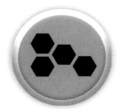 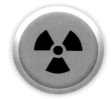 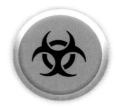 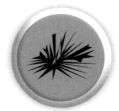

Use of the Nerve Agent Antidote Kit (NAAK)

Chapter Objectives

At the end of this practical skill station you should be able to:

1. **Recognize the signs and symptoms of nerve agent poisoning.**
2. **Recognize a potential nerve agent attack scene.**
3. **Be able to triage nerve agent attack patients into groups with mild, moderate, or severe poisoning.**
4. **From presenting signs and symptoms, be able to decide on the number of NAAKs each patient should receive.**
5. **Correctly use the atropine, 2-PAM, and diazepam (CANA) autoinjectors.**

Nerve agents (organophosphates) are among the deadliest of the chemical agents. They are usually dispersed in the form or a liquid or gas (vapor). They usually enter the body by inhalation or by being absorbed through the skin and eyes. Nerve agents are absorbed rapidly, and the effects are felt immediately upon entry into the body. Nerve agent poisoning can be mild, moderate, or severe. The symptoms vary depending on route of exposure.

GAS EXPOSURE

The general symptoms of exposure to a nerve agent in gas form can be remembered by the acronym "DUMBELS": diarrhea, urination, miosis, bronchoconstriction (dyspnea, wheezing), emesis (vomiting), lacrimation, and salivation. Some prefer the acronym "SLUDGEM": salivation, lacrimation, urination, diarrhea, gastric upset, emesis, and miosis (Table S3.1).

Table S3.1 Range of Symptoms for Nerve Agent Gas Exposure	
Level of Exposure	**Symptoms**
Mild symptoms (require no antidote kit unless they worsen)	Eyes: pinpoint pupils, dim vision, and headache Nose: runny nose Mouth: salivation, possibly drooling Lungs: tightness in the chest or shortness of breath
Moderate symptoms (require one or two antidote kits)	The above plus worsening shortness of breath, weakness, and/or nausea, vomiting, diarrhea
Severe symptoms (require three antidote kits plus diazepam)	Seizing, apnea (stops breathing), cyanosis (blue color to skin), unconsciousness

LIQUID EXPOSURE

Exposure to a nerve agent in liquid form is a more severe hazard, but symptoms may be delayed for several hours. If there is a history of exposure to a liquid nerve agent and the patient has muscle fasciculation (twitching) and sweating at the exposure site, then this is a serious exposure and the patient should be treated and decontaminated immediately.

RECOGNIZE THE SCENE

You should recognize a scene with the potential for nerve agent contamination:
- Bombings
- All explosions of unknown origin
- Suspicious circumstances with an unknown substance, particularly one received by mail or package
- Reports of multiple persons down, especially if seizures are reported
- A scene where a large number of people with the same symptoms (difficulty breathing, tears, coughing, wheezing, etc.) are exiting a building or structure

Before entering such a scene you should take appropriate self-protection steps, ensuring that you have respiratory protection and are wearing at least Level C PPE. It is best if someone (usually a HazMat team) enters the scene and identifies the chemical agent using a chemical agent detector (See Chapter 2 and Practical Skills: 5). While this is going on, your first step is to immediately remove the ambulatory patients from the decontaminated area, have the patients remove their contaminated clothes, decontaminate the patients, perform a brief medical evaluation, and then treat the patients. Victims that are so severely poisoned that they are not ambulatory may have to have the antidotes injected through their clothes before they are removed from the scene.

In a suspected nerve agent attack, the minimum evacuation distance from the scene is 300 feet upwind or 6,000 feet downwind. Nerve agent vapors are heavier than air, so they will accumulate in low areas like drainage ditches, but they will also be blown by the wind.

Unless you have already identified the delivery device for the nerve agent, you should not allow the ambulatory patients to take handbags, briefcases, backpacks, shopping bags, baby carriages, or other articles that could conceal a delivery device for the nerve agent. Because this may separate victims from their identification, they should be tagged with their personal information as soon as possible. If Doff-it kits are available, the patients can put their personal items (jewelry and identification) in the sealed hazardous material bag and take it with them. The contents of the bags will have to be decontaminated or disposed of at some point.

Patients with only mild symptoms (pinpoint pupils, dim vision, headache, runny nose, salivation, possibly drooling, tightness in the chest, or shortness of breath) may be observed for at least 1 hour to see if they worsen. If they worsen, they should receive one NAAK (Note: the NAAK consists of one atropine injector and one 2-PAM injector).

Patients with moderate symptoms (the above symptoms, plus worsening shortness of breath, weakness, and/or nausea, vomiting, diarrhea) should receive one or two NAAKs as soon as their contaminated clothes are removed. The injections can be given through their clothes if there is any delay in getting the patient to the decontamination area. These patients should be observed for possible worsening.

Patients with liquid exposure and any symptoms should immediately receive two NAAKs and have continued observation for worsening.

Patients with severe symptoms (seizing, apnea, cyanosis, unconsciousness) should immediately receive three NAAKs plus diazepam (CANA injector). The autoinjectors will work through two layers of clothes or a chemical suit.

Children with severe symptoms:
2–7 years old—give one NAAK
8–14 years old—give two NAAKs

The NAAK contains two components: the atropine autoinjector (2 mg) and the pralidoxime or 2-PAM autoinjector (600 mg) (Figure S3.1). The ATNAA or

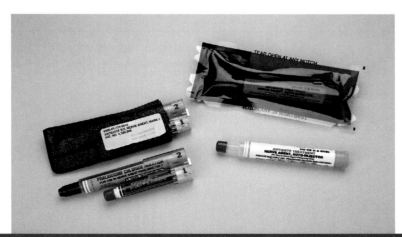

Figure S3.1　The NAAK (left) contains two components: the atropine autoinjector (2 mg) and the pralidoxime or 2-PAM autoinjector (600 mg). The ATNAA (right) Contains both antidotes in the same injector.

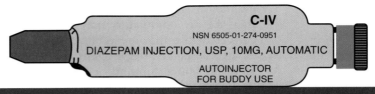

Figure S3.2 Example of a CANA (diazepam) autoinjector found in Mark II Nerve Agent Antidote Kits.

DuoDote has both the atropine and 2-PAM in the same syringe. DuoDote has only recently been made available to civilians. Some kits may also contain a diazepam or CANA injector (Figure S3.2). You must be able to identify the symptoms and signs that require use of the NAAK, select the appropriate dosage, and administer the atropine, pralidoxime, and diazepam as required.

---

1 Locate the NAAK, open the kit, and confirm the dosage and expiration date on the kit. Remove the autoinjector clip using your nondominant hand, and hold it at eye level with the larger 2-PAM autoinjector on top (Figure S3.3a).

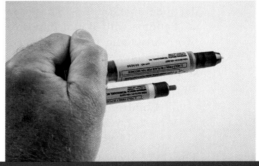

Figure S3.3a Hold the autoinjector clip with the larger 2-PAM autoinjector on top. Hold at eye level with the nondominant hand.

---

2 Grasp the smaller (atropine) autoinjector with the thumb and first two fingers of your dominant hand (like holding a pen or pencil) (Figure S3.3b).

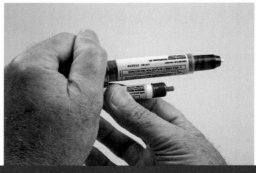

Figure S3.3b Grasp the smaller atropine autoinjector with the thumb and first two fingers of your dominant hand (as if you were holding a pencil).

PRACTICAL SKILLS: 3

3 Pull the atropine autoinjector out of the clip with a smooth motion (Figure S3.3c). Do not cover or hold the green (needle) end of the autoinjector. If you do press on the green end, you may unintentionally inject yourself.

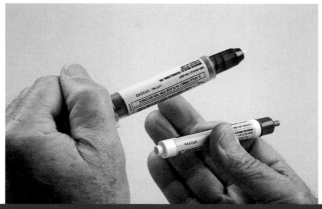

Figure S3.3c   Pull the autoinjector out of the clip with a smooth motion.

4 Close the fingers of your hand. This will place the injector in the correct position to inject (Figure S3.3d).

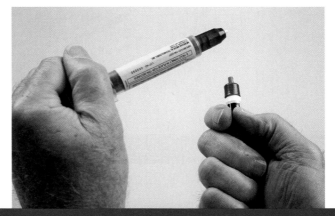

Figure S3.3d   Close your fingers around the injector to put it in the correct position to inject.

5 The injection site is the mid lateral thigh (one hand width below the hip joint and one hand width above the knee) (Figure S3.3e). In very thin patients you can use the upper outer quadrant of the buttocks

(Figure S3.4). To inject the atropine, place the green tip at a 90-degree angle (perpendicular) to the injection site.

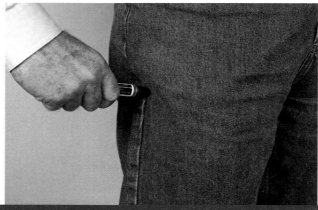

Figure S3.3e The lateral thigh injection site is one handwidth below hip joint and one handwidth above the knee.

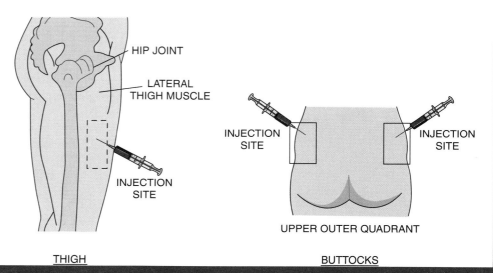

Figure S3.4 For thin patients, you can use the upper outer quadrant of the buttocks.

6 Press (do not jab) the autoinjector firmly against the site until the needle is triggered (clicks). The needle will automatically inject the medication into the muscle. Hold for 10 seconds, counting "One one-thousand,..." etc. while the autoinjector injects its contents.

7 Carefully remove the autoinjector and place it in a sharps container, as the needle will be exposed.

8 Repeat the same process with the pralidoxime (2-PAM) injector, which has a gray end cap and the number 2 (Figure S3.5).

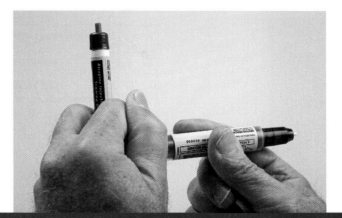

Figure S3.5a Hold the autoinjector clip with the larger 2-PAM autoinjector on top. Hold at eye level with your nondominant hand.

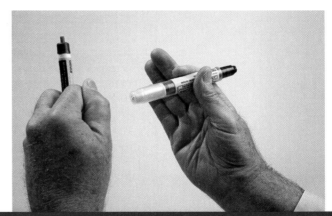

Figure S3.5b Grasp the 2-PAM autoinjector with the thumb and first two fingers of your dominant hand (as if you were holding a pencil).

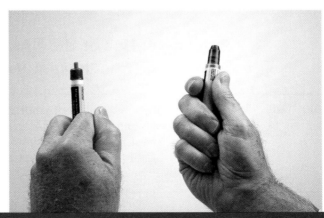

Figure S3.5c Pull the autoinjector out of the clip with a smooth motion. Close your fingers around the injector to put it in the correct position to inject.

9 Make certain you mark the date, time, and amount of drug administered on the patient's triage tag. There are triage tags available for just this purpose (Figure S3.6).

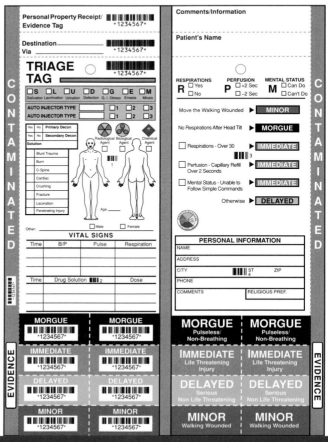

Figure S3.6 Example of a triage tag with a place to record atropine and 2-PAM injections.
Photo: Disaster Management Systems, Inc., www.TriageTags.com.

10 Repeat the entire procedure if you are giving two kits.

Procedure: Use of the NAAK on Patients with Severe Symptoms (Nonambulatory)

1 If the patient is still in the hot (danger) zone, roll the patient onto his or her side and inject the atropine and 2-PAM into the mid-thigh area. Do not kneel beside the patient, because kneeling on contaminated ground may force the chemical agent into your protective suit. Either bend over or squat beside the patient to inject the antidotes.

2 Inject the atropine and 2-PAM following the same procedure as above.

3 Repeat Steps 1 and 2 until you have given three kits (child age 2–7—one kit; child age 8–14—two kits).

4 If you have an autoinjector for diazepam or CANA (convulsants antidote for nerve agent), remove it from its packaging (not for use in children under 14).

5 Grasp the diazepam autoinjector (refer to Figure S3-2) with your dominant hand with the black (needle) end extending beyond your thumb and two fingers (like you held the atropine and 2-PAM injectors—refer to Figure S3-3d).

6 With your other hand, pull the safety cap from the autoinjector base. The injector is now armed. DO NOT touch the black end, because you may unintentionally inject yourself.

7 Position the black end of the injector against the patient's mid-thigh injection site at a 90-degree angle.

8 Apply firm, even pressure (not a jabbing motion) against the site until the needle is triggered (clicks). The needle will penetrate the patient's clothing and automatically inject the medication into the muscle. Hold for 10 seconds, counting "One one-thousand,..., etc., while the autoinjector injects its contents.

9 Carefully remove the autoinjector and place it in a sharps container, as the needle will be exposed.

10 Up to three diazepam injectors may have to be used if the patient continues to have seizures. Wait 10 minutes between injections for convulsions to subside. Diazepam is a sedative, and once it has been given the patient must be monitored closely to be sure he or she does not hypoventilate.

11 These patients should be removed from the danger area, their clothing should be removed, and wet decontamination should be performed if possible. Once decontamination is performed and an IV is started, seizures are better managed with IV diazepam.

12 These patients frequently require aggressive airway support, suctioning, and endotracheal intubation.

Table S3.2 Nerve Agent Exposure Treatment Chart

Symptoms	Number of Mark 1 Kits	Additional Treatment
Ambulatory patients with history of exposure to vapor or liquid and no symptoms	None.	Observe for up to 18 hours for liquid exposure and 1 hour for vapor.
Ambulatory patients with rhinorrhea and miosis and history of exposure to vapor	None.	Observe for increasing dyspnea; if improved, no treatment required.
Ambulatory patients with a history of liquid exposure with localized fasciculation and sweating	One.	Continue to observe and give additional atropine as needed to control symptoms.
Moderate exposure to vapor with continuing dyspnea and/or nausea and vomiting, muscle weakness	One to two (if two NAAKs are given, the victim should also receive one CANA injector of 10 mg diazepam).	Continue to observe and give additional atropine to control dyspnea; administer oxygen and control airway.
Seizing, apnea, post ictal collapse or effects in two or more body systems	Three. Repeat atropine in 2-mg increments as needed. If seizing or post ictal, administer one CANA injector IM. Consider 2–5 mg diazepam IV for seizures. **Children with severe symptoms: 2–7 years old —** 1 NAAK **8–14 years old —** 2 NAAKs	Intubate and ventilate as needed; large amounts of atropine may be needed.

Want to Know More?

Bibliography

National Institute of Justice. *EMS Technician Training, Nerve Agent Antidote Training Series.* 2000.

Internet Sources

www.nbc-med.org/SiteContent/MedRef/OnlineRef/FieldManuals/fm8_285/PART_I/chapter2.htm

ACT Fast Course

http://emc.ornl.gov/CSEPPweb/Act_Fast_2001/Student%20Manual.pdf

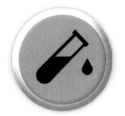 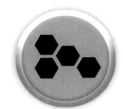 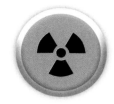 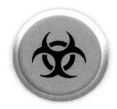 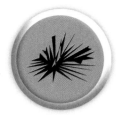

Demonstration of the Anthrax Test Kit

Chapter Objective

At the conclusion of this station, you should be familiar with commercially available or locally assembled test kits to rule out anthrax spores or other biological agents.

You may be called upon to identify whether a powder is anthrax or just a hoax. There are several commercial kits (Figures S4.1 and S4.2) with which to do this, and some manufacturers offer training kits for their tests. The individual tests are relatively inexpensive, but you can also obtain the components of a useful anthrax screening test at your local pharmacy. The active components of the test are simply urine pH and protein test strips (Figure S4.3).

HazMat teams are usually called to evaluate unknown powders but in many places this is done by law enforcement. Remember that this is only a screening test. You should save samples for evidence and for further testing. The value of the test is that if the substance is suspicious for anthrax (you do not have to have positives on all six parts to be suspicious), you will know to quarantine the area until more sophisticated tests can be done to confirm your screening test. If the test is completely negative for anthrax, you would still send a sample for further testing and save a sample for evidence, but you would only need to clean the area, not quarantine it.

Procedure: Use of the Anthrax Test Kit

1   You should identify the situation (suspicious unknown powder) as one requiring an initial field test for a biological agent.

2   Obtain the appropriate kit and assemble the parts before approaching the suspicious powder.

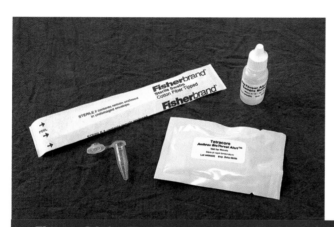
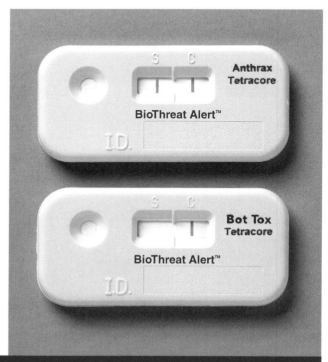

Figure S4.1   The Tetracore Anthrax Biothreat Alert kit is a simple-to-use antigen-antibody test kit that signals a positive test by two pink lines on the test strip.
Photos: Alexeter Technologies, Wheeling, IL.

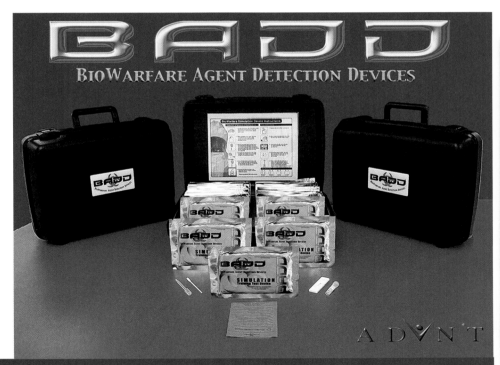

Figure S4.2 advnt Biotechnologies' BioWarfare Agent Detection Device is also an antigen-antibody test kit with test strips that are easy to read.
Photos: www.baddbox.com

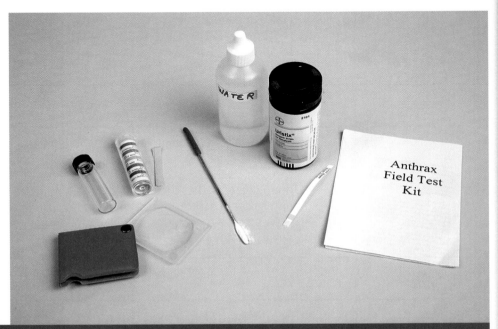

Figure S4.3 Components of a homemade anthrax test kit. Note the white powder on the tip of the spatula.

3

You should select and put on the appropriate PPE (at least Level C). Use of the test requires fine motor use of your hands, so you should choose nitrile gloves rather than butyl rubber.

Preparation of kit. Get everything ready before you start collecting the sample. Get out the following:
- Three glass vials
- One pH test strip
- One protein test strip
- Container of water
- Spatula

4

Using the spatula, fill each of the two vials about half full with the unknown powder. Replace the caps and seal the vials with biohazard tape. Preserve one vial as evidence and the other for confirmatory tests.

5

Observe the unknown powder. The finer the texture and the whiter the powder, the greater the likelihood that it is anthrax spores. A yellow or tan powder would indicate a higher content of the growth medium, so the substance would be less pathogenic. The finer the powder, the greater the possibility the powder is a pathogenic grade of anthrax spores.

6

Collect one spatula of the powder and place it into the third dry glass vial. Replace the top and shake the vial vigorously for 15 seconds. If the powder settles out in the bottom of the vial quickly, it is unlikely to be anthrax. If the powder is suspended in the air after shaking, it is more likely to be anthrax.

7

Fill the vial about half full with water. Invert the vial several times (do not shake yet). Observe the powder. If it completely dissolves and the solution is clear, it is unlikely to be anthrax. If it leaves a heavy precipitate in the bottom of the vial, it has a slight chance of being anthrax, but not a pathogenic grade. If it is suspended in the water and leaves the water with a slightly cloudy appearance, it is more likely to be a pathogenic grade of anthrax.

8

Now shake the vial vigorously for 15 seconds. If foam appears or the solution becomes cloudy, there is a good probability that it contains anthrax.

9 Dip the pH test strip in the solution. Wait 30 seconds and compare the results to the chart on the bottle. If the pH is between 5 and 9 there is a possibility it may contain anthrax. If it is either below 5 or above 9 it is unlikely to be anthrax.

10 Dip the protein test strip in the solution. Wait for 30 seconds and compare the results to the chart on the bottle. The presence of protein indicates a possibility of anthrax. If the protein test is negative, it is unlikely to contain anthrax.

11 The powder is (95%) likely to be anthrax if:
  a. It is very fine and white.
  b. It suspends in the air when shaken.
  c. It suspends in water but does not dissolve.
  d. When shaken in water it becomes cloudy and forms a foam.
  e. It has a pH between 5 and 9.
  f. It is positive for protein.

12 A sample of the powder should be given to the public health department for more sophisticated tests.*

13 If there is a strong possibility the powder is anthrax spores, you should quarantine the area and you must perform decontamination before removing your PPE.

*Note: Although testing for biological agents is still an evolving technology, there are more specific biological detectors that can be used in the field. There are presently two methods. One method uses an antigen-antibody reaction to identify the biological agent. The reaction causes a color change, and each test is specific to one particular agent. The other is a polymerase chain reaction in which the detection device concentrates the DNA from a sample and tags it with a fluorescent dye. An optical reader is then used to determine if the specific biological agent is present. These devices will detect anthrax, tularemia, *Yersinia pestis* (bubonic plague), ricin, staphylococcal enterotoxin B, and *Clostridium botulinum.* In the field setting, they would be most useful for testing a suspicious powder for anthrax or for testing for an aerosol attack of ricin or staphylococcal enterotoxin B. As of this writing they are still evolving and are expensive, but they hold promise for the future.

Want to Know More?

Bibliography

National Institute of Justice. *COBRA Training.* 2003.

Internet Sources

The Guide for the Selection of Biological Agent Detection Equipment for Emergency First Responders, DHS March 2005. The guide, produced for the Department of Homeland Security (DHS), does not make recommendations. It provides you with ways to compare and contrast commercially available biological detection equipment. After registering at the website, type in "DHS AND guide" in the search box. Click on the link to the Bioagent Detector Guide. www.rkb.mipt.org.

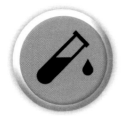 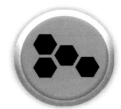 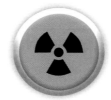 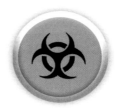 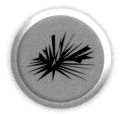

Demonstration of Chemical Agent Detectors

Chapter Objective

At the conclusion of this station, you should be familiar with the different types of chemical detectors available.

CHEMICAL TEST EQUIPMENT

There are multiple types of chemical detectors. Some can only be used to identify the chemical agent, and others are used to determine the concentration of the agent once it is known. Some can do both. This is an area of rapidly expanding technology, and devices will change in the coming years. There are already so many different devices available they cannot all be shown. We will show an example of the different types. If you are interested in a review of all the current chemical detectors available, see *The Guide for the Selection of Chemical Agent and Toxic Industrial Material Detection Equipment for Emergency First Responders*. The link is in the Internet Sources at the end of this chapter.

First responders should know how to notify the local HazMat or Military Civilian Support Team and ask them to assist in identification and management of threat. The most important thing about use of chemical agent detectors is that you *must* be trained in their use and this training *must* occur before you attempt to use one in an emergency situation. The manufacturer's recommendations should be followed in all cases. The procedures may vary from those shown here, depending on the type instrumentation used by your service. Instruments can range from electronic instrumentation using photoionization detectors, colorimetric tests such as the M8/M9 or M256 kits, commercial colorimetric detection kits, or other types of instrumentation.

VOLATILE ORGANIC COMPOUNDS (VOC)

Volatile organic compounds (VOCs) are common and found almost everywhere. They are contained in many household cleaning products, paints, nail polish, nail polish remover, even underarm deodorant. Although they are considered a health risk, in the small quantities you would normally be exposed to during your daily routine (picking up the dry cleaning, putting gasoline in the lawn mower) you are not in danger. Volatile organic compounds are important, not only because they may be present in high concentrations in illegal drug labs, but also because these substances will give false positives when you are using some chemical agent detectors. All positives should be treated as positives until proven to be false, but if you are in an area with especially poor air quality, a high concentration of ozone, many internal combustion engines running, or other fires burning, you can expect a higher ratio of false positives than in an environmentally clean area.

PHOTOIONIZATION CHEMICAL GAS DETECTORS

Photoionization detectors (PIDs) use the response of chemicals to light as a detection method. These devices are accurate and are used not only for identifying chemical agents but also for measuring levels of oxygen, flammable or explosive gases, and volatile organic compounds. The M8A1 automatic chemical agent alarm, the most common chemical agent detector used by the National Guard and the military (though being replaced by the ACADA), is a PID but has been limited to detect only the nerve agents.

Many clandestine drug laboratory settings and other emergency settings such as confined spaces may have an oxygen-deficient atmosphere. These places must routinely be tested for adequate oxygen levels before using an APR/PAPR. APR/PAPRs do not provide you with an adequate air supply; they merely filter impurities/toxins out of the ambient air. If there is not enough oxygen in the air, these devices will not supplement or otherwise enrich the air with oxygen. Whenever possible, use a remote probe to determine that an adequate oxygen atmosphere exists, instead of actually entering the room. If you must enter to test for oxygen level, then you must wear an SCBA (Level A or B PPE). On the opposite extreme, if the environment has a high concentration of oxygen, there is danger that a spark could cause an explosion. In many clandestine drug laboratories, explosive gases are also present, and so you must test for these also. Any flammable gases such as hydrogen, propane, or vapors from flammable liquids can create an explosive atmosphere. If flammable or explosive gases are present or if there is a high oxygen level, the atmosphere must be ventilated to remove the potential for a spark to cause an explosion.

In many settings, especially clandestine drug laboratories, there may be volatile organic compounds that either exceed the protection level of chemical protective clothing or present a flammability hazard or both. Sampling using a PID can determine the presence and level of organic compounds and can identify the compound. Protective clothing can fail in the presence of a high vapor level, exposing the responder to vapor contact with the skin. For this reason testing is required to determine the level of volatile organic compounds. If a high level of VOC is detected, the confined space, structure, or area must be ventilated prior to entry. Once the VOC level is reduced and the specific compound is identified, it should be compared to the rating of the chemical protective suit worn to ensure that the permeation values (levels at which a particular gas or vapor will penetrate the suit) are not exceeded.

PIDs can allow standoff testing by pumping air containing the chemical vapors or gases through tubing, allowing you to be a few feet away from the suspicious source. If a detector wand is used, a PID can also detect many liquid chemicals. Most liquids will emit sufficient vapors to allow the PID to perform a confirmation analysis. Care must be taken, however, to prevent the liquid agent from being sucked into the tubing. In other words, you have to get close to the liquid but be careful not to dunk the sensor tubing in it. These detectors can detect a wide range of chemical agents. They require a warm-up time and usually need a fresh-air calibration prior to use. Periodic calibration of the devices using a standard gas by a trained technician is mandatory. These instruments are expensive and are training and maintenance intensive, but they are the most versatile of available test instruments. These instruments can provide both a qualitative assessment (detection of the presence of the chemical agent) and a quantitative determination (how much agent is present), usually reported in parts per million (ppm).

Procedure: Use of the Photoionization Chemical Test Device to Identify Chemical Agents, Atmospheric Oxygen Levels, Levels of Flammable or Explosive Gases, and Volatile Organic Compound Levels

1

You should recognize that any scene at which multiple people are sick or "down" might be a chemical attack scene. It should, at a minimum, be treated as a HazMat situation. It will be even more suspicious for chemical attack if the victims are complaining of eye pain and difficulty breathing or are seizing. You should also recognize that confined spaces, well-sealed structures, and some exterior settings (such as a leaking gas tank) require testing for flammable gases or vapors, VOCs, and safe oxygen ranges as well as for toxic chemicals.

2 Select the proper instrument for the perceived threat. This will usually be a PID for the broad spectrum of agent detection (Figure S5.1). You must be familiar with the abilities of the instrument and what agents the instrument will measure (qualitative and/or quantitative). Many of these instruments are heat and moisture sensitive and so they should be stored in a dry environment at room temperature.

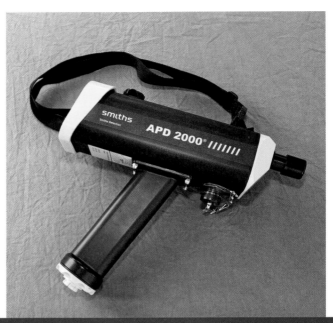

Figure S5.1 Example of a photoionization chemical detector (PID).

a. The level of PPE you should wear will depend on what you expect to find and whether there may be an oxygen-deficient atmosphere. If the oxygen level is low, you must either ventilate the area or wear an SCBA (Level A or B). If in doubt as to the toxic chemical present, it is always best to wear at least Level B attire (if you don't know the identity of the chemical, you might not have the correct filter in your APR/PAPR). Prior to putting on your PPE you should check the equipment for proper function and determine (from its label or self-check) that the instrument is currently calibrated. Most instruments require monthly calibration checks and annual factory-level recertification.

b. Remove the detector from its protective case (Figure S5.2) and review the manufacturer's recommendation for its use. Confirm that this instrument will detect the agent suspected to be present and

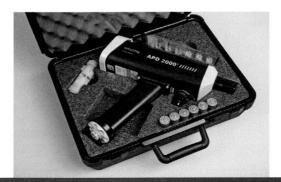

Figure S5.2 Example of PID in protective case.

that the alarm level for LEL (lower explosive limit) has been set for 1%. The concentration of explosive or flammable gases should be less than 1%. Concentration of explosive gases of 10% or greater are critical and require immediate evacuation and ventilation to ensure that the limits fall to less than 1%. The limits for oxygen should be set at a lower limit of 19.5% and an upper limit of 21%. Levels of oxygen permissible for APR/PAPR use are at least 19.5% and no greater than 21%. If the oxygen level is outside this range, ventilation should be undertaken and no entry made until the area has a safe oxygen level. Also set the PID to check for carbon monoxide and VOCs (more commonly found in clandestine drug labs), plus the suspect agent.

c. Remove the battery case and insert the batteries into the instrument (Figure S5-3). Instruments that have rechargeable batteries do not require this step.

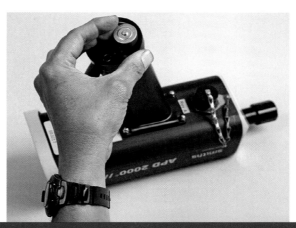

Figure S5.3   Placing batteries into the battery case.

d. Press the instrument's power button to turn it on, and observe the instrument as it performs self-checks (Figure S5.4). *This should be done in a clean area upwind with no vehicle exhausts or other contaminants present.*

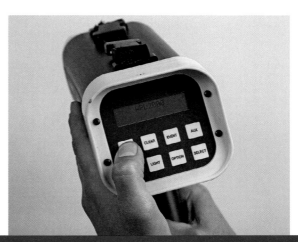

Figure S5.4   Turn on the PID and run a self-check.

e. Confirm that the air-sample pump is active and the air-sample inlet is not blocked (Figure S5.5). Some instruments may require that a filter be inserted prior to connection of a sampling wand or tubing. Be careful not allow any liquids to enter the sample inlet, wand, or tubing. Blocking the sample inlet will result in a shutdown of the instrument.

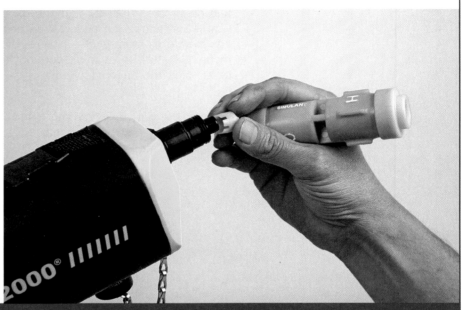

Figure S5.5 Confirm that the air-sample pump is active and the air-sample inlet is not blocked.

f. Observe the self-check and determine that each sensor performs a satisfactory self-check. If the instrument does not self-check properly, it should not be used. Some instruments have a check source to use to test the PID (Figure S5.6).

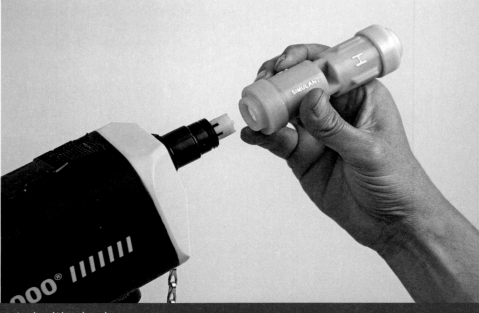

Figure S5.6 PID being tested with check source.

g. Observe the voltage of the batteries. Many instruments will give both a voltage and estimated run time. The run time should be adequate to allow you (or a member of the HazMat team) to enter and depart the hot zone.

h. Perform a fresh-air calibration upwind and away from the hot zone and all vehicles, ensuring that no contaminants are present. The instrument should zero all sensors. Vehicles parked in a cluster, with engines running, as often occurs at disaster sites, especially at night, will often produce multiple types of emissions that will cause false readings and inaccurate calibration of these instruments.

i. Properly protect the instrument from contamination hazards. Place the instrument in a protective bag and tape the plastic around the sample inlet. Some instruments do not require this step. In many instances a sampling wand or plastic tubing may be attached to the sample inlet to give you standoff distance.

j. Approach the contaminated area or suspect containers while observing the PID screen. The oxygen level must be at least 19.5% and below 21% (normal oxygen concentration in air), and the LEL (flammable gas detector) should read below 10% (alarm should sound when above 1%). Any flammable gas is cause for concern, and if the level approaches 10% it is critical and all responders must leave the area. Volatile organic compound readings may vary, but the detection of a VOC is a cause for concern. Other agents that may be detected and are cause for concern **at any level** are nerve agents, halogen gases such as chlorine, toxic industrial chemicals, hydrogen sulfide, cyanide, anhydrous ammonia, and phosphine. If these agents are detected, you should reevaluate the need for entry and the level of PPE being worn by those who do enter the hot zone. If you must enter the hot zone, you should wear Level A or at least Level B attire.

k. By use of this instrument you should correctly identify the agent or agents present and relay the information to the command post. Depending on the gas detected and its level, you may be able to change to a lower level of PPE.

l. You may be required to continue to sample the level of the threat agent to determine if it is decreasing or increasing.

m. When no longer needed you should proceed to decontamination and correctly remove the PPE and shut the instrument down.

n. You should then shower with soap and water.

USE OF COLORIMETRIC SENSORS

Colorimetric sensors use a change of color in a detector to detect the presence of an agent. Some sensors are qualitative; others provide a quantitative measurement. The most commonly used qualitative sensors are attached to the responder's external PPE and provide a color change when an agent is detected. Chemical test equipment comes in a variety of configurations. Some, such as the military M8/M9/M256 kits, use chemical reactions of chemical agents to reagents that give a color change. These are qualitative tests that only indicate the presence of a chemical agent. These tests are also prone to error, as many VOCs will give false positives. M-8 paper and other chemical detection strips will often give a false positive for chemical agents if exposed to common fluids such as coffee or suntan lotion. However, the tests are simple to perform and inexpensive. The downside to these tests is that you must be in immediate proximity of the suspect substance to test it. Most of the detectors will only respond to agents that are volatile and produce vapors or gases, but some detectors, such as the M8 detector, can be used to sample liquid agents. These sensors provide early warning of the presence of the agent. Quantitative instruments provide a reading, usually in PPM, for a specific agent. ***To use a quantitative instrument the identity of the agent must be known.*** Cross-reaction of colorimetric indicators is common because a similar agent or even a VOC may give a false reading. For this specific reason these detectors are not preferred for detection and measurement purposes unless the agents are known. However, this should not prevent the use of early-warning qualitative detectors in low-risk settings. Some agencies use these in settings where there is no known threat, and responders wear them on their normal duty uniforms as an early-warning sensor.

USE OF COLORIMETRIC QUALITATIVE SENSORS

Colorimetric qualitative detectors should not be used as the sole means for the detection of toxic vapors. However, these devices are suitable for use in low-risk settings where they can be worn on the exterior of PPE. Military M9 and M256 kits are examples of kits that will detect gases. The military M8 kit is an example of a kit that will detect chemical liquids.

Procedure: Use of Colorimetric Qualitative Vapor or Gas Detectors

1   Select the proper detector for the perceived threat. This will usually be a colorimetric badge or tape for the broad spectrum of agent detection (Figure S5.7). You must be familiar with the abilities of the detector and what agents it will identify. Because many of these detectors are heat and moisture sensitive, they should be stored in a dry environment at room temperature.

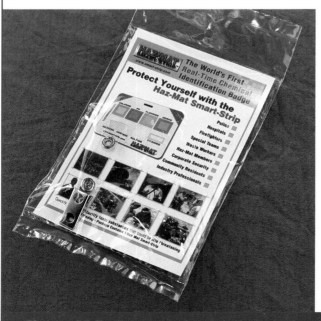
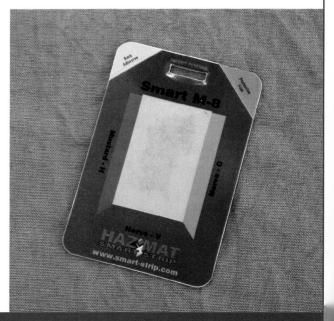

Figure S5.7   Example of a Colorimetric Qualitative Gas Sensor badge.

2 Prior to putting on your PPE, you should check the detector for proper function and determine from its label that its calibration is current and its container is intact. These are one-time-use devices that have an expiration date; many are also sensitive to light and temperature. There should be an expiration date on the detector package. Do not use detectors that are out of date or those whose protective packages are not intact.

3 Remove the detector from its protective container and review the manufacturer's recommendation for its use. Confirm that this detector will detect the agent suspected to be present. Most of these detectors provide broad-spectrum warning of nerve agents, cyanide compounds, halogen gases, some toxic industrial chemicals, and blister agents.

4 *Cross-reaction with other VOCs is common and may give a false positive indication of an agent.*

5 Attach the detector to the outside of your PPE. Some detectors are self-adherent with an adhesive while others have a spring-loaded clip or must be taped in position. Place the detector in a location (usually on the front of your PPE) where you can readily see it but not in a position where it will be torn away as you move around.

6 You must memorize the original color pattern of the detector.

7 Enter the hazard area.

8 Observe the detector frequently and note any color change.

PRACTICAL SKILLS: 5

9 If there is a color change, then a chemical agent has been detected and you should leave the area immediately.

10 Appropriately identify the threat agent from the color chart and report the finding to the command post.

11 Follow-up confirmation of the agent should be made using a PID.

Procedure: Use of Colorimetric Qualitative Liquid Detectors

1 Select the proper detector for the perceived threat. This will usually be a tape or paper detector for broad-spectrum agent detection (Figure S5.8). You must be familiar with the abilities of the detector and what agents it will detect. Because many of these detectors are heat and moisture sensitive, they should be stored in a dry environment at room temperature.

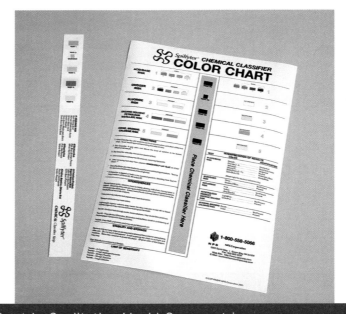

Figure S5.8 Example of a Colorimetric Qualitative Liquid Sensor strip.

2 Prior to putting on your PPE, check the expiration date of the strip. These are one-time-use devices that have an expiration date; many are sensitive to light and temperature. Do not use the detector if it is out of date or if the protective package is not intact.

3 Remove the detector from its protective container and review the manufacturer's recommendation for its use. Confirm that this detector will detect the liquid agent suspected to be present. Most of these detectors provide broad-spectrum warning of nerve agents, cyanide compounds, halogen gases, some toxic industrial chemicals, and blister agents, but some others are made to detect specific agents.

4 *Cross-reaction with other VOCs is common and may give a false positive indication of an agent.*

5 Determine how the detector should be carried to the site to perform sampling of suspect liquids. Most are hand carried or carried in a bag to protect from sunlight.

6 Memorize the original color pattern of the detector in its unused state.

7 Put on your PPE.

8 Enter the hazard area but avoid touching or stepping into the liquid agent to be sampled.

9   Place the detector in the liquid, being careful to avoid any contact with your gloves. You may choose to use a device to obtain a sample that is then placed on the detector.

10   Do not contaminate yourself with the liquid agent!

11   Following the manufacturer's recommendations, observe the detector and note any color change. Most detectors will respond within a few minutes.

12   Color changes indicate that a liquid chemical agent has been detected.

13   Appropriately identify the liquid chemical agent from the color-change chart.

14   Discard the detector.

15   Leave the area and report your findings to the command post.

16   Follow-up confirmation of the agent should be made using a PID.

Want to Know More?

Bibliography

Copenhaver, R. C. *Agent Characteristics and Toxicology First Aid and Special Treatment.* Oak Ridge National Laboratories, 1997.

Marrs, T. C. *Chemical Walfare Agents: Toxicology and Treatment.* John Wiley and Sons, 1996.

Oldfield, K. W. *Emergency Responder Training Manual for the Hazardous Materials Technician,* 2nd ed. Wiley Inter-Science, 2005.

U.S. Army. Chemical and Biological Countermeasures Course, 1997.

Internet Sources

The Guide for the Selection of Chemical Agent and Toxic Industrial Material Detection Equipment for Emergency First Responders, DHS March 2005. The guide, produced for the Department of Homeland Security (DHS), does not make recommendations. It provides you with ways to compare and contrast commercially available Chemical Agent and Toxic Industrial Material detection equipment. After registering at the website, type in "DHS AND guide" in the search box. Click on link to the Chemical Agent and Toxic Industrial Material Detector Guide.
www.rkb.mipt.org

FM17-98: Nuclear, Biological, and Chemical Operations
www.transglobal-aerospace.co.uk/17-98/appb.htm

PRACTICAL SKILLS: 5

Notes

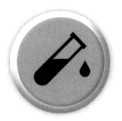 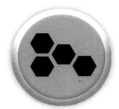 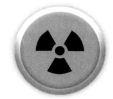 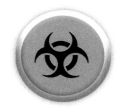 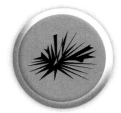

Demonstration of Radiation Detection Equipment

Chapter Objectives

At the conclusion of this station, you should be familiar with:

1.   The use of the various types of radiation detection equipment available
2.   The use of a pencil or ion chamber dosimeter
3.   The use of a low range Beta-Gamma or Alpha radiation detector

Radiation detection equipment operates on the principle that the radiation interacts with gases or crystal within the detector to produce ionization that the instrument electronically converts to a reading. Instruments normally detect only certain types and certain levels of radiation. Most of these devices are not precision instruments, and the error rate can be up to 20%. For this reason, conservative estimates of exposure and dose should be used to ensure that emergency limits are not exceeded.

The emergency limits of radiation exposure established by the Incident Commander should not be exceeded. The rule of thumb is that once the responder is at 50% of the allowable limit, the responder terminates his or her role and departs the hazard area. Emergency limits are set at 5 REM (roentgen equivalent in man) annually for occupational exposure and 25 REM for emergencies representing substantial risk to life and property (some say a limit of 10 REM) with up to 100 REM to save a life (some say a limit of 25 REM). In dangerous situations, rotating personnel should help minimize radiation exposure. Older responders should be used when possible, as they are not as susceptible to radiation injury as younger responders. Any detection of neutron radiation is likely to be associated with a nuclear weapon or radiological dispersion device, and requires immediate departure of all personnel from the hazard area. Notify the FBI immediately if neutron radiation is detected.

Low-range instruments (these normally have a handheld probe) usually detect alpha or beta particles and gamma radiation. These instruments are used to detect contamination (qualitative) and are not useful to measure higher radiation readings.

Higher-range instruments are used to determine radiation levels and dose rates to those exposed, and are not useful for detecting contamination. These instruments are normally handheld with no probe.

Other instruments, such as a badge dosimeter, measure the total amount of gamma radiation to which a person has been exposed (these are worn by hospital X-ray technicians). Some of the electronic types include dose rates of gamma radiation. Some devices, such as the pencil dosimeter, are readable in a field setting and give an ongoing reading. Others, such as thermoluminescent dosimeters (TLD), require instrumentation to determine the dose. TLDs provide a more accurate estimate of exposure than do immediate-reading dosimeters.

Alarming electronic gamma-radiation detectors give a visual/audible alarm when low levels of radiation are detected. Many of these devices are designed to be worn on the person and alert them when they have entered a radiation area. Others alert you when a specific dose has been reached.

You should always wear both a TLD and a responder-readable dosimeter (pencil dosimeter). The pencil dosimeter gives you an immediate but rough estimate of cumulative exposure, while the TLD (calculated later) gives you a more accurate determination of total dose exposure.

Because there are so many instruments available, only the use of the ion chamber dosimeter, thermoluminescent dosimeter (TLD), and the low-range beta-gamma radiation detector will be taught in this station.

Procedure: Use of a Pencil or Ion Chamber Dosimeter Along with a Thermoluminescent Dosimeter

1 You should recognize a scene with potential radioactive contamination. This will include all explosions of unknown origin, bombings, unknown substances (particularly those received by mail or parcel), or other suspicious circumstances with an unknown substance.

2 You must be aware of the limitations of the instrument. Pencil dosimeters detect only gamma radiation.

3 Remove the dosimeter from its container (Figure S6.1). Dosimeters must be stored at room temperature and in a dry environment.

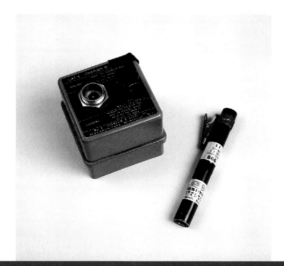

Figure S6.1 Example of a pencil ion chamber dosimeter and charger (calibrator).

4 Check the calibration date of the dosimeter to be sure it is current. Most instruments will be calibrated at least annually (Figure S6.2).

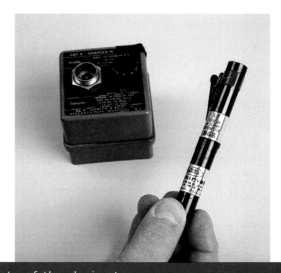

Figure S6.2 Checking the calibration date of the dosimeter.

PRACTICAL SKILLS: 6

5 Remove the dosimeter charger (calibrating device) (refer to Figure S6.1). Most dosimeter chargers will have to be partially disassembled, the battery inserted following the manufacturer's recommendations, and then reassembled.

6 Hold the dosimeter up to a light source with the glass end or top of the dosimeter near the eye and read the dosimeter. The dosimeter should have a line against the scale showing either roentgens or milliroentgens. The dosimeter should read near zero but may have had some drift.

7 Place the dosimeter over the contact on the dosimeter charger and depress it while placing an eye near the end of the dosimeter. You should then turn the knob on the charger to place the filament in the dosimeter at or near zero (Figure S6.3).

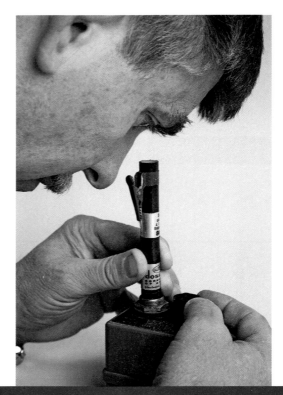

Figure S6.3 Calibrating the dosimeter.

8 Remove the dosimeter and use a light source to read the dosimeter and confirm that it is zeroed. Dosimeters refusing to zero, or ones that drift, should not be used.

9 Log the dosimeter reading and place the dosimeter in a clear plastic bag that can be attached to your PPE.

10 Put on your PPE and attach the dosimeter in a manner that will allow you to read the dosimeter easily while you are in the hazard area. This is usually accomplished by attaching the dosimetry bag to your chest with tape that can be removed (Figure S6.4).

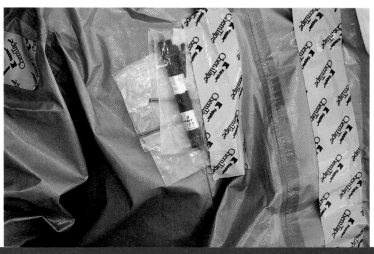

Figure S6.4 Dosimeter in plastic bag attached to PPE.

11 You should frequently check the dosimeter throughout your mission.

12 You should also wear a TLD while in the hot zone. You must be aware of the limitations of the instrument used. Most TLDs will detect only gamma radiation.

13 Remove the TLD from its container. TLDs must be stored at room temperature in a dry environment (Figure S6.5).

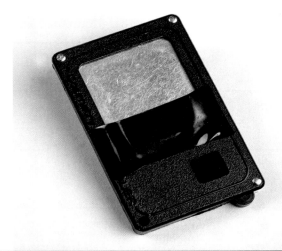

Figure S6.5 Example of a thermoluminescent dosimeter (TLD).

14   Check the calibration date of the TLD to determine that it is current. Most TLDs require calibration at least annually.

15   Place the TLD in a plastic bag or in the bag with the pencil dosimeter or other immediate-reading dosimeter. This bag should be attached to your PPE (Figure S6.6).

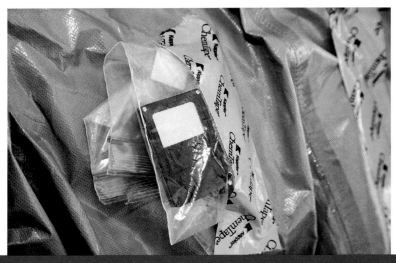

Figure S6.6 Attach the bag containing the TLD to you PPE. You may put the pencil dosimeter and the TLD in the same bag.

16   The emergency limits of radiation exposure established by the Incident Commander should not be exceeded (5 REM annually for occupational exposure, 25 REM for an emergency situation [some say limit of 10 REM] with up to 100 REM to save a life [some say limit of 25 REM]). The rule of thumb is that once you are at 50% of the allowable limit, you should terminate your role and depart the hot zone. Female responders who are pregnant or may become pregnant should not enter the contaminated area, but should be given other assignments outside of the warm or hot zones.

17   Complete your mission.

18   Prior to decontamination, read the pencil dosimeter and record your reading.

19 Remove the pencil dosimeter and TLD, leaving them in their protective bags, and place them in the appropriate location so that the dosimeters can be read for an estimate of your exposure.

20 Go through the decontamination process and remove your protective clothing.

21 You should now be surveyed for radioactive contamination. If any contamination is detected, you should shower with soap and water and be surveyed again. A health physics technician should assess you if any contamination remains.

22 All responders should report their findings to the command post and log their dosimetry readings.

23 Any exposures outside the emergency limits should be evaluated by a health physics technician and a physician knowledgeable in radiation management.

Procedure: Use of a Low-Range Beta-Gamma or Alpha Radiation Detection Instrument

1 You should recognize a scene with potential radioactive contamination. This will include all explosions of unknown origin, bombings, unknown substances, particularly those received by mail or package, or other suspicious circumstances with an unknown substance.

2 You must be aware of the limitations of this instrument. Low-range gamma detectors may not detect alpha, beta, neutron, or high-energy gamma radiation. The shield on a beta-gamma detector will have to be open to detect beta radiation. The shield on the pancake probe must also be removed to detect beta radiation.

3 Check the calibration date of the instrument to be sure it is current. Most instruments will require calibration at least annually (Figure S6.7).

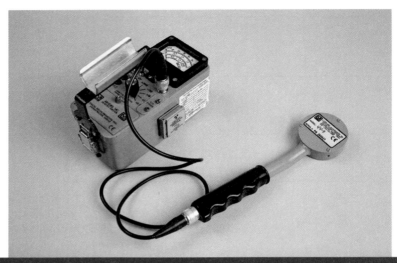

Figure S6.7 Low-range Geiger-Muller-type beta-gamma detector with pancake probe. See calibration recorded on the side of the detector.

4 Most instruments will have to be partially disassembled, the batteries inserted following the manufacturer's recommendations, and then reassembled. This usually includes selecting the correct probe. Normally a pancake probe is used for contamination detection of beta-gamma radiation. There is a specific probe to detect alpha radiation. Some instruments will use a sensitive gamma scintillation probe to detect low levels of gamma radiation. Attach the correct probe as recommended by the manufacturer. This is usually accomplished with a twist-off/on BNC-type connector. Pancake probes are named for their appearance and are used for beta-gamma detection or alpha detection (refer to Figure S6.7). Hotdog probes, named for their appearance (Figure S6.8), are used for higher-level beta-gamma contamination. Gamma scintillation probes shaped like a pipe are used for low-level gamma detection.

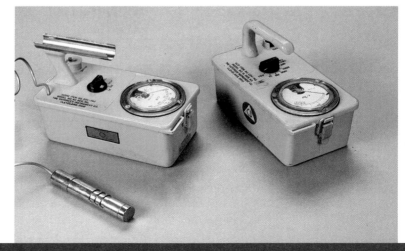

Figure S6.8 Low-range Geiger-Muller-type beta-gamma detector with hotdog probe.

5 Place the batteries in the radiation detector (Figure S6.9).

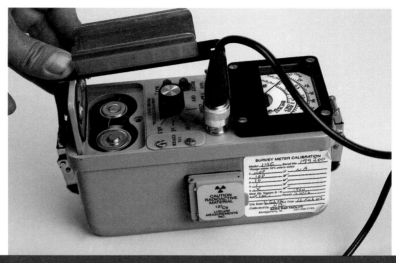

Figure S6.9   Inserting batteries. Note the radiation testing source on the side of the device.

6 Perform battery test (Figure S6.10).

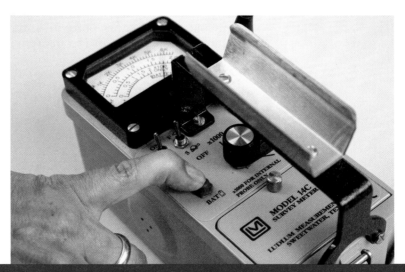

Figure S6.10   Performing a battery test.

7 Follow the manufacturer's instructions to confirm the instrument's response through a check source (radioactive source) or other means prior to use. Most alpha detectors will not have a check source. This check is usually accomplished by turning the instrument on, selecting the correct range, exposing the radiation source, and holding the detector close to it following the manufacturer's recommendations. By observing the instrument dial for appropriate range or needle deflection, you can confirm that the instrument is operating correctly (Figure S6.11). Some instruments will have an audible and/or visual detection capability that can be selected to determine the rate of detection. On some instruments, if a hotdog probe is used, the shield must be open to detect beta radiation.

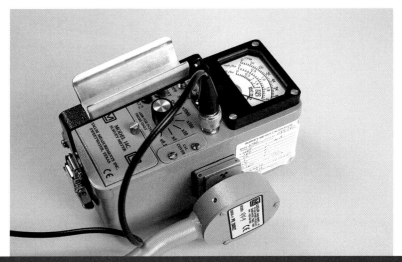

Figure S6.11   Testing the device using a standard radiation source. Note the elevated reading on the dial.

8   Package the instrument or the probe using a plastic bag designed for the application or other protective material such as a rubber glove to prevent contamination of the instrument or probe (Figure S6.12).

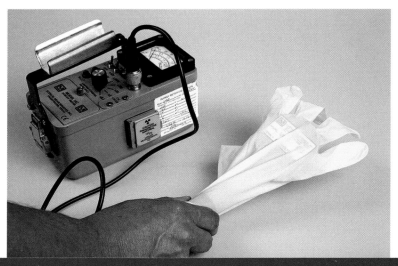

Figure S6.12   Place the probe in a plastic bag or rubber glove to prevent it from becoming contaminated.

9   Obtain your pencil dosimeter and TLDs and place them in protective plastic bags that can be attached to your PPE.

10   Put on the appropriate PPE (at least level C).

11   Attach your pencil dosimeter to your chest so that you can see it (refer to Figure S6.4). The TLD does not have to be in a position where you can see it.

12   You should take a background reading with your beta-gamma detector prior to entering the hazard area. Record this as the normal ambient radiation level.

13   Carry the instrument into the hot zone.

14   Survey potentially contaminated materials by holding the instrument probe, properly protected in plastic, approximately 1 inch from the surface to be surveyed and following a serpentine (S-shaped) pattern over the entire surface. The speed of survey should be no more than 1 inch per second.

15   If there is any radiation present, you will notice an increase above the background reading on the dial. Some instruments give an audible reading also. Any positive reading should be resurveyed to confirm the reading, and then the reading (usually in counts per minute [CPM]) is recorded along with the location of the contaminated area.

16   Low-range contamination instruments may be overloaded and show no readings in high-radiation areas. For this reason you should frequently check your pencil (ion chamber) dosimeter readings to note the dose being absorbed. It is recommended that a high-range survey instrument be used also.

PRACTICAL SKILLS: 6

17 Once you have completed your mission, you should obtain a final reading, leave the contaminated area, turn the instrument off, and place it in the appropriate location for decontamination along with your pencil dosimeter and TLD.

18 You should then go through the decontamination process and remove your protective clothing.

19 You should then be surveyed for radioactive contamination. If any contamination is detected, you should shower and be surveyed for radiation again. You should be assessed by a health physics technician if any contamination remains.

20 You should now record your dosimetry readings and report your findings to the command post.

21 Any exposures outside the emergency limits should be evaluated by a health physics technician and a physician knowledgeable in radiation management.

Want to Know More?

Bibliography

Oldfield, K.W. *Emergency Responder Training Manual for the Hazardous Materials Technician*, 2nd ed. Wiley Inter-Science, 2005.

Radiological Defense Officers Course. FEMA, 1970.

U.S. Army. *TG 244 Med NBC Battle Book.* 2002.

U.S. Army. *Chemical and Biological Countermeasures Course.* 1997.

Internet Sources

A First Responder's Guide to Purchasing Radiation Pagers, available at www.rkb.mipt.org. After registering at the website, type in "DHS AND guide" in the search box. Click on the link to the radiation pagers.

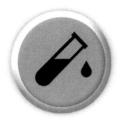 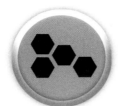 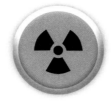 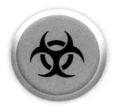 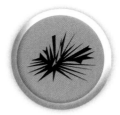

Scenario Review

Objective

At the end of this practical skill station you should be able to:

Review a scenario and determine the type of attack you are dealing with and how to respond to it.

Procedure: As a group or individually, you will be given a practical scenario and will discuss how to evaluate the scene for the type of attack and then how to respond to it. To prepare for this, review Chapter 8, "Putting It All Together."

Notes

Optional Skill: Level B Protective Equipment

Use of Level B Protective Equipment

Although it is not quite as good as Level A PPE, this level provides protection against liquids and most vapors. Unless there is strong evidence of a severe risk, this level is usually adequate. EMS, hospital, and law enforcement personnel require a level of dexterity to perform their duties that precludes the use of Level A PPE. If HazMat evaluation determines that the scene is too dangerous for Level B PPE, then victims will have to be removed from the scene before evaluation by EMS. Level B PPE is a chemical suit with the SCBA worn externally (Figure A.1).

Procedure: Putting on Level B Protective Equipment

You should have a partner to assist you with this.

1. Remove and secure jewelry (including rings, earrings and any body piercings) and other personal items. When possible, remove and secure your clothing and don hospital scrub attire or service clothing. Remember that your clothing should be appropriate to the ambient temperature.

2. If you wear eyeglasses, either secure them with a retaining band or tape them in place. Apply antifogging material to the lenses to prevent fogging or condensation when you sweat. Secure long hair. Check your hydration state. It is recommended that you consume 300–500 ml of water. *Remember that the time to visit the bathroom is prior to putting on PPE.* Also, before you don PPE, you should have your baseline vital signs (pulse rate, respiration rate, oral temperature, and blood pressure) taken and recorded. However, even though this is important, there may be emergency situations when you don't have the time to do this.

3. Select appropriate-sized PPE. Be sure you know your size before the emergency. Confirm that all components are serviceable: inspecting for defects, such as tears or holes, and ensure that the SCBA tanks are full and the regulator is functional. Use chemically rated tape to seal your PPE.

4. While sitting, remove your footwear.

5. Put on a pair of nitrile undergloves. Do not use latex gloves, as they offer no chemical protection (Figure A.2).

6. Step into the legs of the suit, pull up the suit to your waist and then put on chemical boots and tape them in place using chemically rated tape (some suits come with built-in boots). Normally duct tape or paper tape is not used. Make certain to leave a tab so the tape can be easily removed (Figure A.3). Now don your upper suit but do not pull up the hood.

7. Follow the manufacturer's recommendations for the inspection and donning of your SCBA. The usual sequence is this:

   a. Inspect and adjust the harness straps for SCBA tank (Figure A.4).
   b. Make sure that the tank is fitted properly into the harness.
   c. Make sure all hoses are properly attached (Figure A.5).
   d. Check the SCBA tank air gauge to be sure the tank is full of air (Figure A.6).
   e. Attach the regulator hose to the tank (Figure A.7).

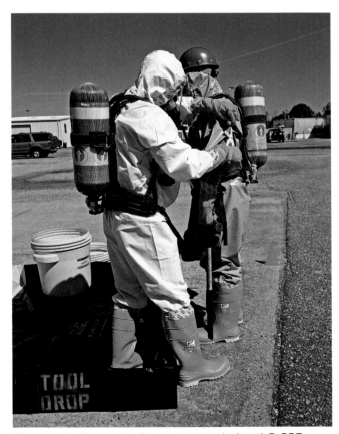

Figure A.1 Example of two rescuers in Level B PPE.

Figure A.2
Donning nitrile
under-gloves.

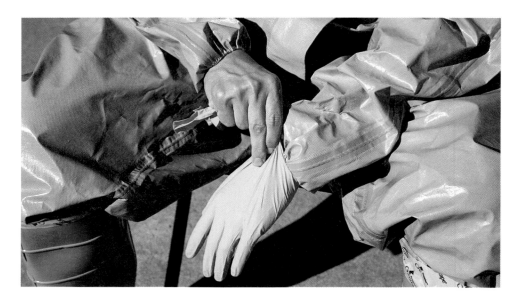

Figure A.3
Tape boots in place using
chemically rated tape.

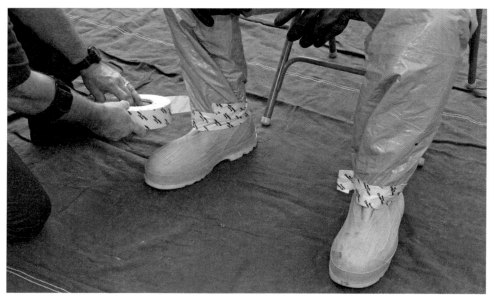

Figure A.4
Checking SCBA harness.

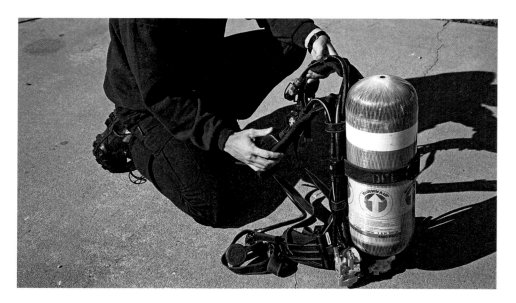

Figure A.5
Checking SCBA hoses.

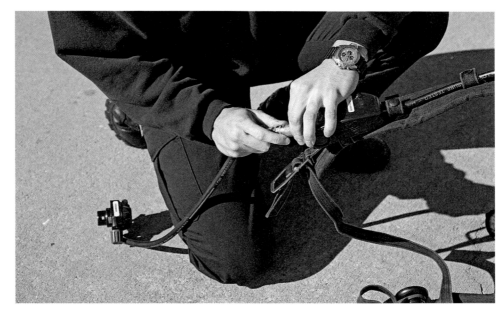

Figure A.6
Checking to be sure tank
is full of oxygen.

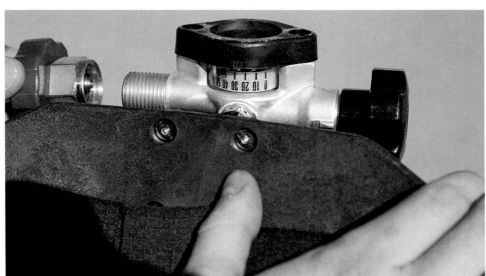

Figure A.7
Attach regulator hose to
tank.

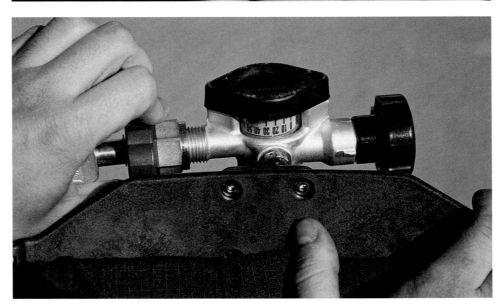

Figure A.8
Turn oxygen tank on.

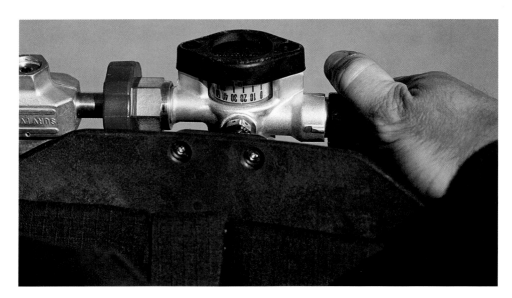

Figure A.9
Compare regulator gauge and tank gauge to confirm they read the same.

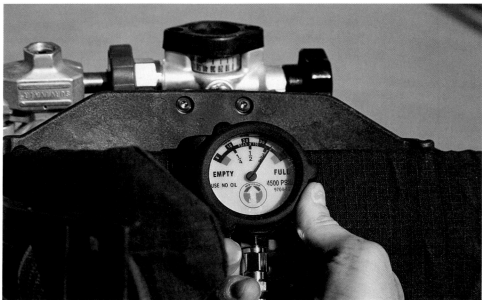

f. Turn on the tank (Figure A.8).
g. Compare the tank gauge with the regulator gauge to be sure they have the same reading (Figure A.9).
h. Activate the emergency bypass valve to confirm that you have emergency air flow (Figure A.10).
i. Turn off the emergency bypass valve.
j. Turn off the main tank.
k. Open the bypass valve again to test the low pressure alarm—the alarm should go off.
l. Have your partner hold your tank and harness behind you while you put on the harness and adjust it for comfort (Figure A.11).
m. Put on the mask (Figure A.12).
n. Do a fit test by inhaling while occluding the intake port. Then hold your breath to make sure there are no leaks around the face area. If a leak is present, readjust the mask and repeat the fit test until there are no leaks (Figure A.13).

o. Confirm that the heads up display (the LED display of the amount of oxygen remaining in the tank) is correctly functioning.

p. Pull up your suit, pull on the hood, and zip up your suit. Get your partner to assist you by sealing the hood to your mask and also sealing the seams of your suit with tape (Figure A.14).

q. While holding your breath, attach the regulator to the mask and seat securely (Figure A.15).

Figure A.10
Activate emergency bypass valve to confirm that you have emergency air flow.

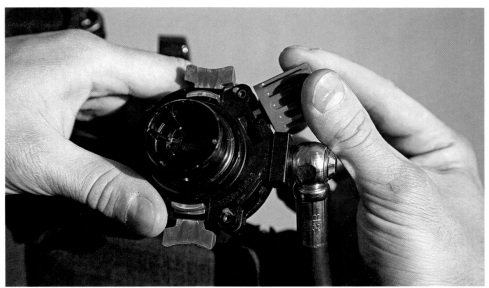

Figure A.11
Put on tank harness and adjust to comfort.

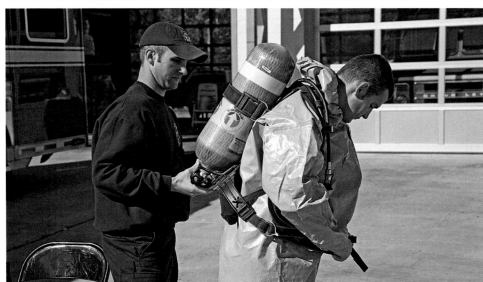

Figure A.12
Put on SCBA mask.

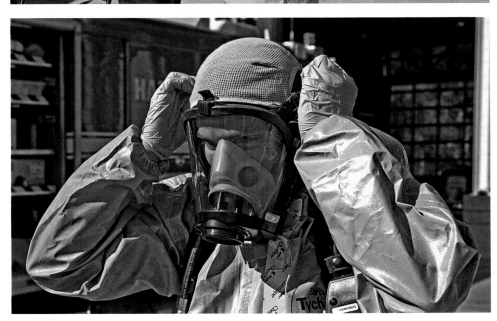

Figure A.13
Perform fit test to confirm
mask does not leak.

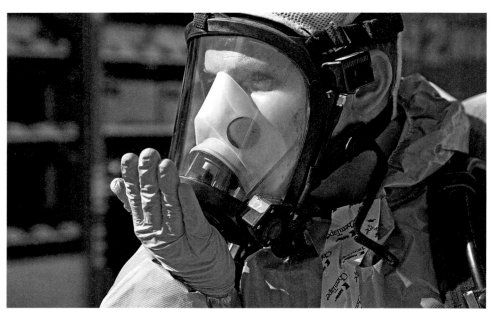

Figure A.14
After donning hood, you
should tape mask to hood
and tape seams of suit.

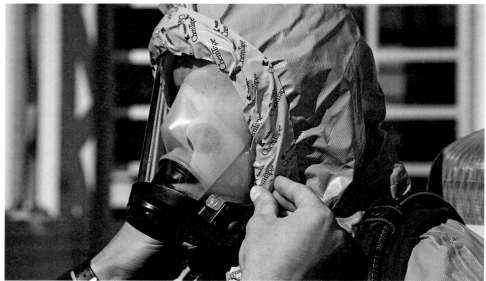

Figure A.15
Attach regulator to the
mask.

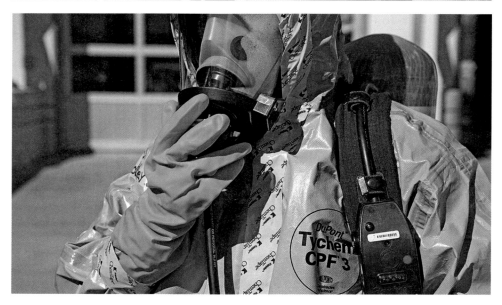

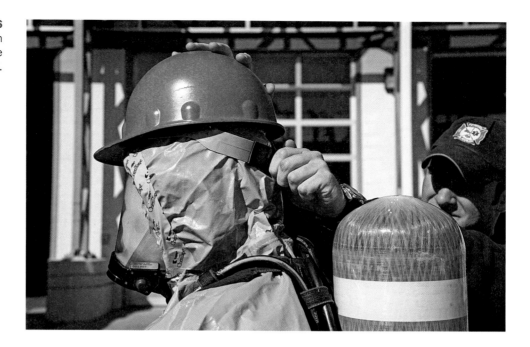

Figure A.16
If needed a hard hat can be taped or otherwise secured in place.

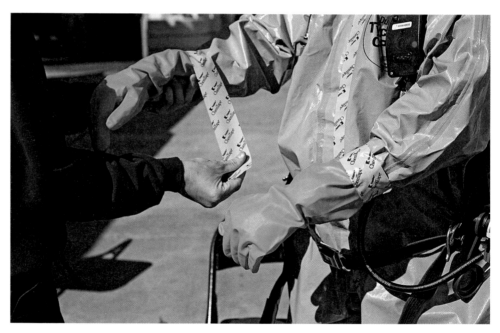

Figure A.17
Put on and tape butyl rubber gloves.

r. Take a breath and confirm that there is no air leak. Retape the mask and hood if needed.
8. It may be appropriate to put on a hard hat and tape it in place or otherwise secure it (Figure A.16).
9. Put on the appropriate gloves and tape them in place, leaving a removal tab. For chemical incidents, the usual recommendation is one set of nitrile gloves followed by a set of butyl rubber gloves. Otherwise two pairs of nitrile gloves are recommended. Avoid ill-fitting vinyl gloves (Figure A.17).

10. Have someone attach a piece of tape with your name on the rear of your suit. If multiple agencies are involved, also note the name of your agency on the tape. Always work in pairs. If one partner becomes disabled, the other can bring help (Figure A.18).
11. Tape a knife or shears to your boot so that if you run out of air you can quickly remove your suit (Figure A.19).

Figure A.18
Place tape with your name
and agency on the sleeve
of your suit.

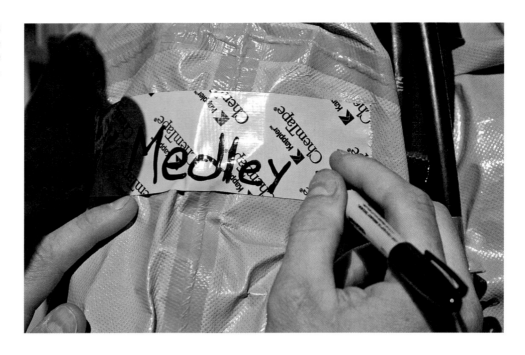

Figure A.19
Tape a knife or shears to
your boot so that you can
quickly remove your PPE in
an emergency.

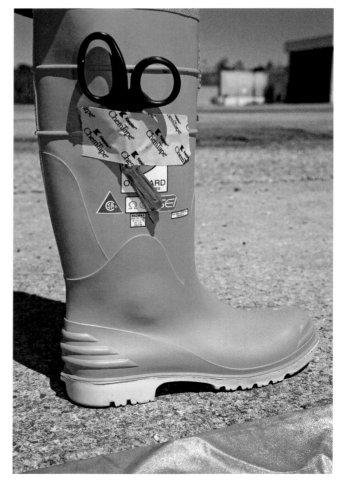

ACRONYMS

ANFO:	ammonium nitrate–fuel oil
APR:	air-purifying respirator (gas mask)
ATNAA:	antidote treatment nerve agent autoinjector (DuoDote)
BAL:	British anti-lewisite
BATFE:	Bureau of Alcohol, Tobacco, Firearms, and Explosives
CAD:	computer aided dispatch
CANA:	convulsants antidote for nerve agent
CBC:	complete blood count
CBRNE:	chemical, biological, radiological-nuclear explosives
CDC:	U.S. Center for Disease Control and Prevention
CDL:	clandestine drug laboratory
CIA:	Central Intelligence Agency
CN:	mace (riot control agent)
COBRA:	Consolidated Omnibus Budget Reconciliation Act
COPD:	chronic obstructive pulmonary disease
CS:	tear gas (riot control agent)
CSEPP:	Chemical Stockpile Emergency Preparedness Program
DHS:	Department of Homeland Security
DUMBELS:	diarrhea, urination, miosis, bronchoconstriction, emesis, lacrimation, salivation
ED:	emergency department
EMA:	Emergency Management Agency
EMS:	Emergency Medical Services
FBI:	Federal Bureau of Investigation
FDA:	Federal Drug Administration
FEMA:	Federal Emergency Management Agency
fps:	feet per second
GHB:	gamma-hydroxybutyrate
GI:	gastrointestinal
HazMat:	hazardous materials
HEICS:	Hospital Emergency Incident Command System
HTH:	high-test hypochlorite
ICS:	Incident Command System
IED:	improvised explosive device
IAEA:	International Atomic Energy Administration
IM:	intramuscular

IV:	intravenous
LD50:	amount of a substance that would kill 50% of those exposed
LOC:	Level of consciousness
LPG:	liquid propane gas
MDA:	3,4-methylenedioxyamphetamine (Ecstasy)
MDMA:	methylenedioxymethamphetamine (Ecstasy)
MICS:	Medical Incident Command System
MTA:	Medical Threat Assessment
NAAK:	Nerve Agent Antidote Kit
NAERG:	North American Emergency Response Guide
NIMS:	National Incident Management System
NRC:	Nuclear Regulatory Commission
OC:	oleoresin capsicum (pepper spray)
OSHA:	U.S. Occupational Safety and Health Administration
PAPR:	powered air-purifying respirator
PCP:	phencyclidine (Angel Dust)
PETN:	pentaerythritetetranitrate
PPE:	personal protective equipment
ppm:	parts per million
RAD:	radiation absorbed dose
RDD:	radiological dispersion device
RDX:	cyclotrimethylenetrinitramine
REACT:	Radiation Emergency Assistance Center/Training
REM:	roentgen equivalent in man
SARS:	Severe Acute Respiratory Syndrome
SCBA:	self-contained breathing apparatus
SEB:	staphylococcal enterotoxin B
SLUDGEM:	salivation, lacrimation, urination, diarrhea, gastric upset, emesis, miosis
SOB:	shortness of breath
TB:	tuberculosis
TNT:	trinitrotoluene
VBIED:	vehicle borne improvised explosive devise
VEE:	Venezuelan equine encephalitis
VHF:	viral hemorrhagic fever
VIG:	vaccinia-immune globulin
WMD:	weapons of mass destruction

Credits

Photos not credited below are:

© McGraw-Hill Higher Education, Inc./Rick Brady, photographer.

Unless indicated Chapter Openers are © McGraw-Hill Higher Education, Inc. & Courtesy of the authors.

Chapter 1:

1.14: Courtesy John Campbell; **1.15:** Courtesy PROTECH Tactical; **1.16:** Courtesy American Body Armor; **1.17:** Courtesy PROTECH Tactical; **1.24:** Courtesy Disaster Management Systems, Inc.

Chapter 2:

2.1a: © Eslami Rad/Gamma Press; **2.1b:** © IRNA/AFP/Getty Images; **2.2:** © AP Photo/Chikumo Chiaki; **2.6:** Courtesy John Campbell; **2.7, 2.9:** Official DoD Photograph; **2.10:** © AP/Robert Mecea; **2.11:** Courtesy Jim Smith; **2.12:** © Dr. Jan Willems; **2.13a:** © AP Photo/Will Kincaid **2.13b**, **2.14:** Courtesy Jim Smith

Chapter 3:

Opener: © Richard Hamilton Smith/CORBIS; **3.1:** Courtesy James Meade, M.D.; **3.2, 3.3, 3.4:** Courtesy CDC/Centers for Disease Control; **3.5:** © Vaughan Fleming/SPL/Photo Researchers, Inc.

Chapter 4:

4.1: Courtesy CDC/Centers for Disease Control; **4.3:** © Mediscan

Chapter 5:

Case Study: © AP/Wide World Photos; **5.5:** © Time Life Pictures/Getty Images; **Case Study Conclusion:** © AP/Wide World Photos

Chapter 6:

Case Study: © AP Photo/Chris Pizzello; **6.1:** Courtesy Jim Smith; **6.4:** © Crown Copyright/Health & Safety Laboratory/Photo Researchers, Inc.; **6.5:** © Charles D. Winters/SPL/Photo Researchers, Inc.; **6.6** b-c: Courtesy Jim Smith; **6.7:** © Les Stone/Sygma/Corbis; **6.9, 6.10, 6.11, 6.12 all:** Courtesy Jim Smith; **6.17:** Courtesy Roy Alson, M.D., FACEP; **Case Study Conclusion:** © AP Photo/Chris Pizzello

Chapter 7:

Case Study, 7.1both, 7.2, 7.3: Courtesy Jim Smith; **7.4 a-b:** NES; **7.5 a-e, 7.6 a-b, 7.7 a-b, 7.8 a-d, 7.9 a-c:** Courtesy Jim Smith; **7.10:** NES; **7.11:** Courtesy Jim Smith; **Case Study Conclusion:** Courtesy Jim Smith

Practical Skills 1:

Opener: © 2006 Asylum Studios

Practical Skills 2:

Opener: © Asylum Studios

Practical Skills 3:

Opener: © 2006 Asylum Studios

Practical Skills 4:

Opener: © 2006 Asylum Studios; **S4.2:** www.badbox.com

Practical Skills 5:

Opener: © 2006 Asylum Studios

Practical Skills 6:

Opener: © 2006 Asylum Studios

Practical Skills 7:

Opener: © 2006 Asylum Studios